To: Tony Rowland

AF691408

With sincere compliments of

stryker Trauma

Chief Editors I. Kempf · K.S. Leung

Co-Editors A. Grosse · H.J.T.M. Haarman
H. Seidel · G. Taglang

Practice of Intramedullary Locked Nails

Scientific Basis and Standard Techniques Recommended by "Association Internationale pour l'Ostéosynthèse Dynamique" (AIOD)

With 239 Figures
and 15 Tables

Springer

Chief Editors

Professor Dr. I. KEMPF
AIOD, 16 Rue du Parc
67205 Straßburg, France

Professor Dr. K. S. LEUNG
The Chinese University of Hong Kong
Department of Orthopaedics
and Traumatology
Shatin, Hong Kong SAR
China

Co-Editors

Dr. A. GROSSE
Centre de Traumatologie et d'Orthopédie
10 Avenue A. Baumann
67400 Straßbourg, France

Professor Dr. H. J. T. M. HAARMAN
Academisch Ziekenhuis
Department of Surgery
De Boelelaan 1117, P.O. Box 7057
1007 MB Amsterdam, The Netherlands

Dr. H. SEIDEL
Allgemeines Krankenhaus Wandsbeck
Abteilung für Unfallchirurgie
Alphonsstraße 14
22043 Hamburg, Germany

Dr. G. TAGLANG
Centre de Traumatologie et d'Orthopédie
10 Avenue A. Baumann
67400 Straßbourg, France

ISBN 3-540-64079-7
Springer-Verlag Berlin Heidelberg New York

Library of Congress Cataloging-in-Publication Data
Practice of intramedullary locked nails: scientific basis and standard technique recommended by AIOD/[I. Kempf, K. S. Leung, chief editors].
p.; cm.
Includes bibliographical references and index.
ISBN 3540640797 (v. 1: alk. paper)
1. Internal fixation in fractures. I. Kempf, I. (Ivan), 1928– II. Leung, Kwok-Sui.
[DNLM: 1. Fracture Fixation, Intramedullary – methods. 2. Bone Nails. 3. Internal Fixators. WE 185 P895 2002]
RD 103.I5 P73 2002
617.1′5–dc21 2001049375

This work is subject to copyright. All rights are reserved, whether the whole or part of the material is concerned, specifically the rights of translation, reprinting, reuse of illustrations, recitation, broadcasting, reproduction on microfilm or in any other way, and storage in data banks. Duplication of this publication or parts thereof is permitted only under the provisions of the German Copyright Law of September 9, 1965, in its current version, and permission for use must always be obtained from Springer-Verlag. Violations are liable for prosecution under the German Copyright Law.

Springer-Verlag Berlin Heidelberg New York
a member of BertelsmannSpringer Science+Business Media GmbH

http://www.springer.de

© Springer-Verlag Berlin Heidelberg 2002
Printed in Germany

The use of general descriptive names, registered names, trademarks, etc. in this publication does not imply, even in the absence of a specific statement, that such names are exempt from the relevant protective laws and regulations and therefore free for general use.

Production: PRO EDIT GmbH, Heidelberg, Germany
Cover design: Erich Kirchner, Heidelberg, Germany
Typesetting: K + V Fotosatz GmbH, Beerfelden, Germany

Printed on acid-free paper
SPIN 10497445 24/3130/Di 5 4 3 2 1 0

Foreword

Medullary nailing is one of the oldest types of surgical fracture treatment. Splinting a fracture by insertion of plugs made of ebony dates back to the ancient Egyptian culture. As for many other types of fracture treatment, some outstanding but lone pioneers performed what was in their hands an art based on intuition. But most of them remained lonely pioneers since they could teach neither the basics nor the surgical art without a deeper understanding of the underlying science. It took the tenacity of Küntscher to establish medullary nailing as an accepted method of treatment world-wide. It is a method that is attractive because of its apparent simplicity and tolerance of the procedures. Küntscher's great achievements were certainly crowned by his success in convincing other pioneers, such as L. Böhler and M.E. Müller, to accept his procedure and to use it in addition to their own special approaches.

It is interesting to note that in respect to what we today understand to be the state of the art in locked medullary nailing. Küntscher had visionary ideas that led the way but did not come to fruition. This gave the next generation the opportunity to made an essential contribution. Küntscher's "detention nail" remained a Cinderella until Klemm and Schellman proved the clinical merits of locked nailing. This technology widened the spectrum of indications for nailing and improved its safety. As impressive as their achievements were, it took the vision and determination of Ivan Kempfs to grasp the idea and to push for its realization. To Arsène Grosse, an ingenious developer and surgeon, we owe a technology that would be accepted and soon find world-wide recognition.

Early on, I was impressed not only by the technology, its simplicity and its safety, but even more so by the school of thought of the Strasbourg team that devised a way of teaching the system to encourage general acceptance. An important factor that contributed to this acceptance was the fact that this school reported clinical experience in a way that did not allow the surgeon to be carried away by enthusiasm. They impressed by reporting merits and pitfalls alike in a very realistic and convincing manner.

When we consider the past, we automatically confront the question, "What is next?" Where are today's problems and what could the solutions be? The present book discusses the view that medullary nailing is able to compensate for the disturbance to blood circulation brought by the fracture, the surgical procedures, the instruments and the implants. On the one hand, it is apparent that there is potential for biological improvements, specifical in terms of avoiding or reducing traumata due to reaming. But this will invariably be achieved at the expense of stability or strength of the fixation. Similar to the possibilities for improving the afferent blood supply, the effects of nailing on a patient local circulation and general, disseminated, microvascular aggregation must be resolved, especially for patients with thoracic trauma. We are convinced that the spirit established by the group in Strasbourg and Hong Kong and maintained by their colleagues and pupils provides good reason to hope that the next step forward is not far beyond the horizon. The present book will not only help the clinically active surgeon and his team, but will serve as a guide to the researcher and developer in the insatiable urge to strive for improvements.

It is obvious that no single method can solve all the problems of fracture treatment. Progress and success depend on clean concepts and optimal employment of each single method. This is where the present book, made with care, deep insight and great experience concerning the important technology of medullary nailing by the authors and editors I. Kempf and K.S. Leung, contributes in an outstanding way.

Stephan Perren
Davos, 16 December 2000

Preface

Following the steps of Gerhard Küntscher, the father of intramedullary fixation of fractures, Dr. Klemm and Dr. Schellmann from Frankfurt am Main, Germany, took up the idea of locking the nail to the bone in the early 1970s. Professor Ivan Kempf and Dr. Arsène Grosse from Strasbourg, France, further developed these concepts, putting intramedullary locked nails into clinical practice in a systemic and scientific manner for the first time. In fact, the introduction of the intramedullary locked nail system to musculoskeletal trauma was considered to be one of the major advancements of the 1970s. Throughout these years, hundreds of training courses were organised to promote the concept and practice of the closed treatment of long bone fractures with this technique. Numerous clinical results have proven the beneficial effect of the technique to patients. Intramedullary locked nail has become an indispensable instrument in fracture management as well as reconstructive surgery in orthopaedics. Fixing long bone fractures with intramedullary locked nails agrees with the modern concept of minimally invasive surgery.

Intramedullary fixation fulfils the biological requirement for fracture healing and minimises surgical trauma. Intramedullary locked nails provide a favourable biomechanical environment, from fracture stabilisation to post-operative rehabilitation. In accordance with the principles of closed biological treatment of fractures and minimally invasive techniques, most long bone fractures can be stabilised using this technique without embarking on more complicated and invasive methods. With many innovative modifications, this technique has been applied to managing difficult trauma conditions as well as a number of other orthopaedic conditions. Today, it is our strong belief that the use of intramedullary locked nails in the management of long bone fractures has become a well-established philosophy of patient management. The principles and applications are universal and far beyond the limit of any particular instrument or implant. Based on this faith, *Practice of Intramedullary Locked Nails* is written in the hope that this technique will evolve further for the betterment of patients.

This book describes the use and relevance of the closed technique of intramedullary locked nails in orthopaedic and trauma surgeries. *The Practice of Intramedullary Locked Nails* comprises of two volumes: Vol. 1 covers the scientific principles and standard surgical techniques of intramedullary locked nails; Vol. 2 covers the advanced surgical techniques in extended indications. This work would not have been possible without the contribution and collaboration of world-leading trauma centres. The contributions from surgeons with different areas of expertise throughout the world are essential in providing international and comprehensive views of these nailing techniques.

Ivan Kempf
Kwok-Sui Leung

Acknowledgements

This book could not have been completed after such an exceptionally long period of preparation without the support and contribution of our friends and colleagues. Our special gratitude goes to:

- Our friends and colleagues who prepared the manuscripts based on the framework proposed by the editorial board. Without their patience and relentless support, this book could never have become a reality.
- Our co-editors and the members of the editorial board who share our vision in promoting the concept and practice of the closed treatment of fractures developed by Prof. Gerhard Küntscher with the intramedullary locked nails.
- Professor Stephan Perren, our dear friend and colleague, for his kind remarks in the Foreword.
- The council members of the AIOD who have supported the project throughout these years of preparation.
- The secretarial staff of the AIOD, especially Mrs. Margot Hamm, Mrs. Michèle Obringer and Ms. Audrey Muller for their patience, endurance and perseverance in making the project progress, for their excellent and professional secretarial support in preparing the manuscripts.
- Mrs. Christiane Schaeffer-Cinqualbre, who prepared the illustrations.
- Mr. Robert Cooley for improving the English of the manuscripts.
- The staff of Springer-Verlag in Heidelberg, especially Mrs. G. Schröder, who supported the project from the very beginning, and for their expertise in producing and publishing this book.

Contents

Contributors

Dr. F. BIGGI
Ospedale Maggiore
Azienda USL Citta di Bologna
40133 Bologna, Italy

Prof. M. BROOKES
68 Lakenheath, Southgate
N14 4RP London, U.K.

Dr. E.N.M. CHEUNG
The Chinese University of Hong Kong
Department of Orthopaedics and Traumatology
Shatin, Hong Kong SAR, China

Dr. D. DAGRENAT
Cabinet de Chirurgie Orthopédique
16 Allée de la Robertsau
67000 Strasbourg, France

Prof. J.-C. DOSCH
Centre de Traumatologie et d'Orthopédie
10 Avenue A. Baumann
67400 Strasbourg, France

Dr. M.G. DUPUIS
Centre de Traumatologie et d'Orthopédie
10 Avenue A. Baumann
67400 Strasbourg, France

Dr. A. GROSSE
Centre de Traumatologie et d'Orthopédie
10 Avenue A. Baumann
67400 Strasbourg, France

Prof. I. KEMPF
Association Internationale
pour l'Ostéosynthèse Dynamique
16 Rue du Parc
67205 Strasbourg, France

Dr. K. KLEMM †
Landgrabenstraße 5
61118 Bad-Villbeck, Germany

Prof. C. LEFÈVRE
Hôpital de la Cavale Blanche
Service d'Orthopédie
29200 Brest, France

Prof. D. LE NEN
Hôpital de la Cavale Blanche
Service d'Orthopédie
29200 Brest, France

Prof. K.S. LEUNG
The Chinese University of Hong Kong,
Department of Orthopaedics and Traumatology
Shatin, Hong Kong SAR, China

Dr. H. SEIDEL
Allgemeines Krankenhaus Wandsbeck
Abteilung für Unfallchirurgie
Alphonsstraße 14
22043 Hamburg, Germany

Prof. D. SELIGSON
School of Medicine
Department of Orthopaedic Surgery
University of Louisville
40292 Louisville, KY, USA

Dr. Ing. A. SPEITLING
Stryker Trauma GmbH
Prof.-Küntscher-Straße 1–5
24232 Schönkirchen, Germany

Dr. G. TAGLANG
Centre de Traumatologie et d'Orthopédie
10 Avenue A. Baumann
67400 Strasbourg, France

CHAPTER 1

Introduction

I. Kempf and H. Seidel

Since time immemorial, man has been the victim of accidents which led to fractures, and it is known that cave men, when faced with this problem, devised ways of immobilization in order to treat and heal injuries which were a threat to survival. Splints made of branches and fixed in place with lianas, applied after an approximate alignment of the fragments, ensured, in line with the still eternal principles of fracture treatment today, the immobilization of the fracture until it healed.

Gradually methods improved, with splints, bandages and different devices and especially with the development of continuous traction and plaster bandages. These methods were used for millennia right down to the first half of the twentieth century with Lorenz Böhler [1] at the height of his career and accomplishments. His treatise *Die Technik der Knochenbruchbehandlung* (*The Technique of Fracture Treatment*) [1] represents an unequaled survey of this field, taken up and improved by Sarmiento with his *Functional Bracing* [9], which freed the joints adjacent to the fracture. The indications for this method should still apply and slow down the current trend in developed countries of operating on everything. It is still the basis of fracture treatment in the developing countries.

Operative treatment of fractures emerged only after the advent of antisepsis and asepsis. Its origins lie in the first half of the nineteenth century and it developed in two directions:

- The open procedure with exposure and open reduction of the fragments followed by internal fixation using the most varied means: bone sutures, wiring, stapling, screws, plates and screws, pegs, pins, nails.
- The closed procedure combining reduction without opening the fracture site and fixation using implants introduced or placed at a distance from the fracture.

As far as the open technique is concerned, development focused mainly on techniques using screws and plates with screws. After the age of the pioneers, Hansmann, Sherman, Hey-Groves, Lambotte – inventor of the expression osteosynthesis – and others, it was with Danis [2], who created the compression plate later taken up and perfected by Müller et al. [8] and the Arbeitsgemeinschaft für Osteosynthesefragen/Association for the Study of Internal Fixation (AO/ASIF), that this technique with the compression screw definitively acquired its position of eminence.

The closed procedure developed more slowly. Using mainly intramedullary implants, pegs made of metal, ivory, bovine cortical bone, etc., are introduced initially through an open site technique. Extra-articular closed nailing of femoral neck fractures devised and implemented by Senn, Delbet, Royal-Whitman, and Smith Petersen opened the way to closed intramedullary nailing of which Küntscher [5, 6, 7] is rightly considered to be the creator. As early as 1940, he set out its principles and the way it could be performed. First he devised the hollow nail with a slot and clover-leaf section, then reaming, which made it possible to use larger nails, and finally, at the end of his life, he laid down the basis for locked nailing.

Küntscher started a revolution in fracture management with this new treatment. He was 40 years old when he published his technique and philosophy of fracture treatment in the 64th volume of the *Deutsche Gesellschaft für Chirurgie* [5] in 1940 in Berlin. His concept was completely new and revolutionary for the establishment. Küntscher reaped a storm of controversy, denial, and personal attacks. His ideas were rejected on the grounds of the existing anatomical science and the accepted standards of fracture treatment. Even today we hear some of these arguments used against the intramedullary nailing technique. However, the clinical background is more advanced than in those pioneering days and there are sufficient experimental data and clinical experience to support the technique. In proposing a direct approach to the medullary canal, Küntscher was running against the widely accepted science of the bone marrow. In the nineteenth century,

Lorenz from Vienna had postulated that one should never touch the marrow because it was considered that the bone marrow is the heart of the bone. Similarly, August Bier in the same century believed that the bone marrow has the main importance for the fracture consolidation. Küntscher himself admitted that he placed the first intramedullary nail with "trembling and quail." The first case was performed in a dog, the results being both spectacular and an overwhelming success with painless anatomical reconstruction of the fracture and full function and weight bearing in a short time. Following these successful animal studies, Küntscher's first human clinical case was a successful femoral nailing in November 1939.

Küntscher was not the first to stabilize a fracture using an intramedullary approach. Such methods had previously been performed by several surgeons. Nicolaysen (1897), Delbet (1906), Lambotte (1907), Schöne (1913), Rush (1927), Müller Mernach (1933), Joly (1935), and Danis (1937) [8] all used intramedullary approaches to fracture management, but their techniques, mainly with opening of the fracture site, were all different from that proposed by Küntscher. They all used different materials for pinning. However, their methods were not functionally stable and were associated with high complication rates.

The principles of Küntscher's new technique are: (a) closed procedure, (b) stable fracture fixation, (c) no external fixation, and (d) early weight bearing. The key to the intramedullary nail designed by Künstcher was that he had extensively studied bone loading and the reaction of the bone once under load. In order to do this, he borrowed the varnish technique developed by two engineers, Dietrich and Leber from Zeppelin industries of Meibach, to visualize the flow of the stretch on the bone. He was able to show the stress lines of the bone during compression and elongation. The conclusion he reached was that new bone, callus, is disturbed during normal loading with the risk of pseudarthrosis. He concluded that only a massive steel implant was capable of neutralizing the bone stress, which he estimated at 10 kg/cm^2 or 1,000–1,500 kg for the femur, and at the same time ensure sufficient stability of the fracture so as to remove the need for external support of the fracture. For such a massive implant, Küntscher considered only the medullary canal capable of accommodating the implant. It was the birth of the intramedullary nail. With his hypothesis deduced from the bone varnish tests, Küntscher's new technique in fracture treatment was the starting point for the development of his ideas. To stabilize the fracture fragments, Küntscher chose a self-locking technique by means of elastic nails with a V-profile – the so-called clover leaf profile. Although surgical colleagues were not convinced of this technique, mechanical engineers adopted the technique and patented the design. The so-called "Schwerspannstift" is widely used in the industry and it is in essence a Küntscher nail. The principal question raised by the technique of intramedullary nailing, blood supply of the bone and the fracture site, remains a topic of discussion at this time. In animal experiments, Küntscher showed that the nutrition of the bone comes from the periosteal supply without any need of internal vessels of the medullary canal. Millions of patients treated worldwide with intramedullary nails are evidence of the efficiency of the technique. Between 1950 and 1954, Küntscher developed his second new technique, nailing by reaming the medullary canal. With this technique a wider range of indications could be treated than with the classic Küntscher nail. The medullary blood supply is completely destroyed with this technique. Küntscher demonstrated the harmlessness of this technique with both animal studies and his subsequent clinical successes. He also found support for his hypothesis in Walterhöfer and Schramm's work. They removed the bone marrow completely without observing subsequent necrosis of the bone in order to stimulate blood regeneration. Also, Dax performed a ligature of the nutrient artery and again he did not observe bone necrosis. Küntscher's animal tests were confirmed by the work of Brookes and Grundnes and their animal studies. The conclusions of both these teams are: (a) no necrosis of bone following intramedullary nailing, (b) the blood flow is rapidly restored, (c) a rich vascularization of the periosteum is increased, and (d) callus consolidation is stimulated.

For a long time, the open and the closed approaches in the treatment of shaft fractures were in conflict.

- For the supporters of the open technique, the latter made it possible to bring about an exact reduction of the fragments and their perfectly rigid fixation with screws and plates which, in the best cases, gave rise to healing per primam without a callus, or primary healing.
- Those in favour of the closed technique thought quite rightly that the small imperfections of the reduction were largely outweighed by the respect of the fracture area and periosteal vascularization. Moreover, the insertion of a support in the neutral axis of the shaft, which, mechanically, is the most efficient one,

thereby enabling a certain flexibility as well as immediate weight bearing in many cases, constituted an undeniable extra in comparison with the open approach.

Since then the dogma of rigid fixation and per primam healing has been called into question and its followers have moved towards a more biological osteosynthesis, even going so far as to imagine the insertion of plates and screws with a minimally invasive percutaneous approach. The idea of the nailing supporter, with a semi-rigid, more flexible and dynamic fixing device enabling healing through the formation of a per secundam periosteal callus, is confirmed by the quality of the results obtained. At the present time, the treatment of large shaft fractures of the femur, tibia, and humerus using Küntscher's intramedullary nailing is in top position despite its drawbacks: imperfection in reduction, the technique's difficulties and risks, danger of radiation, and outcome of endomedullary vascularization. Gradually these drawbacks have been eliminated or reduced:

- The imperfections in reduction, by strict rules of positioning on the fracture table using to a maximum the reduction possibilities of continuous extension – correction of angulation, shortening, rotation – completed if necessary by external manipulation of lateral displacements that cannot be reduced.
- The real difficulties and pitfalls of the technique, through a cautious operating procedure, on a step-by-step basis with great attention paid to the smallest details. Confidence and skill in carrying out intramedullary locking are acquired through a relatively lengthy learning period and protect from technical incidents and complications.
- The dangers of radiation, through the constant improvement in image intensifiers, which emit smaller and smaller doses of radiation, and the wearing of aprons, protective gloves, etc. by the operating staff.

Periodically, reaming is called into question because of its potential dangers: fat embolism and destruction of endomedullary vascularization. The latter, already considerably damaged by the fracture itself, is largely compensated for as a result of the preservation of periosteal vascularization which revascularizes the ischaemic cortex in a short period of time. As for the danger of fat embolism, due to the hyperpressure brought about by reaming but which only exceptionally occurs clinically, this is considerably reduced by the use of appropriately shaped reamers.

Nonetheless, in its standard form, nailing with reaming was relatively limited in application, the ideal indication being the transverse mid-shaft fracture, extended upwards and downwards to 3 cm from the widening of the medullary canal. Many types and locations of fracture could not be repaired by this excellent method, which, in the absence of a sufficiently long and intact medullary canal, could not control rotation, telescoping, or major angulation.

The different attempts to remedy these weaknesses – opening the site with additional insertion of wires, screws, plates, flanged nails, expansion nails, Kaesmann nails, or compression devices, etc., finally led to the better solution of locking. Locked nailing was devised by Küntscher [6] at the end of his life, following both the fundamental principles of static fixing and dynamic fixing as well as the technical implementation with the transfixed nail he called "Detentionsnagel," and was developed by Klemm and Schellmann [4] in Germany under the name "Verriegelungsnagel," then by Kempf and Grosse [3] in France under the name "enclouage verrouillé." The AO/ASIF only presented its "Universal-Nagel" in 1986. Locked intramedullary nailing has made it possible to extend the benefits of the method to types and locations of fractures of the femur and tibia which had, until then, remained inaccessible: proximal and distal fractures from metaphysis to metaphysis, long oblique fractures, spiral, double, and third fragment fractures, and comminuted fractures with bone loss. Then locked nailing was extended to other bones such as the humerus, the ulna, and recently the radius as well as the upper end of the femur, thanks to the Gamma nail.

In elective surgery, nonunions, corrective osteotomies and reconstructions after tumour surgery have all benefited from this method. In biomechanical terms, closed intramedullary nailing with or without interlocking presents obvious advantages over plate fixation: the plate, in an off-centre position, is less efficient mechanically than the nail, which, placed in the central neutral axis of the bone, in most cases permits weight bearing which is often immediate and always early. Moreover, the osteosynthesis plate, far more rigid, brings about bone atrophy with an impairment of mechanical qualities. Unlike the plate which destroys periosteal vascularization, the nail presents satisfactory biological conditions because the closed site respects this vascularization and, unlike the poor, fragile cortical callus, allows the formation of abundant peripheral callus that is mechanically resistant. The immobilization of the site is not rigid but allows for a certain flexibility enabling small movements of intermittent compression during walking and muscular contraction because the nail only neutralizes twisting and flexion movements.

Thanks to this closed dynamic osteosynthesis, both mechanically and biologically healing conditions are better than those offered by open-site osteosynthesis using plates and screws. Thus the practice of rigid osteosynthesis with plating systems is now seriously challenged worldwide.

References

1. Böhler L (1953) Die Technik der Knochenbruchbehandlung, W. Maudrich, Vienna
2. Danis R (1949) Théorie et pratique de l'ostéosynthèse, Manon et Cie Edition, Paris
3. Kempf I, Grosse A, Lafforgue D (1978) L'apport du verrouillage dans l'enclouage centro-médullaire des os longs. Rev Chir Ortho 64:635–651
4. Klemm K, Schellmann WD (1972) Dynamische und statische Verriegelung des Marknagels. Monatschr Unfallklinik 75:568–575
5. Küntscher G (1940) Die Tecknik der Marknagelung des Oberschenckels. Zbl f Chir 1940z:1145
6. Küntscher G (1964) Die Nagelung des Defekttrümmerbruches Chirurg 35:277
7. Küntscher G, Maatz R (1945) Technik der Marknagelung. Georg Thieme Verlag, Leipzig
8. Müller M, Allgöwer M, Willeneger H (1963) Technik der operativen Frakturenbehandlung. Springer, Berlin Göttingen Heidelberg
9. Sarmiento A (1981) Closed functional treatment of fractures. Springer, Berlin

CHAPTER 2

The Biology of Fracture Healing as Related to Intramedullary Locked Nailing

F. Biggi

Introduction

In his original article published in May 1978 [18], McKibbin clearly outlined that: "The healing of a fracture is one of the most remarkable of all the repair processes in the body, since it results not in a scar, but in the actual reconstitution of the injured tissue in something very like its original form. ... A number of factors influence the healing which can be identified from both clinical and experimental work and may be taken into consideration to put treatment on a more rational basis." So a knowledge of the natural history of the fracture healing process is the first and probably the most important step in choosing the right fixation method and technique and also in evaluating all clinical and radiological phases of fracture repair. Research in various fields (developed by histologists, biologists, engineers, radiologists and trauma surgeons) has clarified many aspects of this very complex process, making it possible to say that fracture healing is a multifaceted process characterised by four different but closely interdependent stages: the cellular stage, the vascular stage, the histobiochemical stage, and the biohumoral or mediator stage [4, 5, 7, 8, 10, 14, 21, 26].

The Cellular Stage

The cellular stage is the one leading to the formation of new bony tissue. In the last 20 years, the role of osteoblasts has become better clarified, and it is now known that bone healing requires much more than osteoblasts alone [4, 6, 7, 13]. In this stage we can include *fracture, granulation tissue, provisional callus formation, callus remodelling* and *definitive new bone.*

The *fracture* itself is the immediate reaction that is the first signal-triggering process. The local precursor cells are "sensitised" by biochemical mediators so that activation and proliferation occur [6, 7, 14, 20]. At the same time (Fig. 2.1) macrophages and polymorphs clean up the area

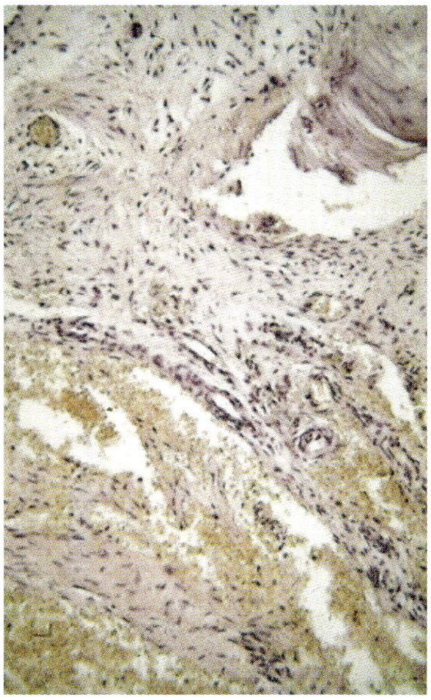

Fig. 2.1. Fracture site immediately after fracture showing macrophages and polymorphs cleaning up the area

by removing all necrotic debris. The haematoma inside and around the fracture site progressively reduces while cellular response is more active. This first biological response probably lasts for 7 days after injury and it is undoubtedly clear that closed reduction respects the fracture site, the haematoma and the surrounding soft tissue, while open reduction does not. This first stage is fundamental since the *mediators* determine if and where fibroblasts, chondroblasts, endothelial cells and osteoblasts will appear; they also determine when and how to nourish them, how many there will be, and how long they will be active. During this phase the system needs stability, and the X-ray appearance shows no-reaction signs (grade 1 callus).

Granulation tissue (Fig. 2.2) represents a true proliferation stage because the sensitised and stimulated cells, reacting to the mediator's signals, produce new cells which develop into fibroblasts, chondroblasts, endothelial cells and the so-called

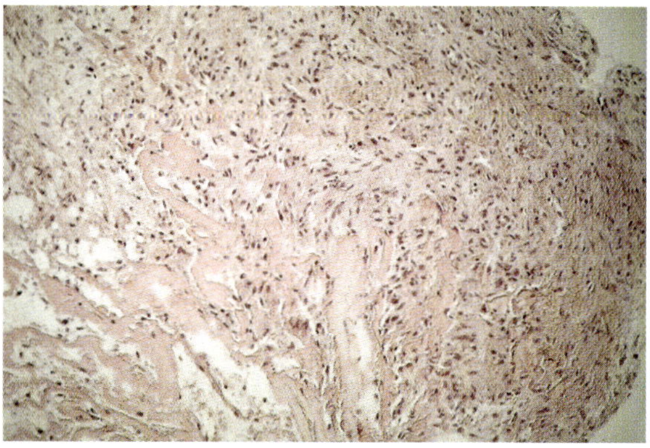

Fig. 2.2. Proliferation of granulation tissue by stimulated cells

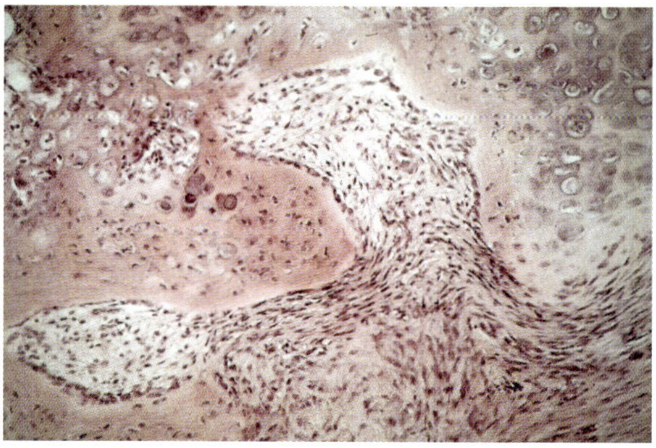

Fig. 2.4. The osteoid tissue with temporary ossification front called the "tide mark line"

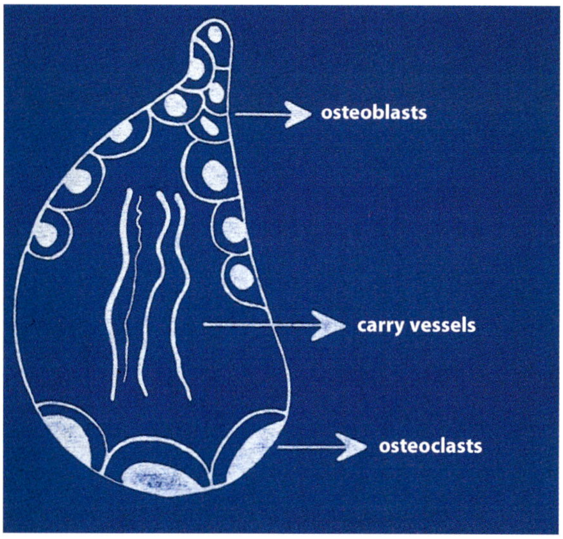

Fig. 2.3. The cutter heads carry vessels, osteoblasts and osteoclasts

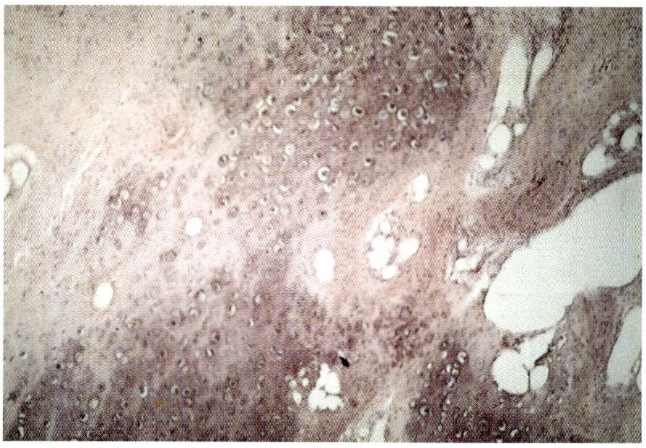

Fig. 2.5. Remodelling during which the woven bone is replaced by lamellar bone

supporting cells (mainly mast cells, and reticuloendothelial cells). These supporting cells, as well as some types of leukocytes and platelets, become the mediator's *producers*. A thin cuff surrounds the bone ends, being an element of intrinsic stability which helps the penetration of cutter heads (Fig. 2.3) carrying vessels, osteoblasts and osteoclasts. At this stage, which lasts about 2 weeks, the system still needs stability. The X-ray appearance corresponds to the grade 2 callus: thin radiopaque trabeculae with no structural appearance, which can be clearly seen by ultrasonography [3].

The *callus*, young and temporary, begins to develop at around the fourth or fifth week. It originates mainly from the periosteum and represents a more specialised granulation tissue which creates new chondroblasts, osteoblasts, the former synthesising extracellular matrix and the latter controlling an immature ossification process. The intercellular matrix begins to calcify at around the fifth or sixth week, and it is strong enough for the patient to resume function with caution. At this moment (Fig. 2.4), the bony tissue is defined as *osteoid*, characterised by the temporary ossification front called the "tide mark line" with no structural orientation. This is the true induced fracture healing, which is certainly encouraged by function and micromotion at the fracture site. The X-ray appearance corresponds to the grade 3 callus that shows at least one periosteal bridge.

Remodelling represents the definitive development of new, well-mineralised bone, with osteoid tissue completely replaced by well-orientated lamellar bone (Fig. 2.5). Osteons are aligned parallel to the compression and traction lines because of weight-bearing and active muscle contraction. Finally, all internal mineralised cartilage is removed in order to restore the medullary cavity.

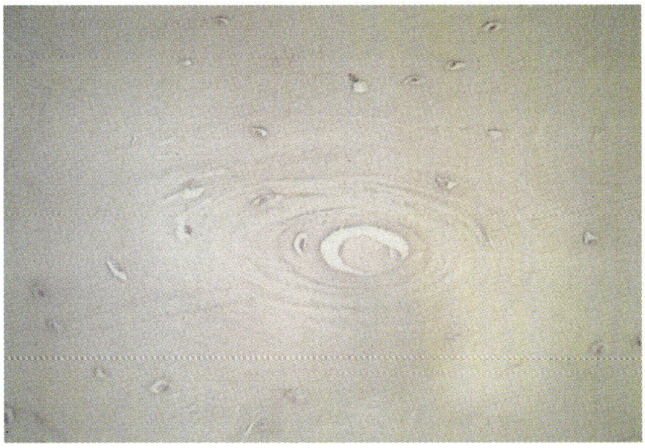

Fig. 2.6. Definitive new bone

All these stages take about 1 year to be completed and are directed by basic multicellular units (BMU) formed by many kinds of cells, intercellular materials, venous and arterial capillaries, which are strictly related to each other for replacing the woven bone with new lamellar bone under the mediator's control [8, 10]. The X-ray appearance corresponds to the grade 4 callus, showing two periosteal bridges and internal radio-opacity. Full weight-bearing and complete function are allowed.

Definitive new bone represents the restoration of the original structure directed by the BMU system (each BMU works over a period of 3–4 months). The final result (Fig. 2.6) is the complete replacement of the callus with mature well-orientated lamellar bone and the restoration of the medullary cavity. The X-ray appearance is defined as grade 5 callus with a typical spindle-shaped cuff. Frost [9], collecting many reports by different authors, emphasized the role played by the RAP (Regional Acceleratory Phenomenon), which acts normally in the tissues and accelerates in special situations, such as fracture and the subsequent healing process. This special research field is investigated by histomorphometrists, showing an increase in metabolic activity a few days after fracture, gaining for a maximum of 1 or 2 months later, decreasing at around 6 months, and ending 1 or 2 years later. (Many techniques were used for evaluating this metabolic increase: Tc-99 bone scan, measurement of regional mitosis, ATP production, pH increase and radiological callus formation.) We can say today that fracture acts like a message, represented by the *cellular stage*; an awakening, sensitising and accelerating of the potentials already present in the tissue.

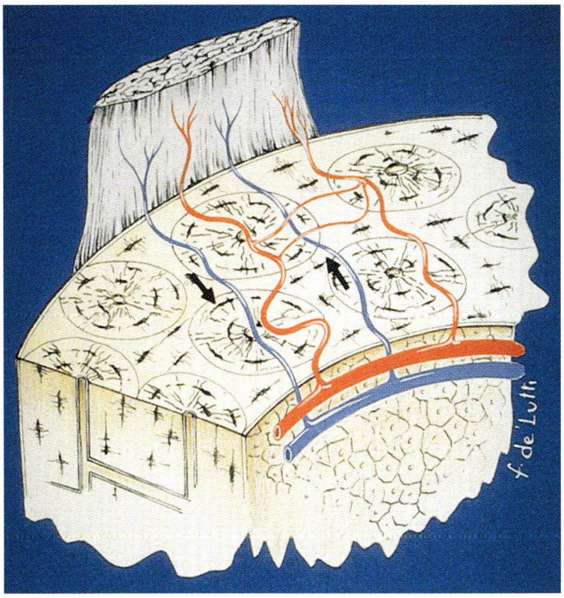

Fig. 2.7. The reversal of the cortical blood flow

The Vascular Stage

The *vascular stage* strongly influences the entire fracture healing process. Diaphyseal bone is equipped with an afferent system supplied by the nutrient medullary artery and by metaphyseal and periosteal arterioles; an efferent system called the internal venous sinus; a microsystem of sinusoid capillaries and arterioles of 8 μm and venules with diameter of 15–60 μm. Any fracture interferes with vascular supply and always damages the central medullary system which supplies the internal two-thirds of cortex [22]. The vascular penetration from the periosteum and surrounding soft tissues, enhanced by reduction and stabilisation, is fundamental to fracture healing [23–25]. Many studies have outlined that the bone vascular system is normally contained by rigid walls that makes compensation difficult after a fracture has occurred. For this reason, a reverse flow starts to accelerate the arterial inflow and the venous outflow (Fig. 2.7) and to activate the so-called resting vessels, which are normally not working. This is a neoangiogenic process arising from reticuloendothelial elements and smooth-muscle cells, triggered by mediators released at the fracture site. Other studies identified an *angiogenic factor* which stimulates the process and a *bone growth factor* secreted by endothelial cells which stimulates the osteogenic precursors. Neoangiogenesis [1, 12, 20] plays a central role in the entire process. Strictly related to the vascular phase of fracture healing is *reaming*. As a result of the consid-

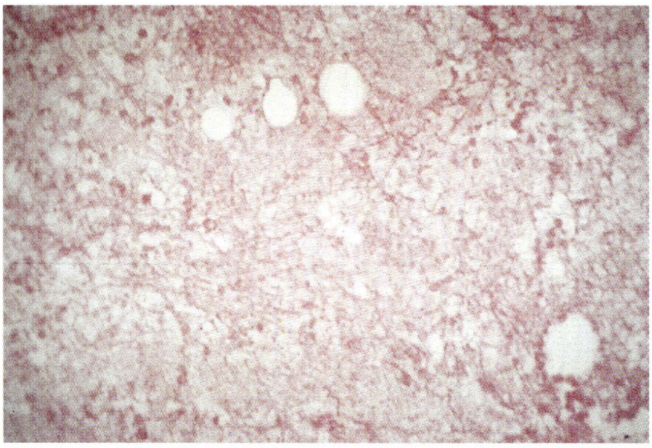

Fig. 2.8. Fibrous tissue covering the endosteum after reaming

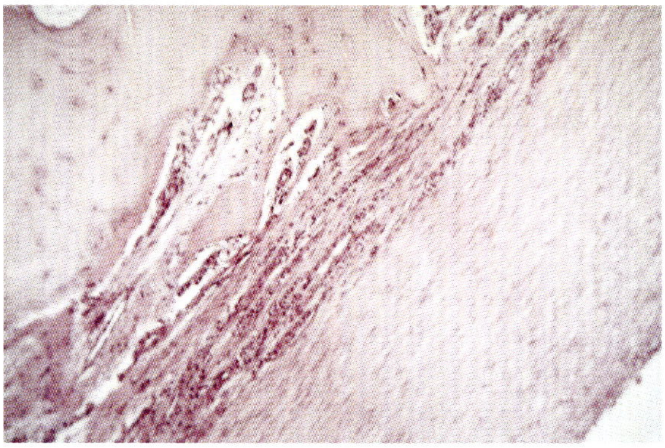

Fig. 2.9. New cortical bone 1 year after fracture

erable mechanical and thermal damage to the endosteal surface and the consequent worsening of vascular supply, the endosteum is covered by fi-

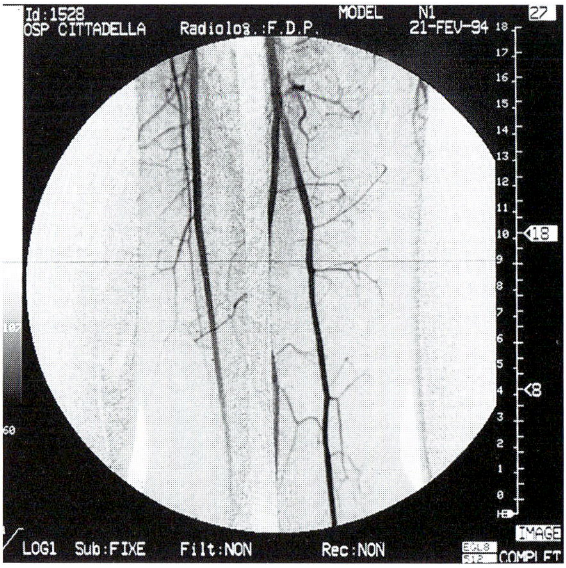

Fig. 2.10. Digitalized angiography showing the vasculature after reamed nailing

brous tissue 4–6 weeks after nailing (Fig. 2.8). One year later, although a thin layer of fibrous tissue still covers the endosteum, a new well-vascularized cortical lamellar bone is present (Fig. 2.9). The vascular response after intramedullary nailing was also investigated with digitalized angiography [3] in order to verify modification in parosteal macro-circulation after reaming. A clearly visible, well-defined vascular tree with branches supplying the new bone bridging the fracture site was observed 8 weeks later (Figs. 2.10, 2.11). No significant differences, in terms of callus formation,

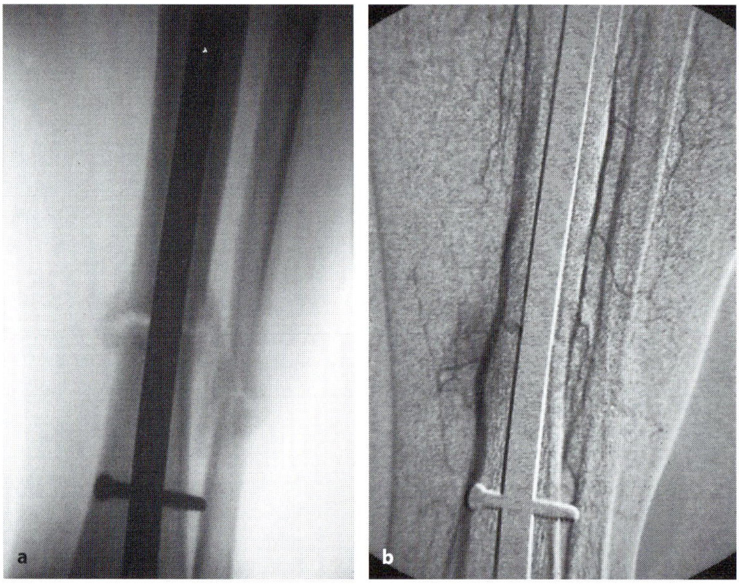

Fig. 2.11 a, b. Vascular supply to the actively repairing fracture site

were found compared with the fracture treated by reamed nails and by external fixator (also by ultrasonography). In conclusion, fracture fixation must ensure stability to allow early function; it must comply with periosteal vascularization, permit new vessel formation and penetration and allow restoration of endosteal circulation.

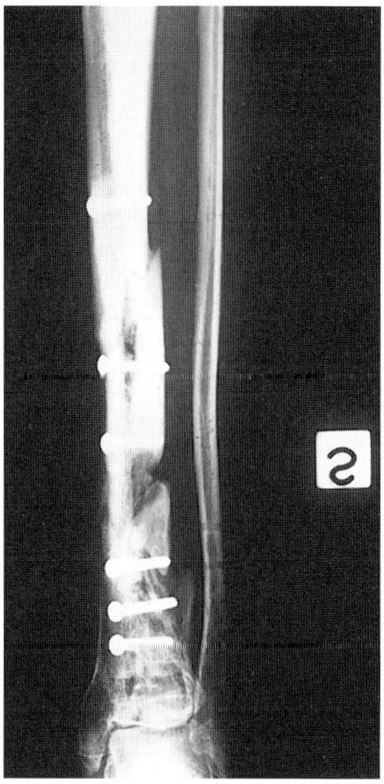

Fig. 2.12. Technical failure

The Histobiochemical Stage

The *histobiochemical stage* concerns the "where, how, when and who" which initiates and controls the calcification process. Research in this field has been focussed by Bonucci [3] on the identification of a *common calcifying factor.* This factor should be present in all calcifying matrix, including the pathological one. It should be an intrinsic component of the matrix and should be present or detectable at the beginning of or during the calcification process. It should be controlled by cells or other factors. In the past, Glimcher and Krone [3, 4], by observing the layout of collagen fibres, identified some points containing chemical groups able to favour the deposition of calcium salts, the so-called "hole-zone" theory. Because it is well known that the deposition of calcium crystals occurs *between* and not *within* collagen fibres, they recognized that something else must be initiating the ossification process. Bonucci identified the *calcifying globules* as positive cellular elements, containing glycoproteins and mucoproteins with alkaline-phosphatase activity, forming hydroxyapatite crystals by fixing calcium ions. These elements have an organic component, the collagen fibres, and an inorganic component, bonding calcium salts. They are isolated only during ossification processes, included pathological ones.

Histobiochemistry emphasizes the role of the intercellular matrix in the ossification processes. Hyaluronic acid is one of most important components. Various studies [16, 17] have demonstrated the abundance of hyaluronic acid in the exudative fluids forming the haematoma cuff at the fracture site, outlining the importance of respecting the haematoma as an important container of mediators.

The Biohumoral or Mediator Stage

The *biohumoral or mediator stage* is the most recent advance [6, 8, 15, 21, 26, 27]. Different substances released after fracture are able to promote the activation and proliferation of pluripotential mesenchymal undifferentiated cells. They are currently being studied in order to evaluate the role they play in this autocrine–paracrine activity, in terms of their influence on producer cells and neighbouring cells. These cells are all connected in a local communication system, triggering the ossification process (a similar process occurs in fracture healing, myositis ossificans, growth plates, algodystrophy and Paget's disease). Mechanical factors, such as compression, traction, and immobilisation, can enhance or inhibit the ossification process. This also applies to bioelectric potentials, magnetic fields, hormones, vitamins, drugs, and surgery [2, 11, 13, 19, 24]. It is possible to divide bone healing problems into *technical failures*, when treatment related problems have impaired the normal biological potential (Fig. 2.12), and *biological failures*, which occur when biological malfunctions have made the correct treatment ineffective. A combination of the two types of failure is also possible. In conclusion, it is possible to say that fracture healing is a highly specialised multi-stage and multifaceted process under the control of a *mediator system.* The fracture itself initiates the process during which fixation stability and vascular supply are absolutely essential. A knowledge of the natural history of fracture healing must be our guide in choosing the best fixation technique.

References

1. Auerbach R, Alby L, Morrissey LW, Joseph J (1985) Expression of organ specific antigens on capillary endothelial cells. Microvasc Res 29:401
2. Bassett CAL, Valdes MG, Hernandez AJ (1982) Modification of fracture repair with selected pulsing electromagnetic fields. J Bone Joint Surg Am 64:888–895
3. Biggi F (1995) The biology of fracture repairing after intramedullary osteosynthesis – Abstract Book, Cours de base sur l'enclouage verrouille centro-medullaire. AIOD, pp 12–15
4. Biggi F, D'Imporzano M (1990) Studio dell'osteogenesi riparativa in rapporto alla sintesi endomidollare. Howmedica, Milano, pp 3–29
5. Chapman MW (1987) Induction of fracture repair: osteoinduction, osteoconduction and adjunctive care. In: Lane JM (ed) Fracture healing. Churchill Livingstone, London, p 81–86
6. Chapman MW (1987) Prostaglandins and secondary injury phenomenon. In: Lane JM (ed) Fracture healing. Churchill Livingstone, London
7. Davidowitch Z, Shanfeld JL, Montgomery PC, Lally E, Laster L, Furst L, Korostoff E (1984) Biochemical mediators of the effects of mechanical forces and electrical currents on mineralised tissues. Calcif Tissue Int 36:586
8. Frost HM (1980) Skeletal physiology and bone remodelling: an overview. In: Urist MR (ed) Fundamental and clinical bone physiology. Lippincott, Philadelphia, pp 208–218
9. Frost HM (1983) The regional acceleratory phenomenon: A review. Henry Ford Hosp Med J 31:3
10. Frost HM (1989) The biology of fracture healing. An overview for clinicians. Part I. Clin Orthop 248:283–293
11. Goldberg VM, Stevenson S (1987) Natural history of autografts and allografts. Clin Orthop 225:7–16
12. Guenther HL, Fleisch H, Sorgente N (1986) Endothelial cells in culture synthesize – a potent bone cell active mitogen. Endocrinology 119:193–201
13. Gustilo RB (1987) Overview of fracture management. In: Lane JM (ed) Fracture healing. Churchill Livingstone, London, pp 3–21
14. Hult A (1980) Fracture healing. A concept of competing healing factors. Acta Orthop Scand 51:5–8
15. Hult A (1981) Fracture healing. More biology than mechanics. Clin Orthop 156:259–261
16. Hult A, Johnell O, Henricson A (1988) The implantation of demineralized fracture matrix yields more new bone formation than does intact matrix. Clin Orthop 234:235–239
17. Maurer PG, Hudack SS (1952) The isolation of hyaluronic acid from callus tissue of early healing. Arch Biochem Biophys 3:49–57
18. McKibbin B (1978) The biology of fracture healing in long bones. J Bone Joint Surg Br 60:150–162
19. Monticelli G, Spinelli R (1981) Distraction epiphysiolysis as a method of limb lengthening. Experimental study. Clin Orthop 154:254–265
20. Oegama T, An KN, Weiland A, Furcht L (1988) Peripheral blood vessel. In: Woo SLY, Buckwalter JA (eds) Injury and repair of the musculoskeletal soft tissues. American Academy of Orthopaedic Surgeons, Park Ridge, Illinois, pp 201–379
21. Parfitt AM (1984) The cellular basis of bone remodelling: the quantum concept re-examined in light of recent advances in the cell biology of bone. Calcif Tissue Int 36 [Suppl]:37–48
22. Rhinelander FW (1974) Tibial blood supply in relation to fracture healing. Clin Orthop 105:34–81
23. Rhinelander FW, Wilson JW (1982) Blood supply to developing, mature and healing bone. In: Sumner-Smith G (ed) Bone in clinical orthopaedics. Saunders, Philadelphia, pp 81–158
24. Sarmiento A (1974) Functional bracing of tibial fractures. Clin Orthop 105:202–219
25. Trueta J (1963) The role of the vessels in osteogenesis. J Bone Joint Surg Br 45:402–412
26. Urist MR (1983) Bone: formation by autoinduction. Science 220:680–691
27. Urist MR, Lietze A, Mizutani H, Takag K, Triffitt JT, Amstutz J, De Lange R, Termine J, Finerman GAM (1982) A bovine low molecular weight bone morphogenetic protein (BMP) fraction. Clin Orthop 162:219–225

CHAPTER 3

Bone Circulation and Effects of Experimental Interventions

M. Brookes

Introduction

Much of the research into the osseous circulation has centred on the long bones of the appendicular skeleton. The evidence gathered from human bone suggests that its vascularity has much in common with the blood supply of mammalian bone. Across the species, there are similar distinctive vascular patterns in the disparate parts of a long bone: in the diaphysis, metaphysis, epiphysis, cortex and marrow, subarticular and juxtaepiphyseal regions. The vascular character of living bone focuses the mind on the microcirculation as an indispensable factor in the production of bone substance, the regulation of bone metabolism and the repair of bone fractures.

Methods of Investigation

Intravascular Injection

At first, coloured dyes were developed for the perfusion of blood vessels in general, followed by histological examination. In 1875, Ranvier [63] employed vermilion, i.e. mercuric sulphide suspensions. A year later, Langer [45] used ferric ferrocyanide, the chief ingredient of his Prussian blue injection mass, and Hoyer, in 1882 [38], used silver nitrate to demonstrate blood capillaries. But while in 1865, Thiersch [77] introduced lead chromate. The latter has stood the test of time for enhancing fine blood vessels in 3D-CT scans [7, 41].

Radiopaque Marker Substances

Perhaps the most successful and unambiguous method for demonstrating the vascular arrangements in bone, whether in mouse or man, is to inject by syringe or simple gravity feed apparatus, radiopaque suspensions such as barium sulphate or lead chromate into the aorta or main artery of a limb. The perfused bones are then removed, fixed in formalin, decalcified and cut in slices from 400 µm to 4 mm thick depending on the size of the object. These are then radiographed, allowing the distribution of the now radiopaque bone blood vessels to be analysed.

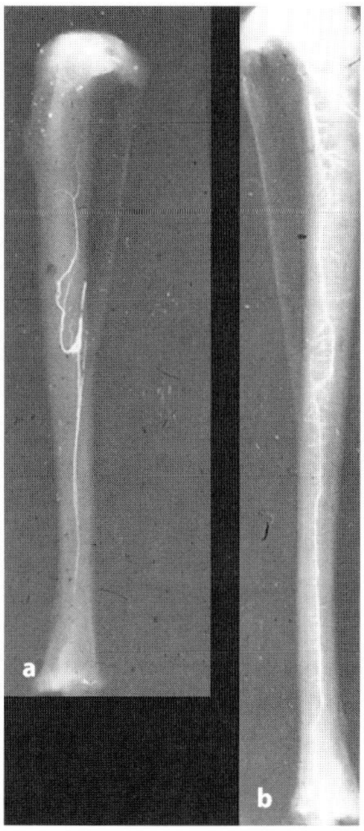

Fig. 3.1 a, b. Rabbit tibial angiograms. **a** Arteriogram showing medullary branches of nutrient artery. **b** Venogram showing central venous sinus and its tributary sinuses

A 45% aqueous suspension of 2 µm barium sulphate particles is excellent for isolating and observing the arterial side of the circulation (Fig. 3.1 a). Because the barium suspension does not fill up the capillary beds, retrovenous injections are necessary to reveal the venous aspect of bone blood vessels (Fig. 3.1 b). For small animal work, a magnification system is imperative. For many years the writer has used a Hilger & Watts microfocal unit with a 10-µm spot X-ray beam source on the tungsten target, and employed it in both contact and projection radiographic modes, using Kodak maximum resolution plates or films [19].

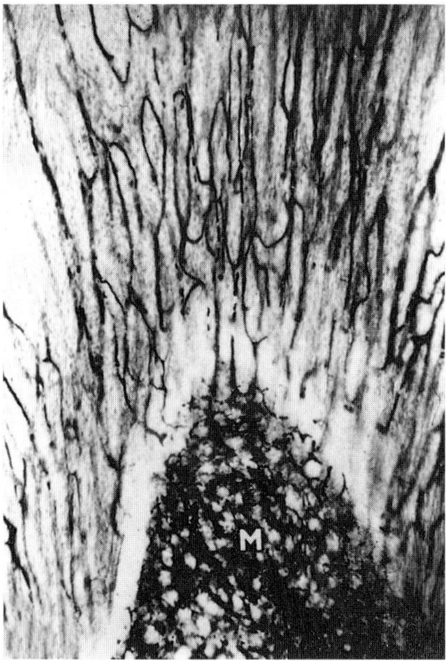

Fig. 3.2. India ink photomicrograph of a histological section through a rat tibia, showing marrow sinusoids (*M*) and cortical capillaries

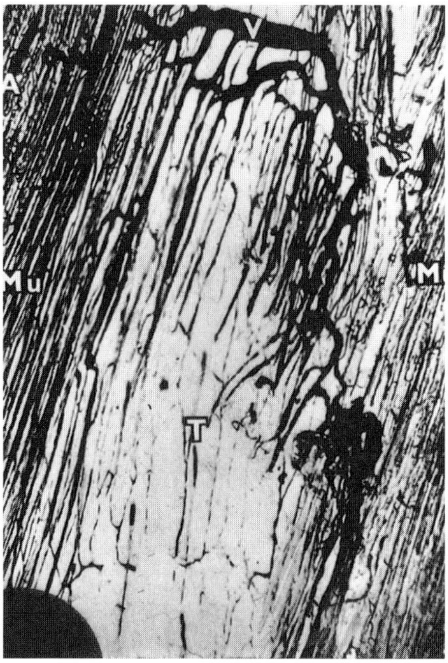

Fig. 3.3. Photomicrograph continuous with Fig. 3.2, showing the tibial crest (*T*), periosteal venules (*V*), and an arteriole (*A*) in muscle (*Mu*)

In the contact mode, the resulting X-ray image is susceptible to photographic enlargement of ×10 to ×25. For most purposes the lower magnification is more than enough for bone vascular studies.

Bone Corrosion Casts

Vascular perfusion with plastic materials followed by corrosion in strong alkali has also contributed to the elucidation of bone vascularization, particularly by indicating the presence of separate vascular territories in whole bone organs [28, 71].

India Ink Suspension

Perfusion with 30% India ink in saline demonstrates osseous capillaries and sinusoids, but the necessary embedding of the bones in gelatin prior to sectioning and examination by light microscopy is time consuming. Nevertheless, the high black and white contrast, and therefore the possibility of higher magnification, gives this method a special utility (Figs. 3.2, 3.3).

Intravital Dyes

The functional blood flow is well demonstrated by the uptake of Disulphine Blue and other water soluble markers such as ferritin and horse radish peroxidase (HRP). These more innovatory methods reveal the functional circulation in vivo and indicate the direction of blood flow in bone.

Bone Structure

In man, fetal cortex is made up of layers of bone trabeculae separated by vascular tissue. In the second year of childhood, the inter-trabecular spaces become filled with primary osteons [32], that is, tiny cylinders of concentric lamellae, each enclosing a central vascular space. Later, secondary, tertiary, and quaternary osteons, otherwise called haversian systems, are formed every 7 years roughly, by the substitution of new concentric lamellae in sites prepared by the local removal of old bone cortex. Circumferential lamellae are deposited at the periosteal and endosteal surfaces at maturity, and have been designated surface bone [72]. As for the blood vessels in bone cortex, multiple vessels occur in the inter-trabecular spaces of fetal cortex; two or three vessels occur in a toddler's primary osteons, but the vascular canals

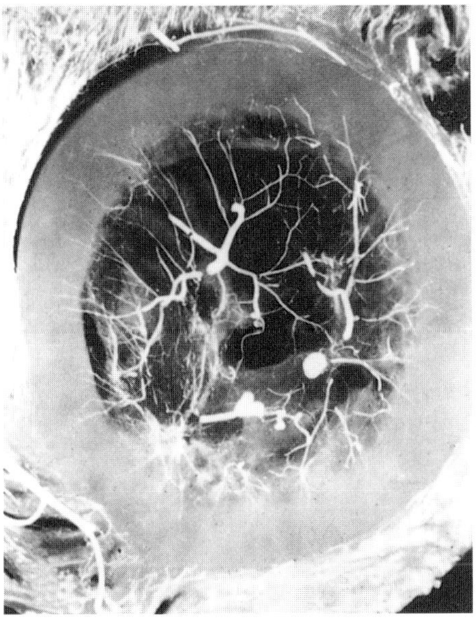

Fig. 3.4. Transverse angiogram through normal canine femur (2 years). The cortex is penetrated by arterioles from the marrow and not from the periosteum

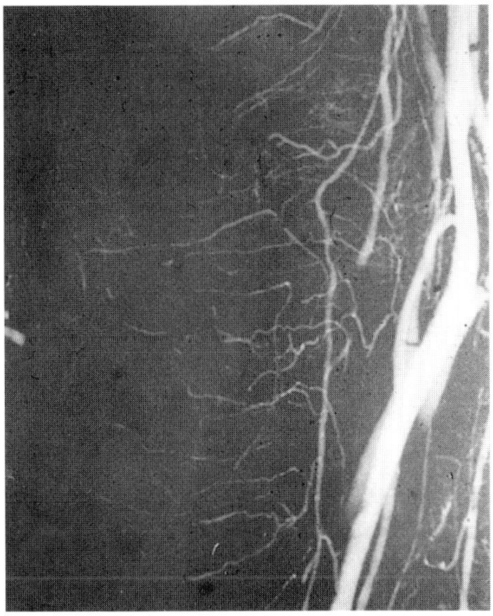

Fig. 3.5. Medullary arterioles seen branching from subcortical arteries in the marrow of a rat. Periosteal arterioles are absent. ×35

in haversian systems generally contain only a single vessel in skeletally mature cortex [18, 56].

Blood Vessels of the Diaphysis

Usually, a single nutrient artery pierces the diaphysis of a long bone. Belonging to the small arteries of anatomical classification, it possesses a tunica media rich in nonstriated myocytes interspersed with elastic and collagenous material. Once in the marrow cavity it breaks up into ascending and descending branches, whose subdivisions lie generally in a subcortical location (Fig. 3.4) and are distributive in function, directing the blood flow to the cortex and marrow. The thick muscular type of arteriole associated with the peripheral resistance of the general circulation, is absent from human and mammalian bone. Instead, the smaller arteries, 250 μm in diameter, abruptly give rise to histological terminal arterioles consisting only of endothelium coated with a few smooth muscle cells [14] acting as precapillary sphincters (Fig. 3.5). These medullary arterioles are the resistance vessels of the osseous circulation, reducing from 100 μm to 5 μm metarterioles in diameter. They end in the cortical capillaries and medullary sinusoids, i.e. the capacitance or reservoir vessels of the cortex and marrow (Fig. 3.2), which regulate the volume of blood in bone.

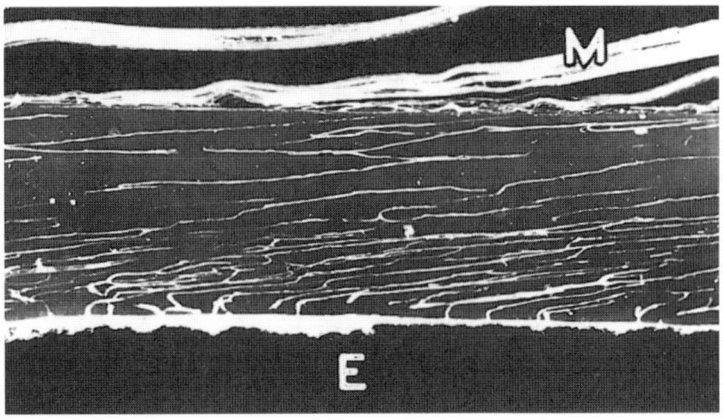

Fig. 3.6. These capillaries in monkey bone cortex largely belong to the periosteal vascular radiation. Those in a thin bony layer close to the marrow cavity (*E*) belong to the endosteal group of cortical vessels. Muscle fasciculi (*M*)

Cortical Capillaries

From the investigations of Testut [75], Weidenreich [83], Marneffe [28], Brookes and Harrison [18], Ham and Leeson [35], Brookes [14], Rhinelander [64], Dillaman [29], Bridgeman and Brookes [8], and many others, the characteristic capacitance vessel to be found in compact bone is a simple endothelial tube of unusual diameter, about 15–30 μm, and can be of unusual length, possibly 2 cm or more in large mammals (Figs. 3.6, 3.7). Cortical vascularization is sparse compared to that in red marrow, but the haversian canals are essentially an extension of the marrow cavity [81]. Indeed, the capillaries of bone cortex

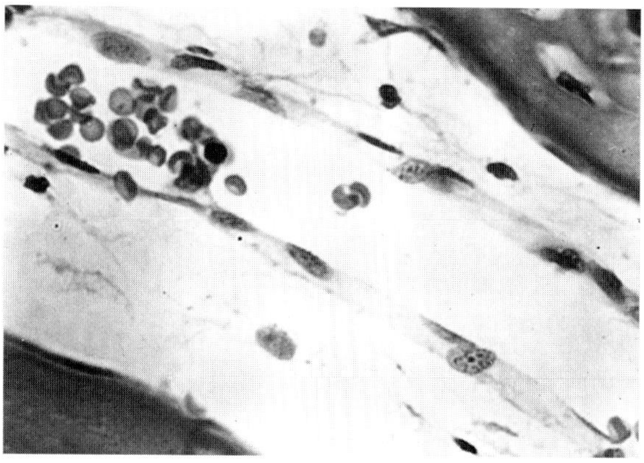

Fig. 3.7. A capillary in the cortex of a human fetal tibia. Its calibre is about 30 μm

are similar to sinusoids, lacking a basement membrane and showing fenestrae in the scanning electron microscope. Although there is a restricted region of the cortex in which the cortical capillaries lie transversely to the long axis of the bone, the general capillary layout is fan-shaped, radiating outwards and obliquely to the surface of the shaft [19]. Short transverse linking vessels unite the unusually long capillaries to form a cortical capillary lattice (Figs. 3.2, 3.3) interposed between the medullary and periosteal circulations, and with a mesh of about 200 μm. This implies that an osteocyte is not more than 100 μm distant from a cortical capillary.

Cortical capillaries become narrower as they approach the periosteal surface (Fig. 3.6). Here, they are continuous with periosteal capillaries, or the interfascicular venules of attached muscle, or the epitendinous vessels at tendon-bone attachments (Fig. 3.8). On the other hand, those situated near the endosteal surface of the bone, where they are continuous with marrow sinusoids, tend to have a wider calibre (Fig. 3.6) than cortical capillaries in general. This does not permit the conclusion that blood flows in the cortex from the periosteal surface into the marrow sinusoids, on the analogy of capillaries widening into venules as in other tissues [24, 37]. The continuity of marrow sinusoids with cortical capillaries gives no indication of the direction of blood flow in the cortex, but is dependent on biomechanics (see p 16).

Arteries of Cancellous Bone

Although perfusion results indicate that the nutrient artery supplies both cortex and marrow of the diaphysis of a long bone, it should be noted that many similar small arteries pierce the cancellous bone extremities. The degree of anastomosis between all these nutrient arterial inputs seems, however, to be sparse. Ablation of diaphyseal [12], metaphyseal [14], or epiphyseal [19] nutrient arteries always leads to some acute zonal necrosis of bone and marrow, which may or may not be corrected in the long term.

Veins

In diaphyseal marrow, the nutrient vein is a branch of the central longitudinal venous sinus (Fig. 3.1 b), confluent with horizontal, radial collecting sinuses draining the medullary sinusoids. Smooth muscle is absent from marrow sinuses. Venous control of the circulation lies in the metarterioles of the cortex, or the small systemic veins outside the bone.

Venous Shunts

The veins accompanying the nutrient arteries outside the bone, lack the valves characteristic of veins lying in intermuscular connective-tissue planes and superficial fascia. Because of this, blood can be shunted down the nutrient veins into the marrow if the great veins of a limb are obstructed. For example, if an Esmarch bandage

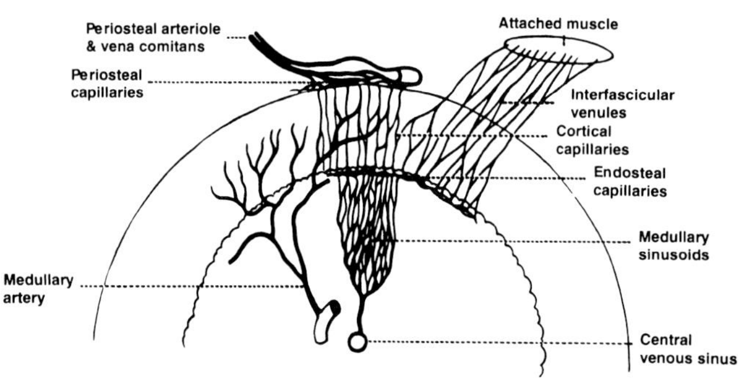

Fig. 3.8. Schema of the blood supply of bone in cross section

is tightly thrown round a cadaveric thigh and a perfusate is propelled into the saphenous vein at the ankle, the perfusion is not obstructed. On amputating the limb above the ligature, the perfusate is seen to pour out of the transected femoral marrow. This explains the incidence of cardiac and CNS toxicity, which complicates intravenous regional anaesthesia (Bier bloc), and why it is possible to demonstrate the venous system of bones by retrograde venography [11].

Young Bone: Medullary Arterial Supply

Cortical arterioles and their metarterioles derived from the medullary arteries, are demonstrable in the inner two-thirds of the cortex (Fig. 3.9) and join the cortical capillaries at an acute angle, pointing outwards to the periosteal surface. Hence, the cortical capillary lattice enjoys a medullary arterial supply.

In particular, terminal arterioles derived from the periosteum have never been convincingly demonstrated in the outer layers of normal bone cortex in the young (i.e. less than 35 years); nor has intra-arterial perfusion with a radiopaque medium ever shown numerous radiopaque streaks entering the cortex from the periosteum in young normal bone. These facts suggest that the direction of flow in bone cortex is normally centrifugal in the young, from the marrow outwards, providing venous escape of cortical blood at the bone surface (Fig. 3.8).

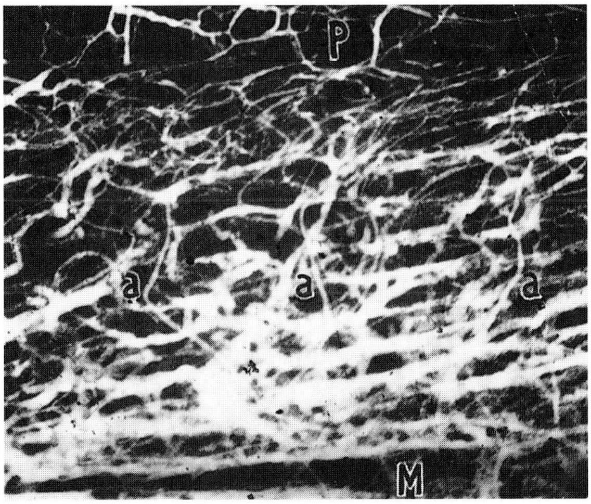

Fig. 3.9. Microangiograph through human fetal cortex. Centrifugal arterioles (*a*) empty into cortical capillaries which join periosteal venules. Marrow (*M*), periosteal vessels (*P*)

Medullary Sinusoids

These characteristic vessels of bone marrow (Fig. 3.2) are varicose in appearance, with a variable diameter of 15–30 μm. Sinusoids are fenestrated endothelial tubes which lack a basement membrane. The cells are held together by junctional complexes and normally permit the passage of blood cells from their extravascular site of development, through the endothelial fenestrae, into the circulating medullary blood. Of course, injected blood-borne cells, particles, and solutes can go the other way, into the haemopoietic extravascular spaces.

Medullary Supply to Cortex

Investigations of the vascular anatomy of long bones are generally confined to youthful rats [10], rabbits [18], and dogs [15], supplemented by human fetal bone [9] and rare adolescent material [11]. Brookes [14, 16, 18] and Rhinelander [64] find that the larger branches of the nutrient artery lie generally in a subcortical situation in the marrow, and supply both cortex and marrow in parallel and not in series. Histologically, these small arteries, with much elastic tissue in the tunica media, give rise to arterioles whose finest branches either end in marrow sinusoids or penetrate the bone endosteally, terminating in the cortical capillary reservoir.

When periosteum and surrounding tissue are perfused, a similar penetration of the external surface of the cortex by periosteal arterioles is not seen. A minor exception is that zygapophyses such as the linea aspera, gluteal tuberosity, and soleal line are pierced by a few periosteal arterioles. Hence, bone angiography suggests that the arterial blood input to the cortex of long bones, in youth, comes overwhelmingly from the marrow, a principle first emphasized by Brookes and Harrison [18]. It is interesting to note that shortly after Wilhelm von Roentgen's discovery of X-rays, for which he won the Nobel Prize, bone angiography demonstrated the absence of an anastomosis between medullary arteries in bone cortex and periosteal blood vessels [33, 73].

Centrifugal Blood Flow

In young bone cortex this is the corollary of the medullary blood supply to bone revealed by angiography. Centrifugal blood flow has been directly observed in normal living human femoral cortex during amputation, after injection of Evans Blue [46], and similarly in rabbit long bones using Disulphine Blue [34]. Also ferritin [29] and horse radish peroxidase (HRP) [51, 30] have demonstrated centrifugal flow of blood in chick and dog bone, and not only blood, but also extravascular bone water [30]. These findings revealed by a method radically different from perfusion and angiography, negate the conclusions of occasional investigators who believe that the arterial supply to bone cortex is centripetal, from the periosteum [77].

The direction of blood and aqueous fluid flow in the cortex depends on biomechanical and haemodynamic factors.

Biomechanical Factors

Muscle Pump

Systemic venous valves are plentiful in the veins lying in the intermuscular spaces. Muscle contraction, aided by diaphragmatic activity inherent in inspiration, empties the veins. The venous valves prevent retrograde flow. It follows that the intermittent contractions of muscle on bone, pumps cortical blood from the bone towards the heart (vis a fronte) [47]. This might well apply to ageing bone. Even with the marrow cavity packed with bone cement and the cortex supplied wholly by periosteal arterioles, centrifugal blood flow in the cortical capillaries still permits venous escape at the periosteal surface. With an extant marrow, venous escape presumably has an ebb and flow action, fluctuating between periosteum and marrow in response to intermittent muscle contractions.

Driving Pressure

Fluid pressure within the marrow cavity is considerably higher at 45-60 mmHg [57, 58] than the 12–15 mmHg in the extraosseous capillaries. A vascular vis a tergo is therefore generated centrifugally across the cortex, from marrow to periosteum.

Pulse Pressure

The iterative pressure of 8–10 mmHg [4, 58, 86] in bone marrow arteries, is confined in an unyielding cortical container. Thus the pulse pressure backs up the driving pressure and promotes centrifugal flow in the cortex at every heart beat.

Impact Forces

These have been demonstrated photographically during human locomotion as a wave of deformation passing up the limb (H. Light, personal communication, 1987). In a simulated laboratory exercise utilizing rabbits, impact forces have been demonstrated manometrically to pass along the bone marrow. These add to the pre-existing medullary pressures, and expel the blood from the marrow as if from a sponge.

Blood Flow Rate

In round figures, 17% of the cardiac output is delivered to the skeleton in the resting adult human. The skeletal perfusion rate as an overall average is 12 ml/100 g per minute [22]. In rats the corresponding values are 10% of the cardiac output and 20 ml/100 g per minute for skeletal flow [13, 22, 23].

Flow Partition

Kelly [43], using hydrogen washout flow measurement in the canine tibia, found that 71% of the nutrient flow went to the cortex and 30% went to the marrow. His dogs were of unstated age. On the other hand, Brookes [14] supplied volumetric data in rat femora, from which it can be calculated that the marrow accounts for 90% of the diaphyseal blood volume in 24-month-old rats, and the cortex receives 10%. Similarly, Okubo et al. [54], using microspheres for blood flow measurement in dogs, found that 88% of the femoral diaphyseal flow went to the marrow and 12% to the cortex.

Haemodynamics of the Osseous Circulation

In round figures, a cardiac output of about 6–8 l of blood per minute is delivered to the skeleton in the resting adult [22, 23] and the perfusion rate of the entire skeleton is about 16 ml/100 g per minute. The diaphysis has a perfusion rate of 5–15 ml/100 g per minute, the higher figure correlating with the presence of haemopoietic marrow and the lower figure with fatty marrow. Representative skeletal blood flow rates in ml/100 g per minute are 19 (rat [22]), 16 (rabbit [86]), and 12 (human [22]). Skeletal weight as a fraction of body weight, however, progressively increases with size: 10% (rat) [22], 11% (rabbit) [26], and

15% (human) [66]. The product of these two variables in the rat (1.9), rabbit (1.7), and humans (1.8 ml/100 g per unit of body weight) suggests that the number 1.8 may be a biological constant. The apparent constancy of skeletal blood flow relative to body weight among the species serves a haemopoietic as well as a mineralization function. Skeletal blood flow is related to erythropoietic activity [50], and most of the blood flow to long bones traverses the marrow rather than the cortex. Under these circumstances, bone extracellular fluid appears to serve as a buffer zone, providing a necessary milieu for mineral homeostasis [22]. This biological constant is also a testimonial to the common vascular anatomy of mammalian bones, with common osseous circulatory functions, i.e. the support of growth, renewal and repair of the skeleton, and maintenance of a constant concentration of calcium in the body fluids. (For further evidence concerning the blood supply to young bone, see Brookes and Revell, pp 116–118 [20].)

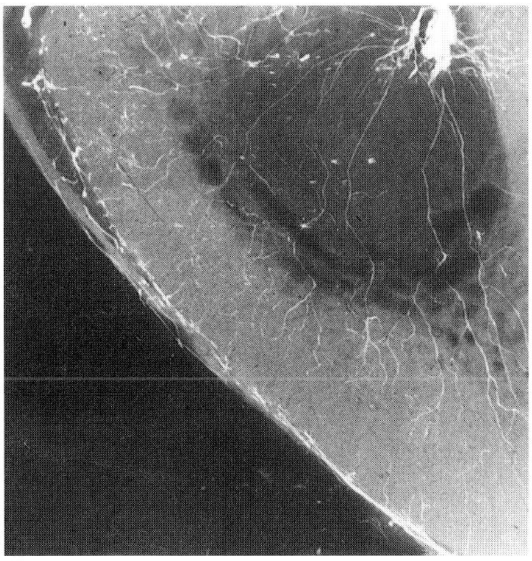

Fig. 3.10. Reserve periosteal and medullary supply to tibial cortex in peripheral occlusive vascular disease (male, 62 years)

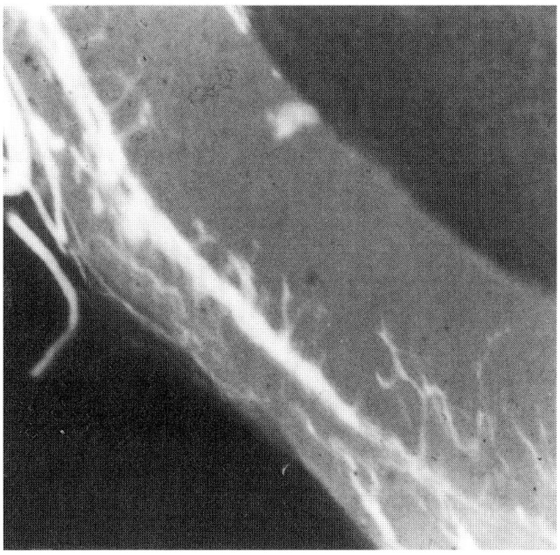

Fig. 3.11. Microradiograph of transverse section of an ischaemic rabbit tibia after ligation of nutrient artery. Note abnormal centripetal blood supply to the cortex and the absence of a medullary supply

Old Bone: Medullary and Periosteal Supply

Descriptions of canals as normally containing arteries, veins, and capillaries [40, 74] are invariably lacking in supporting visual evidence, which appears to stem from Langer's classical account [47] in 1876. He described in detail how periosteal arteries and veins enter the cortex everywhere to participate, together with the medullary vascular system, in the vascularization of compact bone. He insisted that at least two vessels, an artery and a vein, are normally to be found in a haversian canal, and that larger spaces often occur in the cortex which contain a leash of vessels. Stellate vascular figures ("Gefässsterne") were also commonly encountered by Langer in his diligent examination of human bone. The age and source of the material, tibiae in the main, used in Langer's work on adult bone cortex are not, however, given in his essay. His results correspond closely with the findings in ischaemic and ageing material (Figs. 3.10–3.16). It follows that senescence and vascular decline are appropriately linked to those accounts which emphasize a periosteal arterial supply to bone cortex, with multiple vessels in vascular canals, and the frequent occurrence of large vascular spaces.

Both Crock [25] and Trueta [79] illustrated a periosteal supply to human bone cortex, significantly in aged specimens of the seventh decade. Lopez-Curto et al. [49] examined six adult dogs of unstated age and concluded that cortical and medullary vascular beds were largely independent. Transcortical periosteo-medullary anastomoses were also present. It is possible that their use of a silicone elastomer failed, for technical reasons, to demonstrate the continuity between capillary and sinusoid at the osteomyeloid junction. The dogs were probably senescent. Nelson et al. [52] examined 14 human tibiae amputated for femoral cancers. Regrettably the age range again was not supplied, but they described a periosteal arterial supply to the tibia and pointed out the general presence of arterial periosteo-medullary anastomoses and multiple blood vessels in the haversian canals. An osteoporotic cortex and ischaemic bone marrow also illustrate their text, without comment but confirming the aged character of their material.

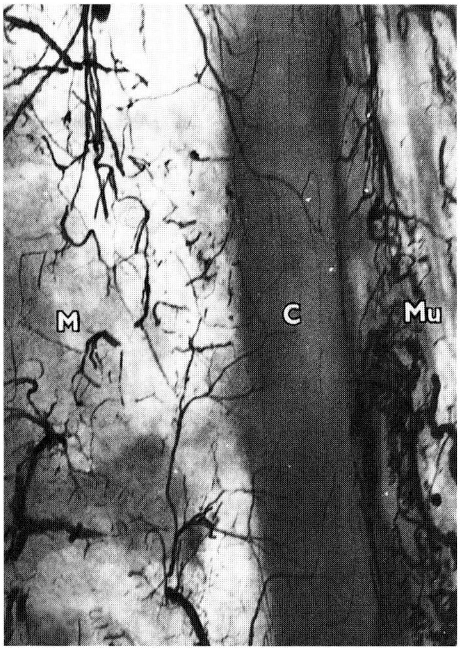

Fig. 3.12. Arteriogram of a longitudinal section of a young normal human tibia. Marrow (*M*), cortex (*C*). The arteries of the attached muscle (*Mu*) do not penetrate the cortex

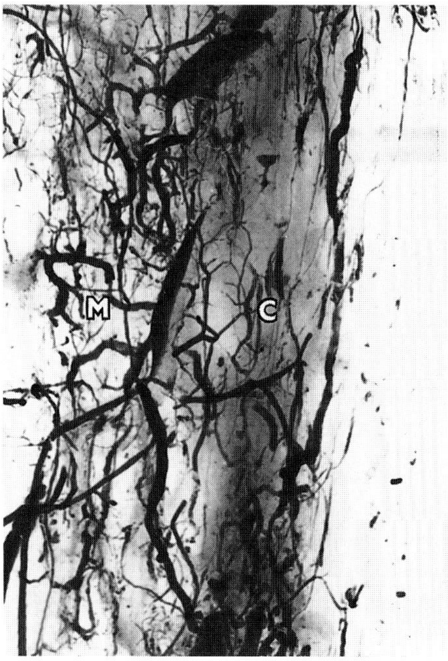

Fig. 3.13. Longitudinal section of human tibia, amputated for peripheral occlusive vascular disease. Periosteal (*C*) and medullary (*M*) vessels are grossly irregular and penetrate the ischaemic cortex

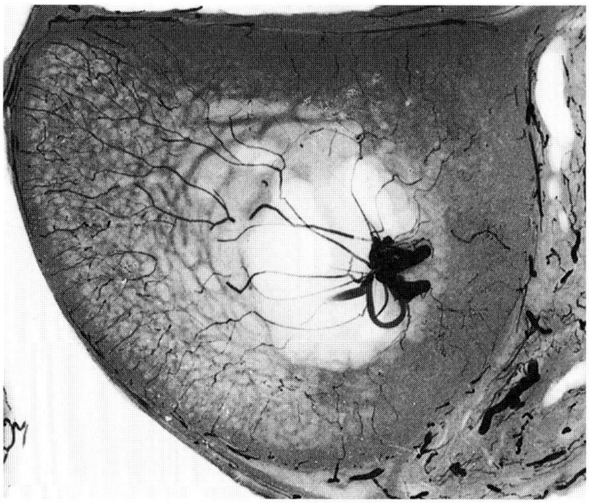

Fig. 3.14. Cross-sectional arteriogram through mid-tibia (male, 59 years). The leg was amputated for pyarthrosis of the knee. Normal appearances of senescence

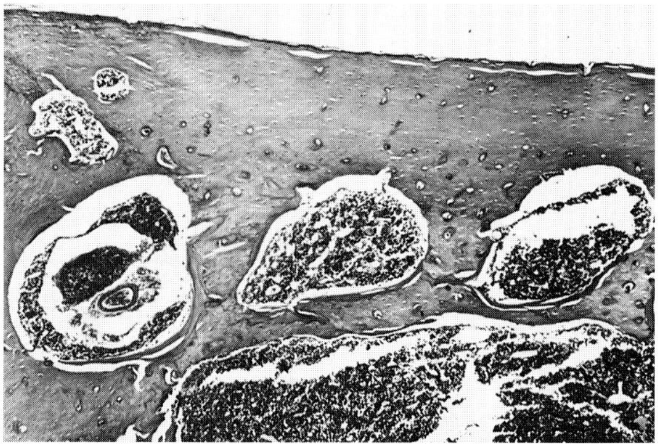

Fig. 3.15. Paraffin section through senescent rat bone showing osteoporotic cavities containing marrow

Brookes [11] demonstrated arterial periosteomedullary anastomoses in 25 human tibiae (59–80 years), amputated for peripheral occlusive atherosclerosis. A periosteal arterial supply to bone cortex was prominent in this material, and contrasted with its absence in a perfused tibia of a 15-year-old youth [19] (leg amputated for femoral sarcoma). Vascular canals in aged bone cortex were irregular in size and contained a variable number of blood vessels. The above features reflect the ageing process in long bones as well as ischaemia (Figs. 3.12–3.14). Experimentally, Brookes [12] produced unilateral marrow ischaemia by nutrient artery section in femora and tibiae of 16 5-month-old rabbits. In contrast to a youthful, medullary supply to the cortex in the contralateral controls, microangiography showed a considerable periosteal blood supply to the ischaemic cortex [12]. Blood volume in rat bone is known to de-

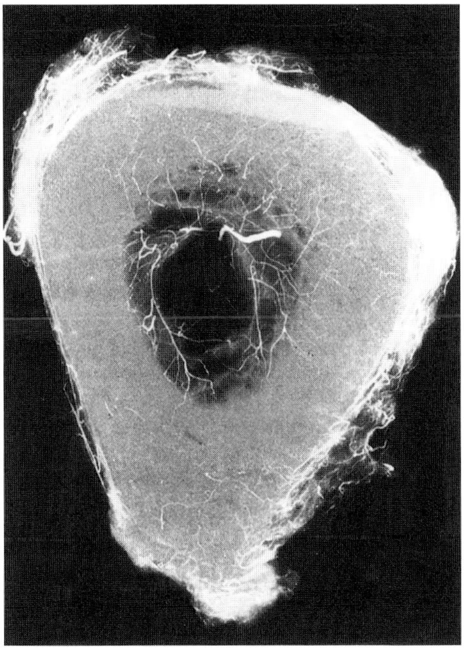

Fig. 3.16. Angiograph of transverse section of a femur perfused 3 days postmortem; youth (21 years) who died by violence. Marrow necrosis is present but medullary arteries are evident, supplying the cortex

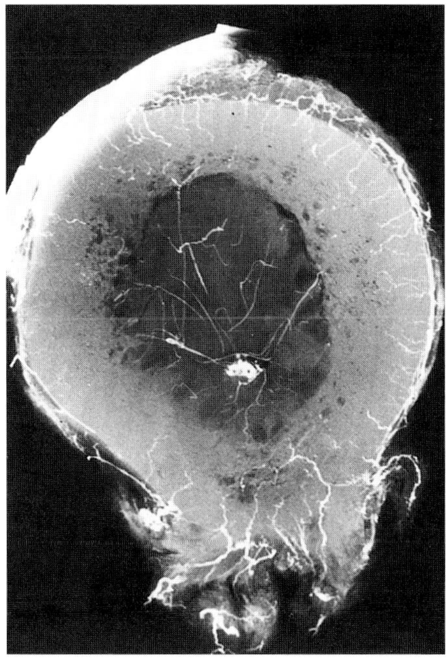

Fig. 3.18. Angiograph of femoral section (male, 65 years). A periosteal supply to the cortex is dominant. The marrow is ischaemic

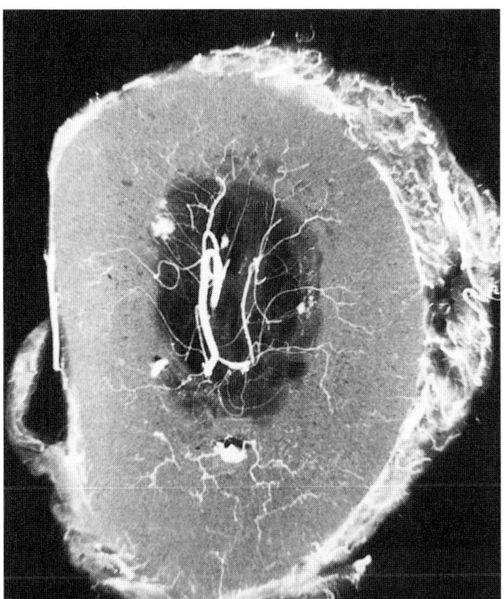

Fig. 3.17. Angiograph of transverse section of femur (male, 42 years). The medullary arteries are robust and largely supply the cortex, except in the right posterior quadrant where periosteal arterial traces are evident

cline semilogarithmically with age from 1–24 months, when it is only a tenth of what it was in youth [14]. Kita et al. [44], in rabbits, demonstrated a falling blood flow in bone marrow of 50, 23, 15 and 12 ml/min per 100 g in immature, mature, middle aged, and aged rabbits, respectively.

Recently, the femoral diaphyses of more than 25 subjects have been perfused postmortem and angiographed. The age at death ranged from 21 to 91 years and death was by violence or supradiaphragmatic disease. The results suggest that below the age of 35 years (Fig. 3.16), the diaphyseal cortex is arterialized from the marrow alone [16]. After this time, a periosteal supply to the cortex slowly develops [16] (Fig. 3.17), and the vascularity of the shaft marrow decreases. In advanced years (60 and older) the periosteal supply is dominant (Figs. 3.18, 3.19), although some medullary supply persists derived from the ischaemic marrow of senescence. Other signs of bone ageing are transcortical arterial anastomoses, linking bone marrow and periosteal arteries.

In a male aged 56 years (Figs. 3.20, 3.21), the upper femur had been reamed 4 years before death and the stem of a hip prosthesis implanted with acrylic cement. Angiography shows that the femoral cortex deprived of all medullary blood supply can be sustained in life solely by the periosteal circulation [16].

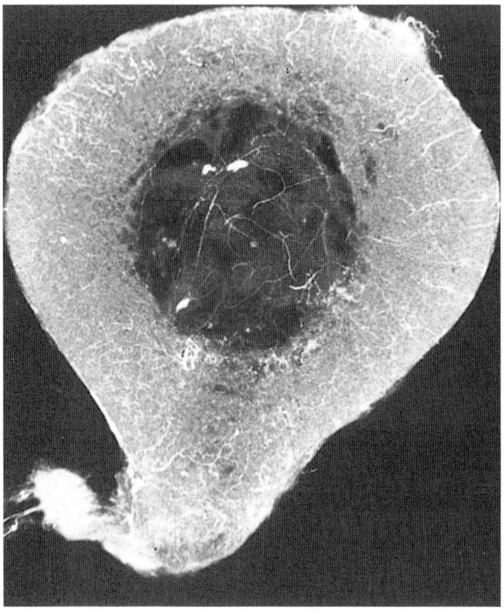

Fig. 3.19. Angiograph of femoral section (female, 72 years). The marrow is ischaemic. The cortex is supplied almost wholly from the periosteum

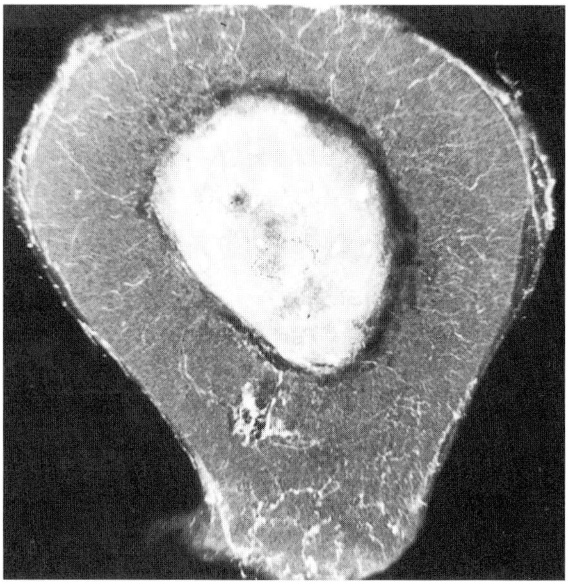

Fig. 3.21. Angiograph of transverse section of the femur below the prosthetic stem. The marrow cavity is blocked with acrylic cement. The entire cortex is vascularized from the periosteum

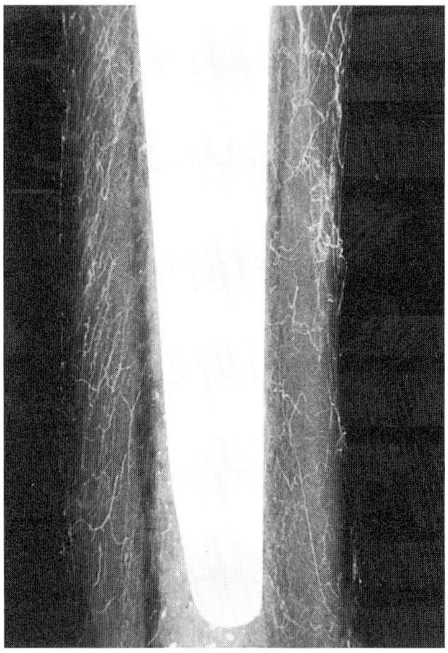

Fig. 3.20. Angiograph in longitudinal section showing the stem of a hip prosthesis held in the femoral diaphysis by acrylic cement. The cadaver (56 years) was perfused 4 years after prosthetic implantation. The cortex is entirely vascularized from the periosteum

Marrow Ischaemia and the Ageing Cortex

In the literature, there is little awareness of marrow ischaemia in long bones, noted here in ageing human femora and in tibiae taken from limbs amputated for peripheral occlusive vascular disease [11]. According to Ramseier [61], the arteries of human bone marrow are subject to atherosclerosis, increasing in severity with advancing years. He reported that grade for grade, vascular disease appears at least 10 years earlier in femoral marrow than in the arteries of the brain, heart, or muscle [61]. Experimentally, ligation of the nutrient artery of the femur in rabbits brings about a periosteal supply to the cortex [12] (Fig. 3.11). A centripetal blood flow in ischaemic marrow is normal in senescence (Fig. 3.10). Ramseier's findings and those of the above-quoted authors indicate that ageing in long bones is normally accompanied by marrow ischaemia.

Bone Cells and Endothelial Cells

Vascular Neogenesis

The vascular patterns of bone cortex, periosteal, endosteal, and endochondral are easy to detect in young bones. Evidence is still wanting which would show with certainty whether they persist in man after maturity, or whether they are superseded in senescence by a longitudinal mesh with transverse cross-connections. The latter process would, of course, entail vascular remodelling as well as internal alteration of the bone structure.

Bone cortex undergoes continual internal remodelling, by forming new generations of osteons throughout the lifetime of an individual [1–3]. Because osteonic renewal involves the near presence of vascular mesenchyme, it seems likely that the cortical vessels, like the mesenchyme in which they are embedded, are not static elements congealed in compact bone substance but are reactive and capable of variation in size and number. This activity is seen in exaggerated form in bone ischaemia [11, 12], and in fracture repair [20, 53, 63, 65].

Evidence for normally occurring vascular neogenesis is found in the writings of Zawisch-Ossenitz [88, 89], Pommer [59], Weidenreich [84], Schumacher [68], Cohen and Harris [24], and Schenk and Willeneger [67]. Two main groups of vascular canals are described in compact bone. In one, each canal on cross-section shows a smooth rounded outline, surrounded by the concentric lamellae of an osteon, or appears interpolated between two circumferential lamellae of surface bone (the interlamellar canals of Weidenreich). The other type of canal is much less common. It has a crenated or jagged border and shows no orderly relationship to lamellae. It simply cuts across them, suggesting the early stage of a new canal breaking through old bone. From such a starting point, Zawisch-Ossenitz described the formation of a new canal, followed by its gradual filling up with lamellae and final obliteration of the contained vessel. She concluded that new bone canal formation required vascular neogenesis and that continual renewal of bone took place based on blood vessels. Later writers then developed the idea of vascular neogenesis and internal erosion of the cortex. In particular, canals with blind endings containing blood vessels were described in detail, supporting the doctrine of continual vascular renewal in bone. In fracture repair, such new vascular canals bring about primary union of the bone fragments following fracture reduction.

It should be emphasized that there are no firm grounds for apportioning an osteolytic function to vascular endothelium. The process of osteonic renewal demands prior removal of bone, but the weight of histological evidence points to this as being carried out by osteoclasts or free mesenchyme cells and not by the blood vessels themselves in the haversian canals.

Syncytial Character of Osteocytes

Since Schwann [69] propounded the cell doctrine in 1839, anatomists have been circumspect before granting a group of cells the status of syncytium. Nowadays this term is being rendered increasingly out of date by electron microscopy, and plasmodium is to be preferred to indicate those cells formed by nuclear division without cytoplasmic division, for example, muscle fibres, giant cells, and the plasmodial trophoblast of the chorion. Leonhardt [48] considers that the term "syncytium" should only be applied in its original meaning to a group of cells, in contact by means of cell processes, whose boundaries, if not obvious in the light microscope, are demonstrable in the electron microscope (EM).

It is held by many that the osteocytes of bone are confluent with each other through their cytoplasmic processes. Suffice it to say that as regards the osteocytes, no EM photograph has ever been published which suggests that these cells form a plasmodium. For the osteocytes, buried alive in hard bone substance, their cytoplasmic processes undoubtedly make a syncytial contact with one another, in the extremely fine canaliculi of bone.

Origin of Bone Cells

Vascular change, the burgeoning and decline of cortical capillaries, at first received emphasis in studies on bone renewal and repair. Originally, osteoprogenitor cells were postulated by Young [87] as the source of osteoclasts, osteoblasts, and osteocytes. Today, it is established that the osteoclasts are derived from mononuclear white blood corpuscles, originating in bone marrow [5, 45]. Later writers have emphasized in this context the origin of osteoclasts from a monocyte-macrophage cell line. Hence the diphyletic proposition that osteoblasts lay down bone and osteoclasts remodel it, but the two are not related.

Oni et al. [55] have used the lectin Ulex europeus I-peroxidase (UEP) which distinguishes tumours of vascular origin from other tumours [38, 82], and also monoclonal antibodies specifically raised against endothelial cell proteins [60]. UEP was used to study lectin binding in early adult human tibial fractures, and osteotomies of adult rabbit tibiae. Monoclonal antibodies were also used on samples obtained from eight adults undergoing open reduction of tibial diaphyseal fractures. Bone trabeculae, osteoblasts, and chondrocytes showed no evidence of lectin binding or antibody uptake, whereas the endothelium of adjacent blood vessels was clearly stained. Osteogenic cells adjacent to endothelial cells were not stained. The total lack of staining of the bone cells opposes the notion that endothelial cells give rise to bone cells, as formerly held by Trueta [78]. Nevertheless, the possibility of extravascular migration of endothelial cells and their transformation into osteoprogenitor cells still finds support [36].

Factors Acting on Blood Flow in Cortex

Vasoactive Drugs

Dohler et al. [31] have studied the effect of these on cortical capillaries. In a well-controlled experiment, they injected a single intravenous bolus of epinephrine, ATP, or insulin in mice, and a piece of tibial diaphysis was removed and examined by transmission EM. Epinephrine increased the luminal width and endothelial thickness. ATP caused endothelial cells to flatten. Injected insulin was associated with a thick endothelium in the haversian canals, possibly as a result of hypoglycaemia. The authors argue that luminal expansion and endothelial thickening reflect a decreased extravascular space in the canals and oedema of cortical bone substance. Intracortical perfusion pressure might then decrease and the bone perfusion rate increase. ATP, on the other hand, increases the extravascular space and reduces transcapillary diffusion time. Importantly, their work suggests that there are specific insulin receptors in bone capillaries.

Prostaglandins

Kapitola et al. [41] have examined bone blood flow in spayed rats. Flows were measured by microspheres in the tibia and distal femur. They found that spaying increased the cortical blood flow rate, as well as the uptake of radiocalcium [47]. Aspirin in the rat feed cake was used to suppress prostaglandin production. They found aspirin abolished the blood flow increase induced by spaying significantly. There was also a decrease in tibial bone density and ash weight. The authors argue for a role for prostaglandins, probably PGE2, to account for the increased bone blood flow in spayed rats.

Heat

The effect on bone blood flow of cooling the knee joint in an ice wrap for 20 min was measured by triple phase technetium bone scans on 21 humans. The opposite knee acted as control. Scans were obtained on completion of cooling. All iced knees demonstrated decreased arterial bone blood flow and decreased bone uptake of 99mTe, reflecting reduced blood flow and metabolism, approximately 40% for flow and 20% for uptake. The reduced flow and cell metabolism might well limit cell death in severe traumatic injury. See also Servelle [70] for the effects of heat on bone growth.

Alcohol Abuse

This is associated with osteopenia and bone fractures, especially in senescence. Bickle et al. [6] studied 27 subjects, aged 26–68 years, with a record of 10 years of alcohol abuse. Seventeen of them were found to have spinal compression fractures by routine X-ray examination. Bone density fell sharply with age; spinal bone density fell two standard deviations in 15 subjects below normal age-matched controls. Osteomalacia was absent, but total surface area of cancellous bone was increased. Although vitamin D metabolites were normal, parathyroid hormone levels in many cases were elevated as shown by urinary cAMP levels.

Smoking

Daftari et al. [27] transplanted autologous cancellous bone into the anterior chamber of the eye in 24 rabbits. Half were given nicotine, the other half received placebos. Revascularization of the implant was followed by slit-lamp and fluorescein angiography. The authors point out that pseudarthrosis after spinal fusion is more frequent in smokers than nonsmokers. Here, the results showed that nicotine caused delayed revascularization of the graft and more grafts became necrotic, as compared with the placebos. Nicotine clearly inhibits revascularization of autologous bone grafts.

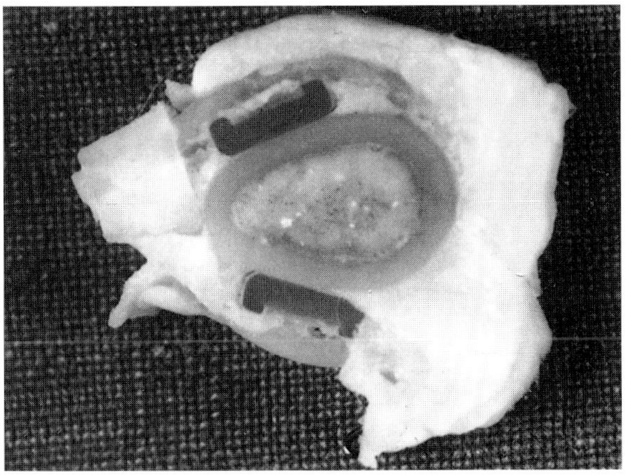

Fig. 3.22. Plating of rabbit femur, showing in cross section two nylon plates applied to the bone. Note external excavation of the plates

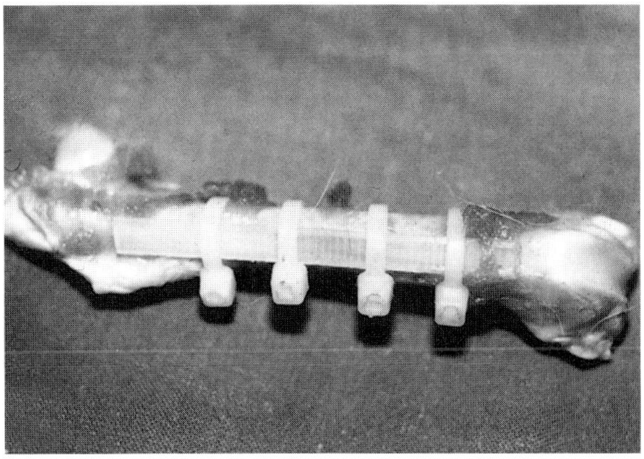

Fig. 3.23. Plating. The two plates are held to the unfractured femur by four nylon ties

Surgical Intervention in Fracture Repair

Vascular Obstruction by Occlusive Plates

The periosteum is a potential source of blood supply to the cortex of mature bone and always a route of venous escape for cortical blood flow. It follows that obstruction of the surface with an orthopaedic plate, in order to fix a bone fracture, can disturb the underlying osseous circulation and therefore bone healing. In order to eliminate reactions dependent on the presence of a fracture, the following experiments were carried out on unfractured bones.

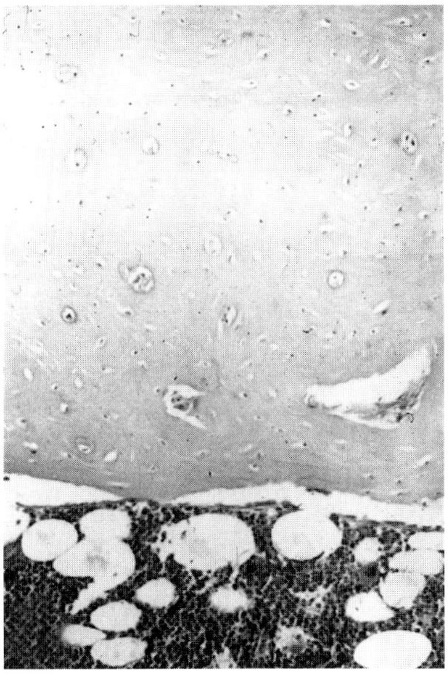

Fig. 3.24. Pyknosis of osteocytes and empty bone lacunae in rabbit cortex, 1 week after plating. The marrow is normal

Materials and Methods

Two flexible nylon plates were applied, one to the medial and the other to the lateral femoral surface, in 18 rabbits. The plastic plates were cut to size from sterile Cerclene bands (Howmedica). The resulting dimensions of the plates were 65 mm×5 mm×1.2 mm.

One surface of the plate was flat and capable of making immediate and obstructive contact with the femoral bone surface (Fig. 3.22). The other side of the plate was excavated by a trough lying between the edges of the plate; it made only a linear contact with the bone surface. The plates were held in place by four nylon cable ties (Fig. 3.23).

In 14 rabbits, the flat surface of the plates was applied to the femoral surface. The plates could not transmit mechanical force. The bones were not fractured. The rabbits were killed serially up to 12 weeks postoperatively by intra-arterial barium sulphate perfusion. Angiographic and histological examination followed.

Results

One week after operation, histology of the cortex of the plated femur showed severe osteocyte pyknosis in the inner third (Fig. 3.24), and the outer two-thirds showed many bone lacunae without a cell nucleus at all. In fine, the osteocytes were largely dead. The dead bone provoked a hyperaemic response.

Four weeks after operation, a marked hypervascularity affected the inner two-thirds of the cortex beneath the plates (Fig. 3.25). Subsequently,

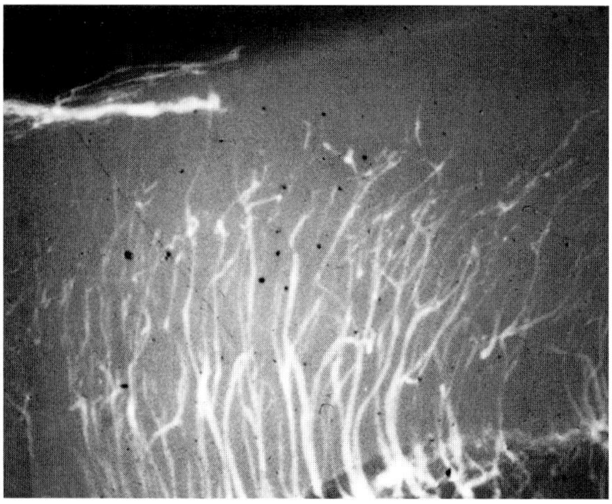

Fig. 3.25. Plating. Cortical vascular congestion deep to an obstructive plate. Arteriogram, 4 weeks after operation

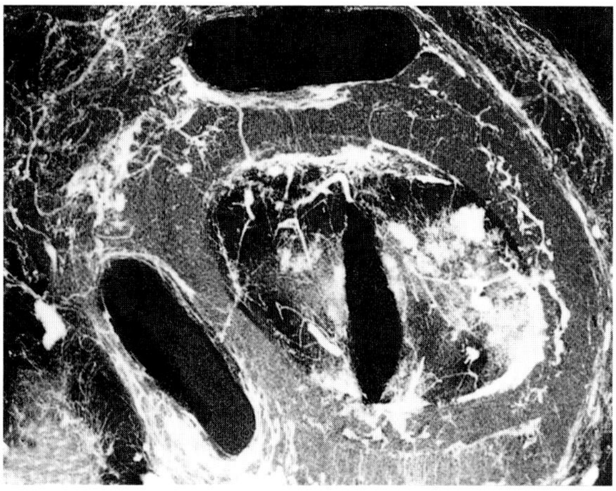

Fig. 3.26. Plating. Bone hyperaemia is generalized after prolonged obstructive plating. Arteriogram, 12 weeks after operation

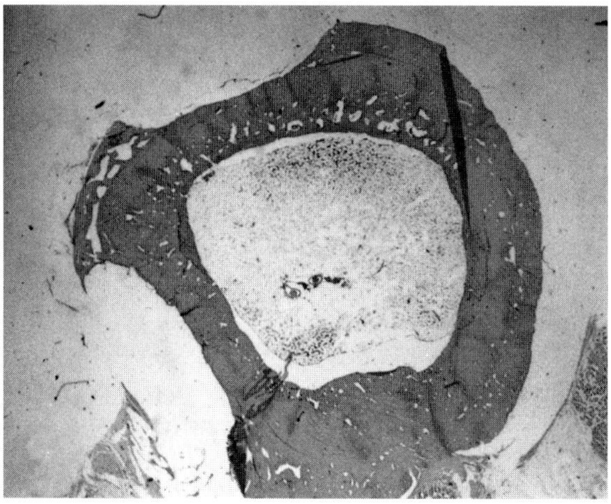

Fig. 3.27. Plating. Osteoporosis in plated rabbit cortex. Photomicrograph (low power), 6 weeks after operation

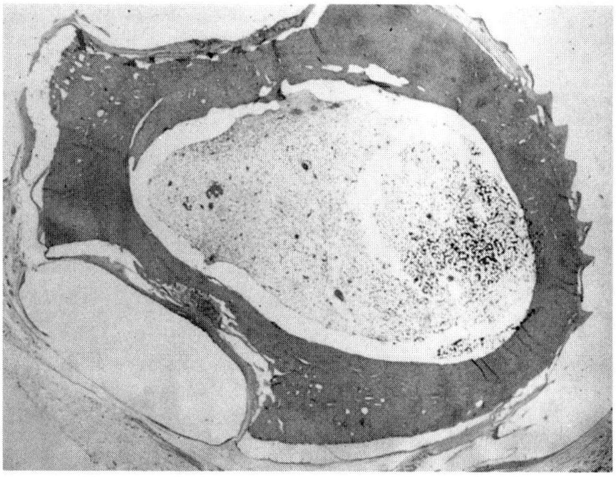

Fig. 3.28. Plating. Severe bone loss after obstructive plating. Photomicrograph (low power) 12 weeks after operation

from 6 weeks onwards, hypervascularity of the cortex became generalized (Fig. 3.26). Erosion cavities were much in evidence, containing medullary tissue (Fig. 3.27). Severe bone removal from the periosteal aspect was also encountered, resulting in thinning of the plated cortex, sometimes in association with endosteal buttressing, deep to the plate (Fig. 3.28). Florid angiographic hyperaemia was present in the osteopenic cortex, and showed no signs of abatement at 12 weeks after operation (Fig. 3.26).

Mock Experiment

In four rabbits, instead of the flat side, the elevated nonocclusive side of the plates was applied. The bones were examined 6 weeks after operation. Where the plates had been inverted and did not obstruct the bone surface, the cortex below the plates 6 weeks after operation was not hyperemic and showed only little osteoporosis. The thickness of the cortex had been maintained.

Discussion

Increased bone fragility following internal fixation of fractures utilizing bone plates has often been attributed to the fracture itself (increased bone remodelling [67]), to the rigidity of the plates, or to stress protection whereby bridging apparatus diverts the transmission of mechanical force across the reparative fracture site. The results here, using flexible nylon plates on unfractured bone, confirm that the consequence of ap-

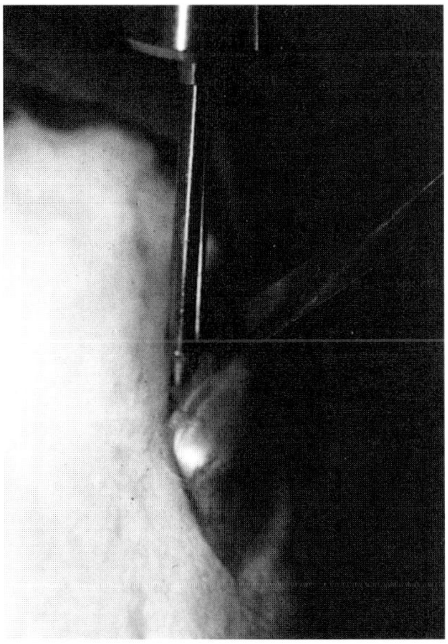

Fig. 3.29. Reaming of rabbit tibia, behind patellar ligament

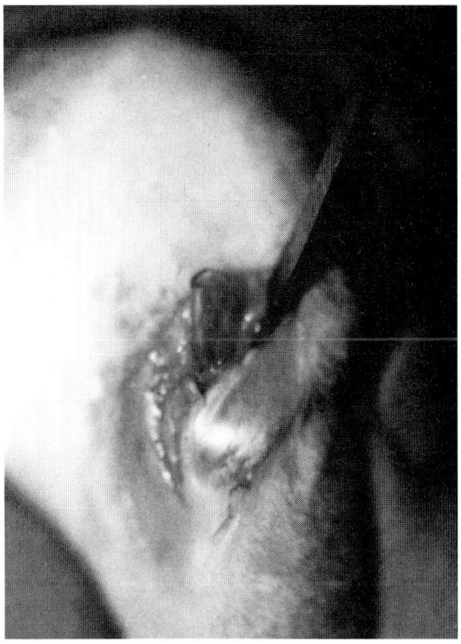

Fig. 3.30. Reaming and nailing. Insertion of polyethylene nail after reaming

plying an obstructive plate to a long bone is to impede the normal centrifugal blood flow in bone cortex in the young, or periosteal supply in the old, and prevents venous escape of blood at the surface whatever the age. This results in a severe and sustained hyperaemia and osteopenia of the underlying cortex, which will not resolve until the plates are removed [80].

Cortical Conservation After Intramedullary Nailing

Intramedullary nailing has obvious mechanical advantages in the reduction and fixation of bone fractures, but initially at least, it is apparently destructive of the medullary circulation. The following investigations were initiated in order to study the effects of medullary reaming on bone cortex, reaming followed by intramedullary nailing, and intramedullary nailing alone. In all cases the bones were not fractured, so that the effects of these procedures on bone cortex might not be obscured by concurrent reparative phenomena.

Materials and Methods

Two similar groups of 12 New Zealand white rabbits were set up. In one, the response of the tibial cortex to reaming alone was studied; in the other group the tibia was reamed and nailed. Reaming of the shaft was performed from a proximal point on the tibial plateau behind the ligamentum patellae (Fig. 3.29). Nailing was simulated only in its volumetric sense, not in its usual mechanical character of an axially situated internal fixator. The nail used was a flexible polyethylene tube which represented a rigid steel intramedullary nail (Fig. 3.30). The bone was not fractured. The investigation was followed at serial intervals up to 12 weeks after operation. The animals were killed by intra-arterial perfusion of barium sulphate. Segments of the tibiae were then studied angiographically and histologically.

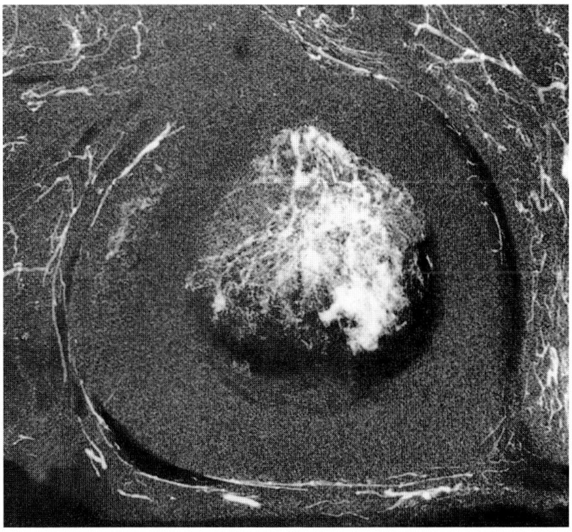

Fig. 3.31. External callus following reaming alone. Angiogram, 2 weeks after operation

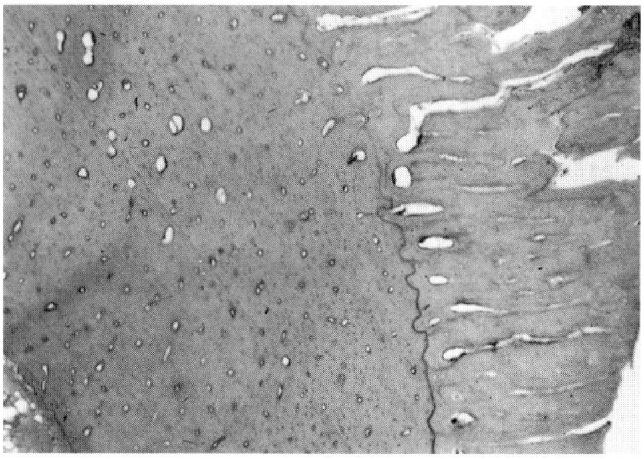

Fig. 3.32. Photomicrograph of reamed tibia 3 weeks after operation, showing external callus histologically

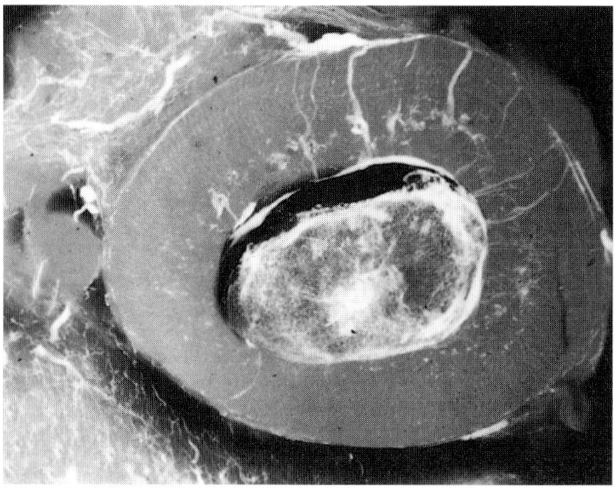

Fig. 3.33. Reaming. Angiogram showing thick substantial cortex, 12 weeks after reaming

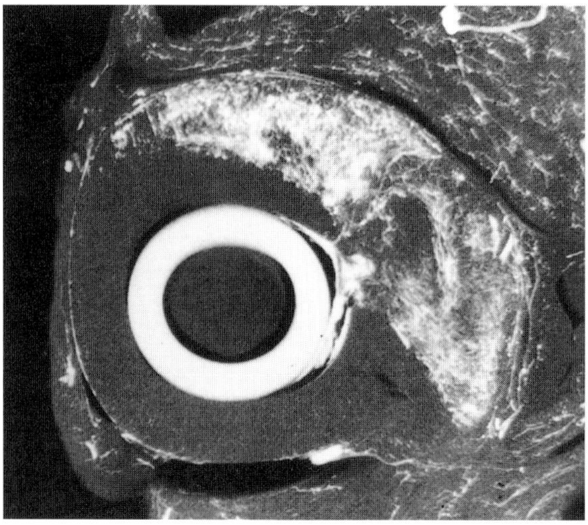

Fig. 3.34. External callus after reaming and nailing. Angiogram, 2 weeks after operation

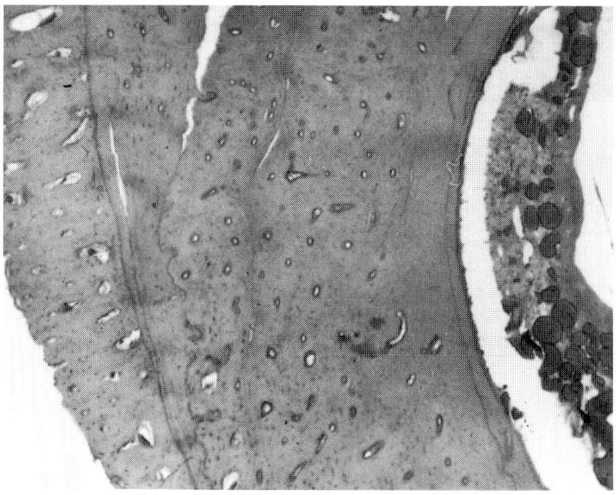

Fig. 3.35. Photomicrograph of reamed and nailed tibia, 3 weeks after operation, showing external callus. Note highly vascular marrow between cortex and site of polyethylene tube

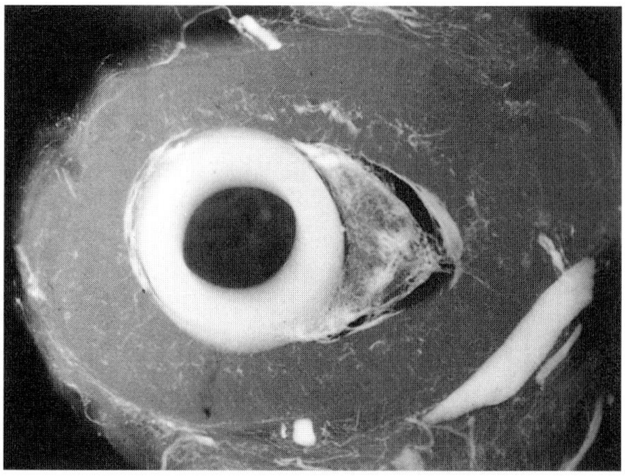

Fig. 3.36. Reaming and nailing. Twelve weeks after reaming and nailing angiography shows a live, thick cortex

Results

Reaming alone stopped the medullary supply to the unfractured cortex for 1 week, but was restored in the 2nd week (Fig. 3.31). The cortex was hardly affected and a periosteal blood supply was in evidence angiographically. A pronounced deposit of external callus was observed from 1–8 weeks, which was supplied by periosteal blood vessels (Figs. 3.31, 3.32). At 12 weeks the cortex was thick, showing only sparse periosteomedullary anastomoses (Fig. 3.33).

Reaming and simulated nailing of rabbit tibiae stopped the medullary supply to the cortex for 1 week, but blood vessels proliferated in the confined space between the tube and endocortex in the second week (Fig. 3.34). Again, the cortex was hardly affected, in spite of the indwelling tube being tightly packed in the marrow cavity. Significantly there was a marked periosteal deposition of external callus on the surface of the bone shaft (Figs. 3.34, 3.35). A thin layer of hard periosteal callus was present at 12 weeks. The cortex was thick, and little osteoporosis was present (Fig. 3.36).

Discussion

Reaming, or reaming with simulated nailing, spares the cortex, following the temporary destruction of the medullary supply in both instances. Frank osteoporosis, reduction in cortical thickness, and medullization of the cortex as seen in ischaemic bone deep to obstructive plates, were absent in both reame and reamed and nailed specimens. The periosteal circulation maintains the cortex alive during marrow regeneration. Compare the dead bone after plating, with the vital cortex after reaming (Figs. 3.24, 3.37).

In addition, external callus deposition is marked, also supplied from the periosteal circulation. This is important in achieving firm bony union and avoiding nonunions. The cause of external callus production following intramedullary nailing is uncertain, but nevertheless useful.

The Unreamed Nail in Experimental Investigations

In fractured bone, medullary nailing without reaming pushes bone marrow and osteogenic precursor cells into the fracture gap, and its immediate environs. In this way, cells are supplied for the production of callus and bony union in a mechanically stable environment. The healing of a bone fracture is intimately associated with, and may be regulated by, orderly sequences of local pH changes in the reparative site [21].

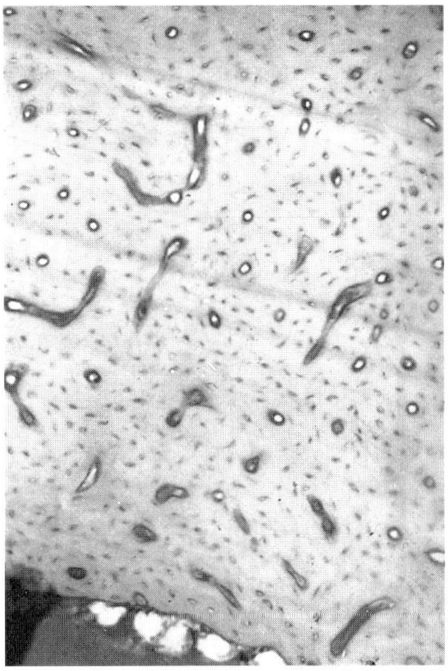

Fig. 3.37. Reamed tibia. Two days after reaming, the cortex of this unfractured bone has a normal lively appearance

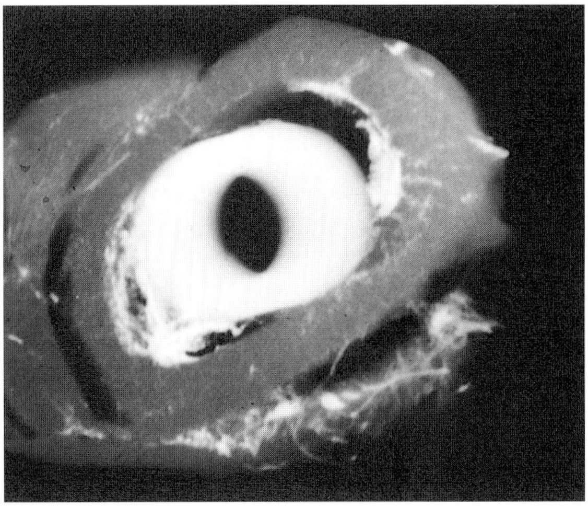

Fig. 3.38. Unreamed nail. Angiogram, 4 weeks after operation, after insertion of a large tube. External callus is absent

In Intact Bone

Recently, the tibiae of four rabbits have been nailed with polyethylene tubing, using either narrow or wide bore tubes. The tibiae were not reamed. At 2 weeks and 4 weeks after operation, whole bone radiography and transverse microradiography of barium-sulphate-perfused material show no sign of external callus deposition (Figs. 3.38–3.41). It follows that after intramedullary nailing in the absence of tibial reaming or some form of internal bone damage, there is a failure of deposition of external callus on the unreamed and intact unfractured bone.

Conclusions

In the surgery of fracture repair, it may be expected that:

- Plating of a fractured bone shaft using obstructive bone plates flat against the surface, inevitably entrains severe cortical ischaemia and osteocyte death. This is followed by a sustained

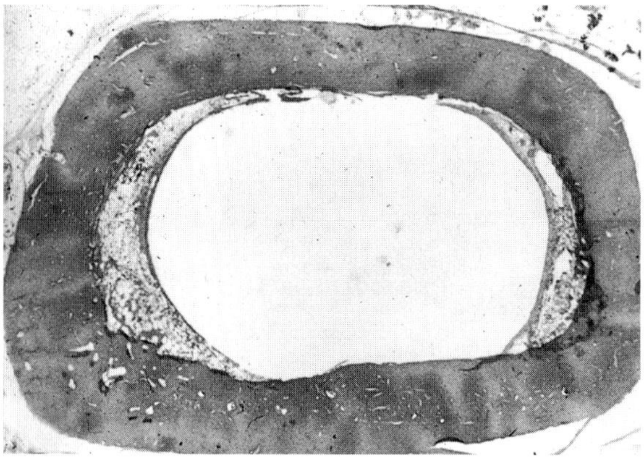

Fig. 3.39. Photomicrograph of histological section after insertion of large tube, showing no external callus

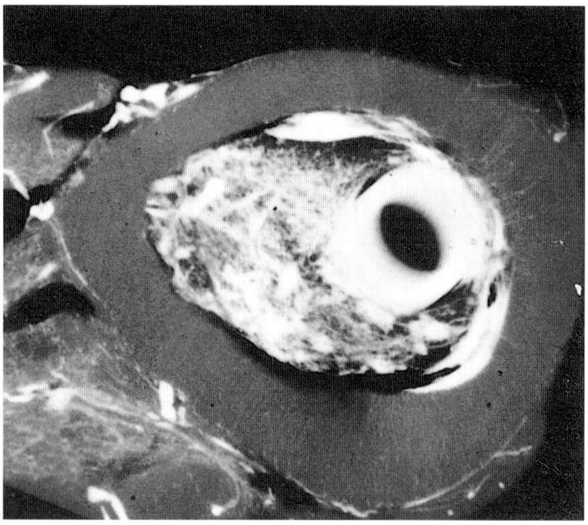

Fig. 3.40. Unreamed nail. Angiogram 4 weeks after operation, after insertion of small tube. No external callus

long-term reactive hyperaemia, osteoporosis, and cortical bone loss.

- Elevated plates, lying somewhat above the bone surface, preserve small arteries and veins and do not provoke these destructive effects, as shown here by the mock plating experiments.
- Intramedullary nailing conserves the periosteal circulation for the repair of bone fractures in both young and old.
  Fractures in the young: intramedullary reaming and nailing provokes an immediate periosteal supply to the cortex, on account of the abolition of normal intramedullary biomechanics. A fall in marrow pressure, and in particular the loss of a centrifugal driving pressure, causes a reversal of the normal flow direction. Conservation of the periosteal circulation prevents osteocyte death and maintains the blood supply to bone cortex, until marrow haemodynamics and normal blood flow patterns are restored.
  Fractures in the elderly: intramedullary reaming and nailing does not have a devitalizing effect on the cortex, inasmuch as a periosteal arterial supply to the cortex is already present. Medullary revascularization is rapid, occurring in 1 or 2 weeks. The periosteal vessels also make possible the production of much external callus, to bridge the fracture gap and fix the bone fragments.

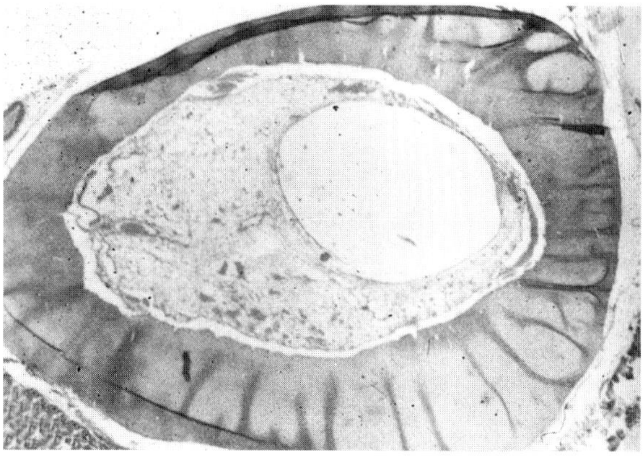

Fig. 3.41. Photomicrograph after insertion of a small tube, showing no external callus

References

1. Amprino R (1955) Struttura microscopica e rinnovamente delle ossa. Atti Soc Ital Patol 4:9–68
2. Amprino R, Bairatti A (1936) Processi di ricostruzione e di riassorbimento nella sostanza compatta delle ossa dell'uomo. Z Zellforsch Mikrosk Anat 24:439–511
3. Amprino R, Sisto L (1946) Analogies et différences de structure dans les différentes régions d'un même os. Acta Anat 2:202–214
4. Arnoldi CC (1994) Vascular aspects of degenerative bone disorders. Acta Orthopaedica Scandinavica Suppl 261:65, 1–82
5. Ashe P, Loutit JF, Townsend KM (1980) Osteoclasts derived from haematopoietic stem cells. Nature 283:669–670
6. Bickle DD, Stesin A, Halloran B, Steinbach L, Recker R (1993) Alcohol-induced bone disease: relationship of age and parathyroid levels. Alcohol Clin Exp Res 17:690–695
7. Bachmann G, Pfeifer T, Spies H, Katthagen BD (1993) 3D-CT and angiography of cast preparations of pelvic vessels: demonstration of arterial blood supply of the acetabulum. ROFO 158:214–220
8. Bridgeman G, Brookes M (1996) Blood supply to the human femoral diaphysis in youth and senescence. J Anat 188:611–621
9. Brookes M (1958a) The vascular architecture of tubular bone in the rat. Anat Rec 132:25–47
10. Brookes M (1958b) The vascularization of long bones in the human foetus. J Anat 92:261–267
11. Brookes M (1960a) The vascular reaction of tubular bone to ischaemia in peripheral occlusive vascular disease. J Bone Joint Surg Br 42:110–125

12. Brookes M (1960b) Sequelae of experimental partial ischaemia in long bones of the rabbit. J Anat 94:552–561
13. Brookes M (1970) Arteriolar blockade: a method of measuring blood flow rates in the skeleton. J Anat 106:557–563
14. Brookes M (1971) The blood supply of bone: an approach to bone biology. Butterworth, London
15. Brookes M (1986) An anatomy of the osseous circulation. Bone 3:32–35
16. Brookes M (1990) Blood flow in the diaphysis of long bones. ARCO (Toulouse) News Letter 2:75–85
17. Brookes M (1993) Morphology and distribution of blood vessels and blood flow in bone. In: Schoutens A et al. (eds) Bone circulation and vascularization in normal and pathological conditions. Plenum Press, New York pp 19–28
18. Brookes M, Harrison RG (1957) The vascularization of the rabbit femur and tibiofibula. J Anat 91:61–72
19. Brookes M, Revell WJ (1998) Blood supply of bone: scientific aspects. Springer, London
20. Brookes M, Richards DJ, Singh M (1970) Vascular sequelae of experimental osteotomy. Angiology 21:355–367
21. Brueton RN, Revell WJ, Brookes M (1993) Haemodynamics of bone healing in a model stable fracture. In: Schoutens A et al. (eds) Bone circulation and vascularization in normal and pathological conditions. Plenum Press, New York, pp 121–128
22. Charkes ND, Brookes M, Makler PT (1979) Studies of skeletal tracer kinetics: II. Evaluation of a 5-compartment model of [18F] fluoride kinetics in rats. J Nuc Med Tech 20:1150–1157
23. Charkes ND, Makler PT, Brookes M (1980) Radiofluoride kinetics. In: Colombetti LG (ed) Principles of radiopharmacology. CRC Press, Boca Raton, Florida, pp 225–242
24. Cohen J, Harris WH (1958) The three-dimensional anatomy of haversian systems. J Bone Joint Surg Am 40:419–434
25. Crock HV (1967) The blood supply of the lower limb bones in man. Livingstone, London
26. Cumming JD, Nutt ME (1962) Bone marrow blood flow and cardiac output in the rabbit J Physiol 162:30–34
27. Daftari TK, Whitesides TE, Heller JG, Goodrich AC, McCarey BE (1994) Nicotine in the revascularisation of bone graft. An experimental study in rabbits. Spine 19:904–911
28. De Marneffe R (1951) Recherches morphologiques et expérimentales sur la vascularisation osseuse. Brussels: Acta Med Belg Supp:7–80.
29. Dillaman RM (1984) Movement of ferritin in the 2-day-old chick femur. Anat Rec 209:445–453
30. Dillaman RM, Roer RD, Gay DM (1991) Fluid movement in bone: theoretical and empirical. J Biomech 24 (suppl 1):163–177
31. Dohler JR, Hennig FF, Hughes SP (1995) Reactivity of cortical bone capillaries. Functional TEM analysis with adrenalin, ATP and insulin. Langenbecks Arch Chir 380:176–183
32. Gebhardt W (1901) Ueber funktionell wichtige Anordnungsweisen der grösseren und feineren Bauelemente des Wirbeltierknochens. Arch Entw-Mech Org 11:383–498
33. Grégoire R, Carrière C (1921) Circulation artérielle intra-osseuse du fémur et du tibia. CR Assoc Anat 16:179–185
34. Gunst MA (1980) Interference with bone blood supply through plating of intact bone. In: Uhthoff HK (ed) Current concepts of internal fixation of fractures. Springer, Berlin, pp 268–276
35. Ham AW, Leeson TS (1964) Ham's histology, 4th ed. Lippincott, New York
36. Hansen ES (1993) Microvascularization, osteogenesis and myelopoiesis in normal and pathological conditions. In: Schoutens A, Arlet J, Gardeniers J, Hughes S (ed) Bone circulation and vascularization. Plenum, London, pp 229–242
37. Heřt J, Hladíková J (1961) Die Gefässversorgung des Haversschen Knochens. Acta Anat 45:344–361
38. Holthofer H, Virtanen I, Kariniemi AL, Hormia H, Linder E, Miettinen A (1982) Ulex europeus I lectin as a marker for vascular endothelium in human tissues. Lab Invest 47:60–66
39. Hoyer H (1882) A silver nitrate gelatin mass. Biol Centralbl ii:19–22
40. Johnston TB, Davies DV, Davies F (1958) Grays Anatomy 32nd edn. Longmans, London
41. Kapitola J, Andrie J, Kubickova J (1994) Possible participation of prostaglandins in the increase in the bone blood flow in oophorectomized female rats. Exp clin endocrinol 102:414–416
42. Katthagen BD, Spies H, Bachmann G (1995) Arterial vascularization of the bony acetabulum. Z Orthop 133:7–13
43. Kelly PJ (1973) Comparison of marrow and cortical bone blood flow by 125-labeled 4-iodoantipyrine(1-Ap) washout. J Lab Clin Med 81:497-505
44. Kita K, Kawai K, Hirohata K (1987) Changes in bone marrow blood flow with aging. J Orthop Res 5:569–575
45. Ko JS, Bernard GW (1981) Osteoclast formation in vitro from bone marrow mononuclear cells in osteoclast-free bone. Am J Anat 161:415–425
46. Lamas A, Amado D, da Costa JC (1946) La circulation du sang dans l'os. Presse Med 54:862–863
47. Langer K (1876) Über das Gefässsystem der Röhrenknochen, mit Beiträgen zur Kenntnis des Baues und der Entwicklung des Knochengewebes. Denkschr K K Akad Wiss Wien 37:217–240
48. Leonhardt H (1967) Histologie und Zytologie des Menschen. Thieme, Stuttgart
49. Lopez-Curto JA, Bassingthwaite JB, Kelly PJ (1980) Anatomy of the microvasculature of the tibial diaphysis of the adult dog. J Bone Joint Surg Am 62:1362–1369
50. Michelson K (1969) Haemodynamics in the bone marrow of anaemic rabbits with increased haematopoiesis. Acta Physiol Scand 77:52–57
51. Montgomery RJ, Sutker BD, Bronk JT, Kelly PJ (1988) Interstitial fluid flow in cortical bone. Microvasc Res 35:295–307
52. Nelson GE, Kelly PJ, Peterson LFA, Janes JM (1960) Blood supply of the human tibia. J Bone Joint Surg Am 42:625–634
53. Nilsonne U (1959) Biophysical investigations of the mineral phase in healing fractures. Acta Orthop Scand Suppl 37:1–81
54. Okubo M, Kinoshita M, Yukimura T, Abe Y, Shimazu A (1979) Experimental study of measurement of regional blood flow in the adult mongrel dog using radioactive microspheres. Clin Orthop Rel Res 138:263–270
55. Oni OA, Dearing S, Pringle S (1993) Endothelial cells and bone cells. In: Schoutens A (ed) Bone Circulation and Vascularization in Normal and Pathological Conditions. Plenum Press, London, pp 43–48
56. Peterson LFA, Neher M, Janes JM, Kelly PJ (1959) A stereoscopic microradiographic camera with vacuum filmholder and a stereomicroscope. Proc Staff Meet Mayo Clin 34:283
57. Petrakis NL (1954) Bone marrow pressure in leukaemic and non-leukaemic patients. J Clin Invest 33:27–35
58. Polster J (1970) Zur Haemodynamik des Knochens. Ferdinand Enke Verlag, Stuttgart
59. Pommer G (1927) Ueber Begriff und Bedeutung der durchbohrenden Knochenkanäle. Z Mikrosk Anat Forsch 9:540–584

60. Pringle S, De Bono DP (1988) Monoclonal antibodies to damaged and regenerating vascular endothelium. J Clin Lab Immunol 26:159–162
61. Ramseier E. (1962) Untersuchungen über arteriosklerotische Veränderungen der Knochenarterien. Virchows Arch Pathol Anat 336:77–86
62. Ranvier L (1875) Traité technique d'histologie. Savy, Paris
63. Rhinelander FW (1968) The normal microcirculation of diaphyseal cortex and its response to fracture. J Bone Joint Surg Am 50:784–800
64. Rhinelander FW (1980) Vascular proliferation and blood supply during fracture healing. In: Uhthoff HK (ed) Current concepts of internal fixation of fractures. Springer, Berlin, pp 9–14
65. Richards DJ, Brookes M (1969) Physico-chemical sequelae of experimental osteotomy. Calc Tiss Res 2[Suppl]:93
66. Recommendations of the International Commission on Radiological Protection (1975) Report of the task group on reference man (vol 23). Pergamon Press, New York
67. Schenk R, Willenegger H (1964) Zur Histologie der primären Knochenheilung. Langenbecks Arch Klin Chir 308:440–452
68. Schumacher S (1935) Zur Anordnung der Gefäßkanäle in der Diaphyse langer Röhrenknochen des Menschen. Z Mikrosk Anat Forsch 38:145–160
69. Schwann T (1839) Mikroscopische Untersuchungen über die Uebereinstimmung in der Struktur und dem Wachstum der Thiere und Pflanzen. Sander, Berlin
70. Servelle M (1948) Stase veineuse et croissance osseuse. Bull Acad Nat Med 132:471–474
71. Skawina A, Litwin JA, Gorczyca J, Miodonski AJ (1994) The vascular system of human fetal long bones; a scanning electron microscope study of corrosion casts. J Anat 185:369–376
72. Smith JW (1960) Collagen fibre patterns in mammalian bone. J Anat 94:329–344
73. Soulié A (1904) Sur les applications de la radiographie stéréoscopique à l'étude des artères des os. (Note technique.) CR Assoc Anat 6:172–174
74. Steinbach HL, Jergeson F, Gilfillan RS, Petrakis NL (1957) Osseous phlebography. Surg Gynecol Obstet Am 40:215–226
75. Testut L (1880) Vaisseaux et nerfs du tissu conjonctif fibreux et osseux; anatomie et physiologie. Thèse d'agrégation
76. Thiersch K (1865) Thiersch Graft: lead chromate for perfusion. Arch Mikrosk Anat 149
77. Trias A, Fery A (1979) Cortical circulation of long bones. J Bone Joint Surg Am 61:1052–1059
78. Trueta J (1963) The role of the vessels in osteogenesis. J Bone Joint Surg Br 45:402–418
79. Trueta J (1968) Studies of the development and decay of the human frame. Heinemann, London
80. Uhthoff HK, Dubuc FL (1971) Bone structure in the dog under rigid internal fixation. Clin Orthop Rel Res 81:165–170
81. von Leydig F (1856) Histologie des Menschen und der Thiere, von Meidinger Verlag, Frankfort-am-Main
82. Walker RA (1985) Ulex europeus I-peroxidase as a marker of vascular endothelium: its application in routine histo-pathology. J Pathol 146:123–127
83. Weidenreich F (1923) Knochenstudien. I. Teil. Ueber Aufbau und Entwicklung des Knochens und den Charakter des Knochengewebes. A Anat EntwGesch 69:382–466
84. Weidenreich F (1930) Das Knochengewebe. In: von Möllendorf W (ed) Handbuch der mikroskopischen Anatomie des Menschen (2nd series, part 2) Springer, Berlin
85. White NB, Ter-Pogossian MM, Stein AH (1964) A method to determine the rate of blood flow in bone and selected soft tissues. Surg Gynec Obstet 119:535–540
86. Wilkes CH, Visscher MB (1975) Some physiological aspects of bone marrow pressure. J Bone Joint Surg Am 57:49–63
87. Young RW (1962) Cell proliferation and specialization during endochondral osteogenesis in young rats. J Cell Biol 14:357–370
88. Zawisch-Ossenitz C (1926) Histologische Untersuchungen über Gefässeinschluss und Gefässentwicklung im knochen. Z Mikrosk Anat Forsch 6:76–161
89. Zawisch-Ossenitz C (1927) Ueber Begriff und Bedeutung der durchbohrenden Knochenkanäle. Z Mikrosk Anat Forsch 9:585–606

CHAPTER 4

Biology and Physiology of Intramedullary Reaming in the Fixation of Fractures

K.S. Leung and E.N.M. Cheung

Introduction

The biology of fracture healing with closed intramedullary nailing follows the process of natural bone healing. The classic three phases of fracture healing are observed with haematoma formation, callus formation and callus remodelling. With this technique, the fractures are fixed with adequate stability without external immobilisation, which facilitates functional recovery of the injured limbs. This natural bone healing, which is considered to be the preferred way of fracture healing in the modern concept of fracture repair, can only be possible with the fracture haematoma preserved. The importance of fracture haematoma preservation has been proven [20, 21, 49] and is further confirmed with the continuous discovery of the presence of the numerous growth factors in the haematoma. Together with the presence of the progenitor cells at the fracture site, cellular differentiation leads to the well-orchestrated process of callus formations and remodelling. Intramedullary fixation provides early mechanical stability that promotes revascularisation, which is vital for fracture healing. The change in the direction of cortical blood flow after nailing and the preservation of the periosteum with the closed technique further enhances the revascularisation process with the intact periosteal blood flow [68, 82, 89].

Reaming of the medullary canal was first proposed by G. Küntscher in order to have an elastic fixation of the bone with his original design of nail, which had a clover leaf cross section [41] (Fig. 4.1). Although this concept of intramedullary fixation of fractures has been seriously challenged today, reaming is still widely practised and remains the essential part of the operation during intramedullary nailing. Reaming does increase the number of the contact points as well as the total area of contact surface between the nail and the undulating surface of the medullary cavity. This provides stability in fixation. This interference fitting is most important in nails without interlocking design. Biomechanically, fracture stability in-

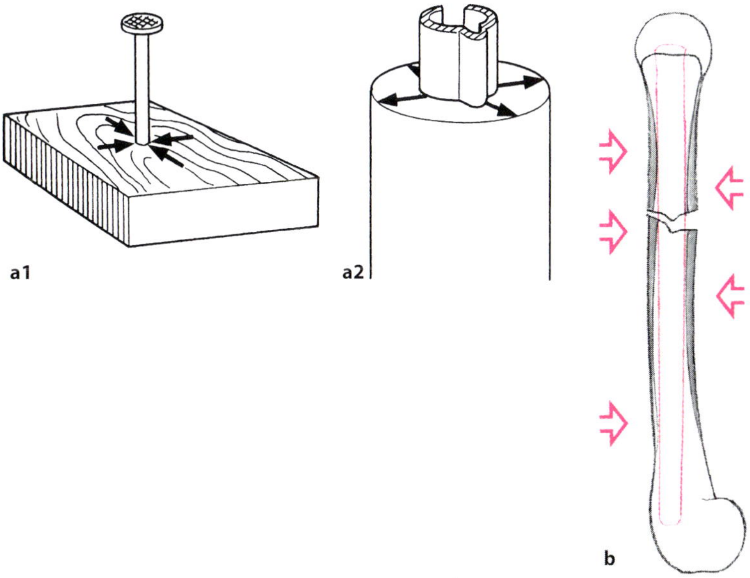

Fig. 4.1 a, b. Küntscher's concept of elastic impingement of the nail in the intramedullary canal for fracture fixation. **a** Cloverleaf cross section of the nail and the elastic jamming. **b** Elastic impingement

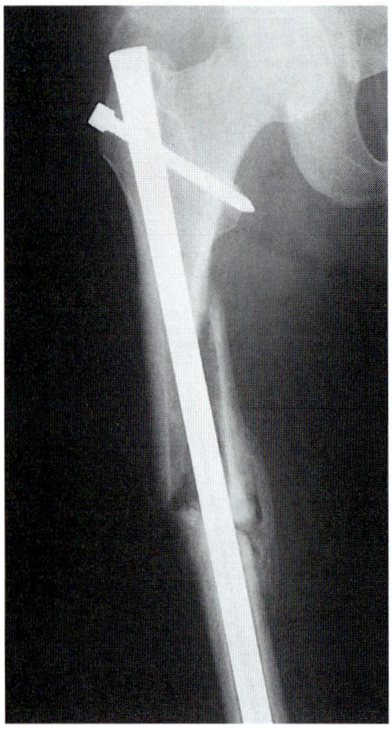

Fig. 4.2. Iatrogenic fracture of the medial cortex of the femur due to insertion of a rigid unslotted nail

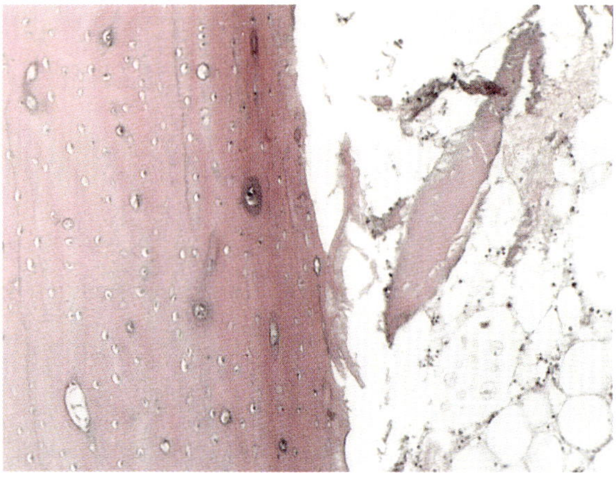

Fig. 4.3. Histomorphological study revealed that inner cortex, endosteum and intramedullary structure were destroyed immediately after intramedullary reaming. Bone fragments were found inside the medullary cavity. (H&E staining, ×100)

creases exponentially with the increase in the diameter of the nail inserted. Reaming is thus needed to fulfil this mechanical requirement by providing a larger passage for the optimal diameter of the nail to be inserted. From the practical aspect, reaming is also needed to facilitate the insertion of the relatively more rigid structure into the bone so as to decrease the chances of iatrogenic fractures during nail insertion. Studies have shown that reaming significantly affects the axial force required to insert the nail [34, 53]. By over-reaming 1 mm in the proximal femur and 0.5 mm in the distal segment of the femur, both the axial and push-out forces decrease in the order of magnitude [83]. Today, with the use of the more rigid designs such as unslotted nails, reaming is even more necessary for these similar reasons (Fig. 4.2).

Effect on Cortical Circulation

Reaming increases the inner diameter of the medullary canal by removing the inner cortex and at the same time destroying the other intramedullary structures (Fig. 4.3). Of these structures, the disturbance in the intramedullary circulation is one of the major concerns after reaming. The effect on the blood supply of the remaining cortex and the alteration of the blood flow are discussed in Chap. 3 of this volume. Though much has been studied about the change in the blood flow and the regeneration of the intramedullary blood vessels after the reaming procedure [9, 17, 56, 67, 75], not all of these processes are fully understood. The post-reaming changes in the cortical circulation typically go through the stages of extensive cortical ischaemia and necrosis followed by regeneration of the medullary blood supply and reversal of the centripetal cortical blood flow to centrifugal blood flow from the intact periosteal circulation [67].

The cortical necrosis is much more extensive than that which can be observed in the fracture ends [13, 44, 57]. It is due to the destruction of the medullary vessels and embolisation of the cortical vessels by the intravasated marrow content and the generation of heat during reaming of the cortical bone. The subsequent replacement of the necrotic bone by creeping substitution is a very slow process. On the other hand, the regeneration of the medullary vessels has been shown to be excellent and rapid from the intact metaphyseal vessels [68, 69] with stable skeletal fixation [23]. The total bone and cortical blood flow increases as the fractures heal after reaming [22]. The increase in the blood in these regenerated vessels and the periosteal blood vessels enhances the bony resorption and result in the generalised osteoporotic histological picture in the early phase of fracture healing. This again explains the decrease in the bone mineral content as well as bone mineral density in the early phase of fracture healing after intramedullary fixation [43] (Fig. 4.4). The destruction of the medullary circulation stimulates the periosteal circulation and the opening up of the many latent vasculatures in the periosteum. The blood flow thus changes from the normal centripetal to the centrifugal direction

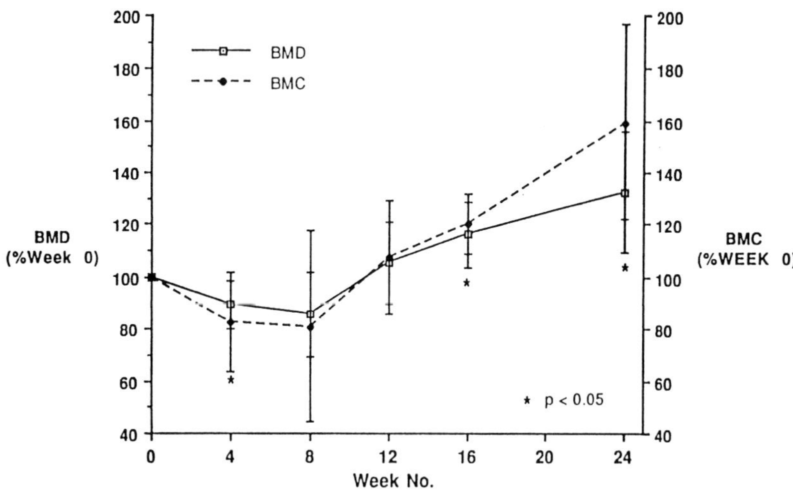

Fig. 4.4. Changes of the bone mineral content (*BMC*) and the bone mineral density (*BMD*) in the healing of femoral fractures fixed by intramedullary locked nails

[67]. The reactive changes in the periosteal blood vessels and blood flow lead to the final revascularisation of the cortex under stable fixation. Ultimately this leads to the re-establishment of the connection between medullary, cortical and periosteal circulation by the regeneration of the new vessels along and across the cortex [62]. Since the blood supply of the cortices depends on intact periosteal circulation [10, 87, 93], the presence of the more vascular structures, such as the muscles and tendon attachment in the cortex, will definitely enhance this process. This may explain the predictably good results in fixing femoral fractures with reamed intramedullary nails when compared with those from fixing tibial fractures. This is particularly evident in treating open fractures where soft tissue injury is common and where the blood supply of the bony structure is critical. The treatment of open femoral fractures with intramedullary locked nails thus illustrates the importance of the periosteal blood supply from the surrounding musculature and the mechanical stability provided by the locked nail in facilitating early regeneration of the cortical circulation. For open fractures of the tibia, the place of reamed intramedullary locked nails remains to be explored because of the less favourable periosteal circulation from the surrounding soft tissue envelope.

Effect on Fracture Healing

One of the most interesting observations concerning the healing of fractures that are treated with reamed intramedullary fixation is the extensive proliferation of the periosteal blood vessels. These lead to exuberant subperiosteal callus formation as observed both in clinical practice and in animal experiments [16]. This results in an increase in the mechanical strength, both in bending and torsion, of the bone with the healed fractures [22, 31]. The callus forms by membranous ossification with the trabecular structure orientated obliquely or perpendicular to the cortical surface [14]. As the callus quality depends on the mechanical stability of fracture fixation, endochondral ossification is uncommon in this subperiosteal osteogenesis, which indicates that the mechanism of callus formation is very different from that observed in fractures fixed with methods other than intramedullary nailing. At least two mechanisms have been proposed for this positive finding in fracture healing. One of the theories put forward is the stimulatory effect of the cortical ischaemia, which induces periosteal blood vessel proliferation. This triggers a similar process of fracture healing in response to the cortical ischaemia [88] and results in extensive callus formation in the cortex. However, this proposed explanation is not universally accepted due to conflicting evidence from animal experiments. The other proposed mechanism is the expulsion of the reaming material from the medullary cavity through the fracture sites into the fracture haematoma and the periosteal space during the rise in the intramedullary pressure from reaming. The expulsed material acts like marrow and bone grafts which react with the fracture haematoma and result in extensive bone formation. This autologous bone graft is very often observed in clinical practice (Fig. 4.5) and is one of the definite advantages of the intramedullary fixation of fractures with reaming [22, 39, 95]. This effect is particularly advantageous in fractures with bone loss where bone grafting has to be performed if open methods of fracture fixa-

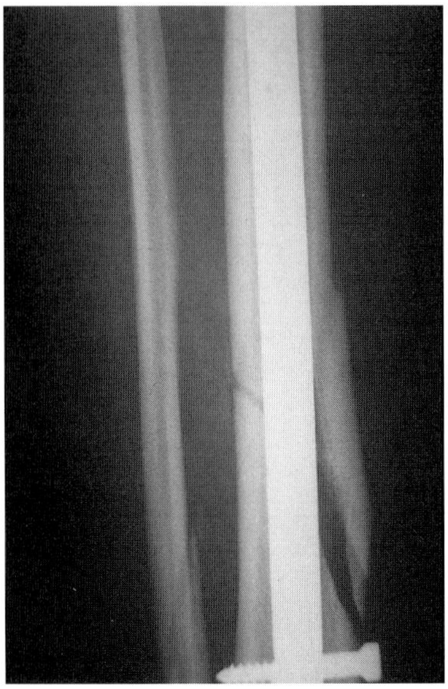

Fig. 4.5. Immediate post-operative X-ray film of a tibial fracture fixed with reamed intramedullary nail showing reamed bony debris dispersed around the fracture site

tion are chosen. However, the biological activity of this reamed material needs further studies, as the heat and pressure generated during reaming is quite substantial. Although the interaction between reaming material and the fracture haematoma in the process of fracture healing is a most interesting topic for future study, the role of periosteal osteogenesis in the healing of fractures fixed with intramedullary nails is obvious.

Intramedullary reaming has been demonstrated to increase the circulation of the intact soft-tissue envelope. The increased extraosseous circulation may have implications for fracture healing. Reamed intramedullary fixation of long bone fracture significantly reduces rates of non-union in comparison with non-reamed nailing [6]. The stimulatory effect on fracture healing after reaming is also well demonstrated when this technique is applied to the delayed union and non-union of fractures [24, 25, 35, 100]. Predictable good results are obtained in cases with hypertrophic non-union where additional bone graft is unnecessary. Reaming stimulates the osteoblastic activities around the fracture sites as well as in the periosteal activities. Intramedullary nail fixation provides good mechanical stability which allows load transfer across the fracture sites. In treating atrophic non-union by intramedullary nailing, the result is non-uniform and secondary bone grafting, often required to enhance fracture union, although the reamed products may act as an osteoinductive agent in the formation of endosteal callus [28].

Mechanical Effect of Reaming

The original indication for reaming in intramedullary nailing was based on mechanical considerations. The effect of this mechanical procedure on the biological tissue has been the subject of many studies in the past years. Reaming is performed in order to increase the fixation stability by increasing the surface contact and allowing the insertion of a larger diameter nail. Fixation stability of interlocking nails is achieved by locking screws in the proximal and distal segments rather than by surface contact between the nail and inner cortex. Biomechanically, the change from the use of the less flexible, pliable nails to more rigid, stronger nails is important in providing stability in fractures. Reaming is therefore applied for different indications. The most frequently observed local effects are thinning of the cortex, heat generation and an increase in intramedullary pressure during reaming. Apart from the direct injury imposed on the intramedullary blood vessels and the weakening of the cortex, systemic complications can be observed in certain groups of patients with predisposing conditions [19, 60].

The Effect on Bone Mineral Content of the Cortex

Reaming removes a certain portion of the cortical bone which may account for the decrease in the bone mineral content (BMC) in the early post-fixation period. This also corresponds to the decrease in the bone mineral density (BMD) observed in clinical studies (Fig. 4.4) [43]. Although these observations still need further study with a better animal model, the hypothesis that the early suppression of the osteoblastic activities immediately after injury may well be one of the mechanisms that explains the delayed and persistent decrease in the bone mineral content [42]. The reactive osteoporosis in the cortex after reaming is one of the causes for this observation, as the decrease in the BMD also affects the regions of the normal cortical bone away from the fracture site. The BMD increases to significantly higher levels during the course of fracture healing, indicating the excellent stimulatory effect of reaming on fracture healing with intramedullary fixation [92]. This effect may also be due to the better mechanical environment of the load-sharing property with intramedullary fixation for fracture callus mineralization, according to Wolff's law. The vascular insult theory in the production of osteoporosis after plate fixation of fractures has been seriously challenged [90, 91]. Experimentation further proves the importance of the load-shielding effect of plating in the production of osteopenia [91]. The use of a load-sharing device such as intramedullary nails is much preferred, based on biomechanical considerations as well as callus mineralization.

The Effect of Heat Production

A rise in local cortical temperature is considered to be detrimental to fracture healing, as the enzymes involved in the healing process are damaged by the heat generated [66]. Animal experiments have also shown that the rise of the local cortical temperature of 3°–4 °C while reaming in rabbit tibiae [78] gave rise to subsequent complications of fracture healing as a result of thermal damage during intramedullary reaming. During intramedullary reaming, this rise in cortical temperature is directly proportional to the radius of the reamer head used, the speed of reaming, the pressure exerted during reaming process, the sharpness of the reamer heads and the cooling effect of the body fluid [54]. The relatively poor heat conductance of the bony cortex also contributes to the thermal injury. However, the biological effect of the increase in temperature during reaming must be considered together with duration of exposure, the maximum temperature reached, the cooling effect of the fluid flow inside the medullary canal and the susceptibility of the cortical bone to high temperature. According to Eriksson, the threshold temperature for damage to occur in the bone cortex is 47 °C with an exposure time of 1 min [18]. In clinical practice, the production of heat due to the increase in the friction that is caused by the large radius of the reamer heads, particularly with blunt reamer heads [3, 54], seldom reaches such high levels and the duration is usually only a few seconds. Thermal necrosis of cortical bone occurs after reaming of a narrow intramedullary canal [44, 57]. Nevertheless, careful observation of reaming technique and the use of sharp reamers is recommended in order to prevent complications caused by the rise in the local temperature.

The Effect of an Increase in Intramedullary Pressure

Intramedullary pressure rises during reaming as well as during nail insertion [26]. The piston effect of the reamer movement is the major cause of the increase in intramedullary pressure (Fig.

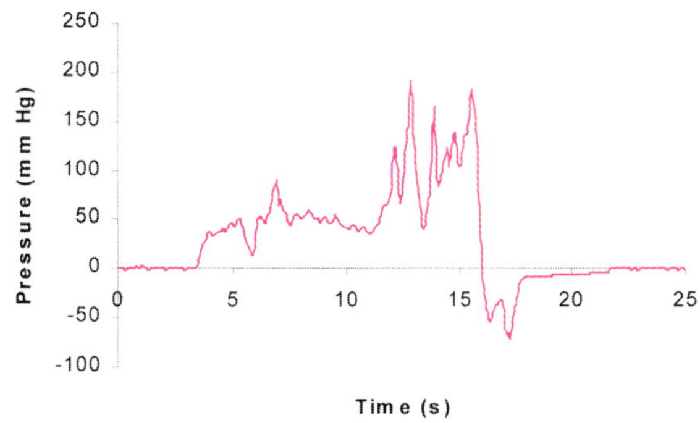

Fig. 4.6. Changes of intramedullary pressure were measured during reaming of goat's femur. The pressure increased with several peaks when inserting a reamer head into the intramedullary canal. Negative pressure was also generated when removing reamer from the canal

4.6). Mechanically, the distance between the reamer head and the cortex, the viscosity of the medullary content and the relative centricity of the reamer in the medullary cavity also contribute to the rise in intramedullary pressure [52, 78]. In clinical practice, the size of the reamer shaft and reamer head, the magnitude of the pushing force during reaming and the length of the intact diaphyseal bone are the factors contributing to this increase in pressure. Intramedullary pressure has been found to increase to significantly high values, well above the systolic pressure during reaming. In animal experiments, values as high as 1500 mmHg were recorded during the reaming of sheep tibiae [79]. The increase in intramedullary pressure has both local and systemic effects.

The Local Effect of an Increase in Intramedullary Pressure

Reaming destroys the medullary circulation and causes cortical necrosis. However, the extent of the cortical necrosis after reaming cannot be explained purely by the destruction of medullary circulation alone because the extent is much greater than that predicted by the vascular study [79]. The high intramedullary pressure created during reaming also contributes to local damage. Under increased intramedullary pressure, the reamed material is forced into the minute cortical channels. These are opened up by the reaming process. The piston effect of the reamer causes the dispersion of the medullary content, clots, and bone debris into the haversian canals, the Volkmann canal and blocks the nutrient arterioles. The clogging of these channels impairs the venous drainage, which takes place through the

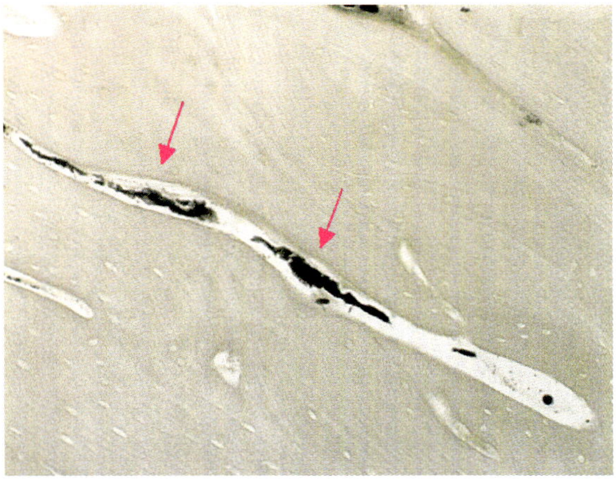

Fig. 4.7. Immediately after intramedullary reaming of goat's femur, fat particles (*arrows*) were found inside the haversian canal of cortical bone. (Osmium, ×100)

periosteal route. This destructive effect of reamed material clogging can be explained by its harmful effect on the intracortical perfusion. The observation of a pulsatile physiological medullary cavity pressure supports the theory that the nutrition of the osteocytes and venous drainage of the cortical circulation depend on this centripetal pressure gradient [2, 45]. Animal study has shown the presence of marrow fat inside the canaliculi of the cortex (Fig. 4.7) [11]. The blockage of the intraosseous circulation and the destruction of the medullary blood supply disturb the intracortical transport system of the osteocytes and thus result in extensive cortical necrosis after reaming.

The other local effect on the injured limb is the risk of a rise in the compartmental pressure during reaming. The extrusion of the marrow content and the bleeding induced during reaming may lead to an increase in the compartmental pressure [47, 50, 51, 58]. Clinical study has shown that the rise is transient and related to the forward movement of the reaming procedure [80]. A decrease in pressure is observed following the backing out of the reamer head and after reaming [86]. Nailing also increases the compartmental pressure transiently [48, 50], the compartmental pressure returns to normal quickly after operation. The risk of compartment syndrome is related to the type of fracture, the severity of soft tissue injury and the delay in undertaking the nailing procedure. However, compartmental pressure increases more significantly in those patients undergoing prolonged operations or with excessive traction during operation [84]. Unsatisfactory positioning of the injured limb during and after operation also increases the compartmental pressure. It is therefore advisable to monitor the compartmental pressure in patients undergoing a prolonged surgical procedure during reaming. It is obvious that patients must be positioned properly for nailing, especially for tibial fractures (see Chap. 10, this volume).

The Systemic Effect of an Increase in Intramedullary Pressure

The clinical finding of marrow content in the circulation during intramedullary nailing has been reported for some time. Marrow content was also collected from the cannulated femoral-vein blood samples during reaming in animal experiments [15]. This intravasation of the marrow content is thought to be caused by the increase in the intramedullary pressure generated during reaming. A rise in intramedullary pressure of about 50 mm Hg has been demonstrated to be the threshold value of marrow fat intravasation [97]. The demonstration of emboli inside the right atrium by the trans-oesophageal echocardiography is another vivid proof [63, 97]. Showers of emboli were detected with this method during and after the reaming procedure, lasting for 4–11 days after surgery. Although emboli may be detected in all stages of the operation, starting from fracture manipulation for closed reduction to the insertion of the nail, the largest showers of emboli are observed during reaming and nail insertion [99]. Morbidity and mortality have been reported and attributed to this embolic phenomenon [55, 73]. However, apart from the description of paradoxical embolism in patients with patent foramen ovale, which leads to developing systemic fat embolism syndrome [46, 63], the effect of the intravasated bone marrow is mostly described in the pulmonary tissue (Fig. 4.8) [12]; the effect on the other organs in the body is not so well defined.

Many hypotheses have been put forward to explain the role of intravasated bone marrow in the pathogenesis of these systemic complications, particularly the development of the post-traumatic adult respiratory distress syndrome (ARDS). The hypothesis that there is massive occlusion of the pulmonary vessels by the emboli has been much challenged. The amount of marrow fat intravasation is found to be insufficiently large for the occlusion of pulmonary circulation [64]. Simple mechanical blockage of the pulmonary arteries by marrow fat cannot completely explain the clinical presentation and laboratory findings. Local release of humoral factors, as well as the stimulation of the pressure receptor due to hypoxia, may also partly contribute to the pulmonary response

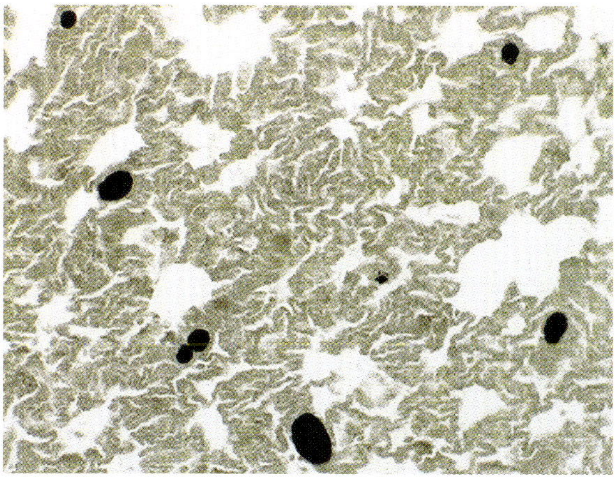

Fig. 4.8. Fat droplets (*black*) were demonstrated in pulmonary tissue after reamed intramedullary nailing in goat's femur. (Osmium, ×100)

to acute embolisation of marrow fat content [40]. The toxic effect of bone marrow fat on other tissues may also contribute to the pathogenesis of ARDS. Injecting bone marrow into the systemic circulation activates coagulation [8] and leads to increasing the size of the fat emboli by inducing aggregation of thrombi around the fat emboli [74]. Platelets as well as fibrinogen levels are decreased by the introduction of marrow fat in the systemic circulation [5]. Together with the activation of neutrophils [94, 96] and the other complement systems in patients with severe trauma and hypovolaemic shock, the intravasation of the bone marrow may be responsible for deterioration in lung function.

It is certain at this stage that reaming does not cause fat embolism syndrome in all patients [30, 63]. Pulmonary injury after severe trauma is not caused by the presence of marrow fat in the systemic circulation alone. Instead, a combination of the mechanical effect of emboli, a modulation of the mechanical changes by the reflectory mechanism and the effect of the circulatory humoral mediators after injury must play a part to induce the complex reactive changes in the pulmonary parenchyma, which lead to the full-blown pictures of ARDS in patients with multiple injuries. The effect of initial lung injury [85, 98] and the effect of intramedullary reaming are cumulative in the pathogenesis of ARDS. On the other hand, early stabilisation of the skeletal injuries has been shown to decrease the intravasation of marrow fat into the circulation and its advantages in the management of patients with multiple injuries are well established [1, 4, 7, 32, 71, 72, 81]. The judicious use of intramedullary fixation in long bone fractures is recognised as one of the most efficient ways to provide fracture stability in polytrauma patients. The recognition of a particular group of patients at risk is very important in the total management of polytrauma patients. Special precautions must be taken in fixing multiple long bone fractures in these patients. The conditions associated with high post-traumatic complications are hypovolaemic shock with massive transfusion [101] and pulmonary contusion [33]. It is therefore very important to prevent hypovolaemic shock by supplying energetic fluid replacement and detecting the presence of pulmonary contusion, which may sometimes be difficult at the acute stage of injury [60].

As the intravasation of the marrow content into the circulation contributes to the development of pulmonary complications and since this occurrence is partly caused by the increase in intramedullary pressure during the process of reaming, the use of either unreamed nails or minimal reaming are the logical solution deduced from the currently available information. However, interference to the cortical circulation is still observed after the insertion of unreamed nails [38]. Similarly, a transient increase in the intramedullary pressure is recorded during the insertion of unreamed nails [27, 59]. Alteration of pulmonary function [28] and fatal fat embolism syndrome have been seen after unreamed nailing [65]. Furthermore, mechanical failure is common in unreamed nails [70] and its role in the management of long bone fractures needs further study. The mechanical advantage of nails with large diameters is well recognised and thus reaming still remains an essential part of the operation. Another approach has been tried to decrease the intramedullary pressure generated during reaming. This can be done by further improvement of reamer heads [77] to allow better transport of reamed bone chips by having larger flutes between the cutting edges [61]. The use of smaller diameter reamer shafts which can provide enough torsional rigidity mechanically also generates less pressure [52, 76]. Controlling the advancing speed of the reamer also prevents a substantial rise in intramedullary pressure (Fig. 4.9) [12].

Other theoretical approaches to decrease the pressure include the creation of a vent hole in the distal femur. This has been shown to be ineffective [36]. The postulation of abnormal circulation in patients with bony metastasis and the demonstration of a shunting mechanism between arterial and venous systems in animals may also explain the failure of such modification. Suction irrigation systems have been designed to provide continuous flushing of the reamed debris and removal by

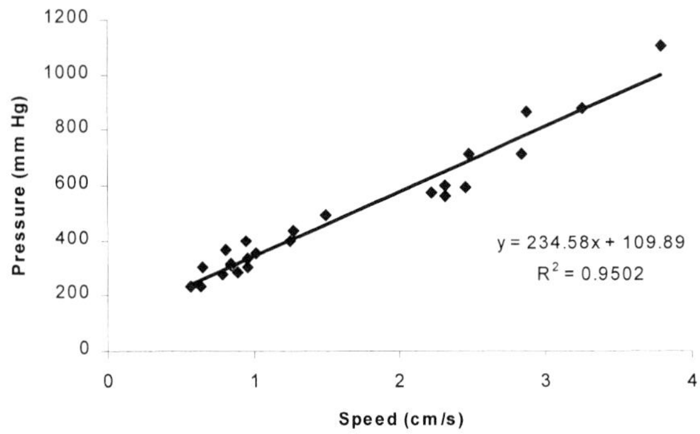

Fig. 4.9. The relationship between the reamer's advancing speed and the rise in intramedullary pressure from a laboratory test. The rise in intramedullary pressure correlates with the reamer's advancing speed

suction in the proximal end of the medullary cavity. These systems have been shown to decrease the pressure to a negative one, lower the temperature and significantly increase the survival of the bony cortex in animal experiments [79]. The disadvantages are the loss of the reaming product as well as the clearing of the fracture haematoma, which may have a negative effect on callus formation and fracture healing. Furthermore, blood loss is expectedly increased with this set-up. It must be stressed at this point in time that this design has not been applied in clinical practice. Removal of bone marrow fat by intramedullary suction alone prior to intramedullary reaming has been demonstrated to effectively reduce the rise in intramedullary pressure and in the amount of pulmonary embolic fat in animal studies [12]. This technique may be beneficial for the prevention of fat embolism syndrome.

Future Directions in Research

As we understand more about the biological effects of intramedullary reaming on fracture healing and its role in the pathogenesis of pulmonary complications in susceptible patients [60], it is necessary to evaluate the clinical situation regarding the choice of skeletal fixation in patients. Reaming is important in the provision of stable fixation and helps to decrease the complications of closed intramedullary fixation of fractures. It is obvious that improvements in reaming instrumentation and in the design of intramedullary nails are essential for further reduction of the complications related to this surgical procedure, thus improving the outcome of fracture treatment in the future. More studies are needed to define the quantitative relationship between the rise in intramedullary pressure and the embolic phenomenon [99], to define the role of the marrow fat emboli in the pathogenesis of the systemic embolic phenomenon and to improve the surgical technique in the practical use of the instruments during operation. Until this stage is reached, reaming must be performed with sound surgical principles and meticulous technique [29] to reduce the deleterious effect of marrow embolisation. The following recommendations should be followed while treating long bone fractures with closed intramedullary locked nailing:

- Reaming should be carried out with the use of sharp reamer heads.
- Reaming should be carried out without excessive pushing force.
- Reaming should be carried out with a slow rhythm.

Special precaution must also be taken with:

- Patients with long segments of intact cortex and multiple long bone fractures
- Patients with concomitant lung injury, where reaming may have to be delayed
- Patients undergoing an episode of post-traumatic hypovolaemic shock
- Patients with pathological fractures in multiple long bones

References

1. Amis JA, Grank DJ, Burkhead WZ, Bucholz RW (1989) The role of medullary reaming in closed nailing of femur fractures. Intramedullary rods: clinical performance and related laboratory testing. In: Harvey JP, Daniels AU, Games RF (eds) Intramedullary rodes: clinical preformance and related laboratory testing, ASTM, pp 108–118
2. Ascenzi A (1972) Physiological relationship and pathological interferences between bone tissue and marrow. In: Bourne GH (ed) The biochemistry and physiology of bone. Academic Press, New York, pp 403–444
3. Baumgart F, Kohler G, Ochsner PE (1998) The physics of heat generation during reaming of the medullary cavity. Injury 29(suppl 2):11–25
4. Behrman SW, Fabian TC, Kudsk KA, Taylor JC (1990) Improved outcome with femur fractures: early vs. delayed fixation. J Trauma 30:792–797
5. Bergentz SE, Gelin LE, Rudenstam CM (1960) Intravascular aggregation of blood cells following intravenous infusion of fat emulsions. Acta Chir Scand 120:115–120
6. Bhandari M, Guyatt GH, Tong D, Adili A, Shaughnessy SG (2000) Reamed versus nonreamed intramedullary nailing of lower extremity long bone fractures: a systematic overview and meta-analysis. J Orthop Trauma 14:2–9
7. Bone LB, Johnson KD, Weigelt J, Scheinberg R (1989) Early versus delayed stabilization of femoral fractures. A prospective randomized study. J Bone Joint Surg Am71:336–340
8. Bradford DS, Foster RR, Nossel HL (1970) Coagulation alterations, hypoxemia, and fat embolism in fracture patients. J Trauma 10:307–321

9. Brinker MR, Cook SD, Dunlap JN, Christakis P, Elliott MN (1999) Early changes in nutrient artery blood flow following tibial nailing with and without reaming: a preliminary study. J Orthop Trauma 13:129–133
10. Chanavaz M (1995) Anatomy and histophysiology of the periosteum: quantification of the periosteal blood supply to the adjacent bone with 85Sr and gamma spectrometry. Author J Oral Implantol 21:214–219
11. Cheung NME (2000) The study of pathogenesis of pulmonary fat embolization after intramedullary reaming and possible improvement in reaming technique (PhD Thesis). The Chinese University of Hong Kong
12. Cheung NME, Leung KS (2000) Factors affecting intramedullary pressure during intramedullary reaming (abstract no. 6C). ISFR-2000, September 2000, Hong Kong
13. Curtis MJ, Brown PR, Dick JD, Jinnah RH (1995) Contaminated fractures of the tibia: a comparison of treatment modalities in an animal model. J Orthop Res 13:286–295
14. Danckwardt Lillieström G, Lorenzi GL, Olerud S (1970) Intramedullary nailing after reaming. An investigation on the healing process in osteotomized rabbit tibias. Acta Orthop Scand Suppl 134:1–78
15. Danckwardt Lillieström G (1969) Marrow embolism as a cause of circulation block after surgery to the medullary cavity. Proceedings of the European Society of Experimental Surgery Congress, p 4
16. Danckwardt Lillieström G (1969) Reaming of the medullary cavity and its effect on diaphyseal bone. A fluorochromic, microangiographic and histologic study on the rabbit tibia and dog femur. Acta Orthop Scand Suppl 128:1–153
17. El Maraghy AW, Humeniuk B, Anderson GI, Schemitsch EH, Richards RR (1999) Femoral bone blood flow after reaming and intramedullary canal preparation: a canine study using laser Doppler flowmetry. J Arthroplasty 14:220–226
18. Eriksson AR, and Albrektsson T (1983) Temperature threshold levels for heat-induced bone tissue injury: a vital-microscopic study in the rabbit. J Prosthetic Dentistry 50:101–107
19. Goris RJA, Meek RN, Bone LB, et al. (1990) Fracture management and pulmonary failure. In: Border JR (ed) Blunt multiple trauma. Marcel Dekker, New York, pp 77–91
20. Grundnes O, Reikeras O (1993) The importance of the hematoma for fracture healing in rats. Acta Orthop Scand 64:340–342
21. Grundnes O, Reikeras O (1993) The role of hematoma and periosteal sealing for fracture healing in rats. Acta Orthop Scand 64:47–49
22. Grundnes O, Utvag SE, Reikeras O (1994) Effects of graded reaming on fracture healing. Blood flow and healing studied in rat femurs. Acta Orthop Scand 65:32–36
23. Grundnes O, Utvag SE, Reikeras O (1994) Restoration of bone flow following fracture and reaming in rat femora. Acta Orthop Scand 65:185–190
24. Gualdrini G, Rollo G, Montanari A, Zinghi GF (1996) Aseptic nonunion of the tibia treated by intramedullary osteosynthesis. Chir Organi Mov 81:275–278
25. Hak DJ, Lee SS, Goulet JA (2000) Success of exchange reamed intramedullary nailing for femoral shaft nonunion or delayed union. J Orthop Trauma 14:178–182
26. Heim D, Schlegel U, Perren SM (1993) Intramedullary pressure in reamed and unreamed nailing of the femur and tibia – an in vitro study in intact, human bones. Injury 24(suppl 3):56–63
27. Heim D, Schlegel U, Perren SM (1994) Intramedullary pressure in intramedullary nailing of the femur and tibia. Helv Chir Acta 60:605–610
28. Heim D, Regazzoni P, Tsakiris DA, Aebi T, Schlegel U, Marbet GA, Perren SM (1995) Intramedullary nailing and pulmonary embolism: does unreamed nailing prevent embolization? An in vivo study in rabbits. J Trauma 38:899–906
29. Hopf T, Gleitz M, Hess T (1994) Intramedullary pressure in the femur during boring and nailing with modern compression interlocking nails – risk of fat embolism? Unfallchirurg 97:458–461
30. Hughes SP, Reichert IL, McCarthy ID (1993) Biological effects of intramedullary reaming. J Bone Joint Surg Br 75:845–847
31. Indrekvam K, Gjerdet NR, Engesaeter LB, Langeland N (1991) Effects of intramedullary reaming and nailing of rat femur. A mechanical and chemical study. Acta Orthop Scand 62:582–586
32. Johnson KD, Cadambi A, Seibert GB (1985) Incidence of adult respiratory distress syndrome in patients with multiple musculoskeletal injuries: effect of early operative stabilization of fractures. J Trauma 25:375–384
33. Johnson JA, Cogbill TH, Winga ER (1986) Determinants of outcome after pulmonary contusion. J Trauma 26:695–697
34. Johnson JA, Berkshire A, Leighton RK, Gross M, Chess DG, Petrie D (1995) Some basic biomechanical characteristics of medullary pressure generation during reaming of the femur. Injury 26:451–454
35. Kempf I, Grosse A, Rigaut P (1986) The treatment of noninfected pseudarthrosis of the femur and tibia with locked intramedullary nailing. Clin Orthop 212:142–154
36. Kerr PS, Jackson M, Atkins RM (1993) Cardiac arrest during intramedullary nailing for femoral metastases. J Bone Joint Surg Br 75:972–973
37. Kessler SB, Hallfeldt KK, Perren SM, Schweiberer L (1986) The effects of reaming and intramedullary nailing on fracture healing. Clin Orthop 212:18–25
38. Klein MP, Rahn BA, Frigg R, Kessler S, Perren SM (1990) Reaming versus non-reaming in medullary nailing: interference with cortical circulation of the canine tibia. Arch Orthop Trauma Surg 109:314–316
39. Klemm KW (1986) Treatment of infected pseudarthrosis of the femur and tibia with an interlocking nail. Clin Orthop 212:174–181
40. Kroupa J (1986) Fat globulemia in early diagnostics of traumatic fat embolism. Czech Med 9:90–108
41. Küntscher G (1965) Intramedullary surgical technique and its place in orthopedic surgery: my present concept. J Bone Joint Surg Am 47:809–818
42. Leung KS, Fung KP, Sher A, Liu P (1993) Bone specific alkaline phosphatase activities during fracture healing and callotasis in rabbit. SIROT 93 Seoul, 6th General Meeting, Seoul, Korea
43. Leung KS, Poon KM, Chan WS, Lee S (1993) Bone mineral changes in fractures fixed with intramedullary locked nails. SIROT 93 Seoul, 6th General Meeting, Seoul, Korea
44. Leunig M, Hertel R (1996) Thermal necrosis after tibial reaming for intramedullary nail fixation. A report of three cases. J Bone Joint Surg Br 78:584–587
45. Lopez Curto JA, Bassingthwaighte JB, Kelly PJ (1980) Anatomy of the microvasculature of the tibial diaphysis of the adult dog. J Bone Joint Surg Am 62:1362–1369
46. Lung TK, Leung TY, Leung KS (1997) Mortality after reamed intramedullary nailing of acute fractures in patient with patent foramen ovale. Hong Kong J Orthop Surg 1:74–77
47. Mawhinney IN, Maginn P, McCoy GF (1994) Tibial compartment syndromes after tibial nailing. J Orthop Trauma 8:212–214
48. McQueen MM, Christie J, Court Brown CM (1990) Compartment pressures after intramedullary nailing of the tibia. J Bone Joint Surg Br 72:395–397
49. Mizuno K, Mineo K, Tachibana T, Sumi M, Matsubara T, Hirohata K (1990) The osteogenetic potential of fracture haematoma. Subperiosteal and intramuscular transplantation of the haematoma. J Bone Joint Surg Br 72:822–829

50. Moed BR, Strom DE (1991) Compartment syndrome after closed intramedullary nailing of the tibia: a canine model and report of two cases. J Orthop Trauma 5:71–77
51. Moehring HD, Voigtlander JP (1995) Compartment pressure monitoring during intramedullary fixation of tibial fractures. Orthopedics 18:631–636
52. Müller C, Frigg R, Pfister U (1993) Effect of flexible drive diameter and reamer design on the increase of pressure in the medullary cavity during reaming. Injury 24(suppl 3):40–47
53. Müller C, McIff T, Rahn BA, Pfister U, Perren SM, Weller S (1993) Influence of the compression force on the intramedullary pressure development in reaming of the femoral medullary cavity. Injury 24(suppl 3):36–39
54. Müller C, McIff T, Rahn BA, Pfister U, Weller S (1993) Intramedullary pressure, strain on the diaphysis and increase in cortical temperature when reaming the femoral medullary cavity–a comparison of blunt and sharp reamers. Injury 24(suppl 3):22–30
55. Müller C, Rahn BA, Pfister U, Meinig RP (1994) The incidence, pathogenesis, diagnosis, and treatment of fat embolism. Orthop Rev 23:107–117
56. Nakamura T, Itoman M, Yokoyama K (1999) Cortical revascularization after reamed and unreamed intramedullary nailing in the rabbit femur: a microangiographic histometric analysis. J Trauma 47:744–751
57. Ochsner PE, Baumgart F, Kohler G (1998) Heat-induced segmental necrosis after reaming of one humeral and two tibial fractures with a narrow medullary canal. Injury 29(suppl 2):1–10
58. Ovre S, Hvaal K, Holm I, Stromsoe K, Nordsletten L, Skjeldal S (1998) Compartment pressure in nailed tibial fractures. A threshold of 30 mmHg for decompression gives 29% fasciotomies. Arch Orthop Trauma Surg 118:29–31
59. Pape HC, Dwenger A, Regel G, Schweitzer G, Jonas M, Remmers D, Krumm K, Neumann C, Sturm JA, Tscherne H (1992) Pulmonary damage after intramedullary femoral nailing in traumatized sheep – is there an effect from different nailing methods? J Trauma 33:574–581
60. Pape HC, Regel G, Dwenger A, Sturm JA, Tscherne H (1993) Influence of thoracic trauma and primary femoral intramedullary nailing on the incidence of ARDS in multiple trauma patients. Injury 24(suppl 3):82–103
61. Pape HC, Dwenger A, Grotz M, Kaever V, Negatsch R, Kleemann W, Regel G, Sturm JA, Tscherne H (1994) Does the reamer type influence the degree of lung dysfunction after femoral nailing following severe trauma? An animal study. J Orthop Trauma 8:300–309
62. Pazzaglia UE, Andrini L, Di Nucci A (1997) The reaction to nailing or cementing of the femur in rats. A microangiographic and fluorescence study. Int Orthop 21:267–273
63. Pell AC, Christie J, Keating JF, Sutherland GR (1993) The detection of fat embolism by transoesophageal echocardiography during reamed intramedullary nailing. A study of 24 patients with femoral and tibial fractures. J Bone Joint Surg Br 75:921–925
64. Peltter LF (1956) Fat embolism. I. The amount of fat in human long bones. Surgery 40:657–660
65. Peter RE, Schopfer A, Le Coultre B, Hoffmeyer P (1997) Fat embolism and death during prophylactic osteosynthesis of a metastatic femur using an unreamed femoral nail. J Orthop Trauma 11:233–234
66. Povacz F (1979) Thermal damage to the tibial diaphysis caused by intramedullary reaming. Unfallheilkunde 82:126–128
67. Reichert IL, McCarthy ID, Hughes SP (1995) The acute vascular response to intramedullary reaming. Microsphere estimation of blood flow in the intact ovine tibia (see comments). J Bone Joint Surg Br 77:490–493
68. Rhinelander FW (1973) Effects of medullary nailing on the normal blood supply of diaphyseal cortex. In: The American Academy of Orthopedic Surgeons, Instructional course lectures (vol 22) CV Mosby, Saint Louis, MO, pp 161–187
69. Rhinelander FW (1974) Tibial blood supply in relation to fracture healing. Clin Orthop 105:34–81
70. Riemer BL, DiChristina DG, Cooper A, Sagiv S, Butterfield SL, Burke CJ 3rd, Lucke JF, Schlosser JD 1995) Nonreamed nailing of tibial diaphyseal fractures in blunt polytrauma patients. J Orthop Trauma 9:66–75
71. Riska EB, von Bonsdorff H, Hakkinen S, Jaroma H, Kiviluoto O, Paavilainen T (1976) Multiple injuries. Injury 8:110–116
72. Riska EB, von Bonsdorff H, Hakkinen S, Jaroma H, Kiviluoto O, Paavilainen T (1977) Primary operative fixation of long bone fractures in patients with multiple injuries. J Trauma 17:111–121
73. Robert JH, Hoffmeyer P, Broquet PE, Cerutti P, Vasey H (1993) Fat embolism syndrome. Orthop Rev 22:567–571
74. Saldeen T (1970) Fat embolism and signs of intravascular coagulation in a posttraumatic autopsy material. J Trauma 10:273–286
75. Schemitsch EH, Kowalski MJ, Swiontkowski MF, Senft D (1994) Cortical bone blood flow in reamed and unreamed locked intramedullary nailing: a fractured tibia model in sheep. J Orthop Trauma 8:373–382
76. Speitling A (1994) Results of the evaluation of flexible reamers. Technical notes. AIOD Technical Committee, internal document
77. Speitling A, Harder HE (1995) Evaluation of IM – Reamer Design. Newsletters of The Association International Osteosynthesis Dynamic 2:3
78. Stanwyck ST (1985) Fracture healing and medullary nailing. In: Sibilson D (ed) Concepts in intramedullary nailing, Grune and Stratton, Orlando, FL, pp 27–49
79. Stürmer KM (1993) Measurement of intramedullary pressure in an animal experiment and propositions to reduce the pressure increase. Injury 24(suppl 3):7–21
80. Taglang G, Grosse A (1992) Compartment syndrome. International Symposium on Recent Advances in Locking Nails, Hong Kong, pp 58–59
81. Talucci RC, Manning J, Lampard S, Bach A, Carrico CJ (1983) Early intramedullary nailing of femoral shaft fractures: a cause of fat embolism syndrome. Am J Surg 146:107–111
82. Tarr RR, Wiss DA (1986) The mechanics and biology of intramedullary fracture fixation. Clin Orthop 212:10–17
83. Tencer AF, Sherman MC, Johnson KD (1985) Biomechanical factors affecting fracture stability and femoral bursting in closed intramedullary rod fixation of femur fractures. J Biomech Eng 107:104–111
84. Tischenko GJ, Goodman SB (1990) Compartment syndrome after intramedullary nailing of the tibia. J Bone Joint Surg Am 72:41–44
85. Todd TR, Baile E, Hogg JC (1978) Pulmonary capillary and permeability during hemorrhagic shock. J Appl Physiol 45:298–306
86. Tornetta P 3rd, French BG (1997) Compartment pressures during nonreamed tibial nailing without traction. J Orthop Trauma 11:24–27
87. Triffitt PD, Cieslak CA, Gregg PJ (1993) A quantitative study of the routes of blood flow to the tibial diaphysis after an osteotomy. J Orthop Res 11:49–57
88. Trueta A, Caladias AX (1964) A study of the blood supply of the lone bones. Surg Gynecol Obstet 118:485–498
89. Trueta J (1974) Blood supply and the rate of healing of tibial fractures. Clin Orthop 105:11–26
90. Uhthoff HK, Foux A, Yeadon A, McAuley J, Black RC (1993) Two processes of bone remodeling in plated intact femora: an experimental study in dogs. J Orthop Res 11:78–91

91. Uhthoff HK, Boisvert D, Finnegan M (1994) Cortical porosis under plates. Reaction to unloading or to necrosis? J Bone Joint Surg Am 76:1507–1512
92. Utvag SE, Reikeras O (1998) Effects of nail rigidity on fracture healing. Strength and mineralisation in rat femoral bone. Arch Orthop Trauma Surg 118:7–13
93. Utvag SE, Grundnes O, Reikeraos O (1996) Effects of periosteal stripping on healing of segmental fractures in rats. J Orthop Trauma 10:279–284
94. Vedder NB, Winn RK, Rice CL, Harlan JM (1989) Neutrophil-mediated vascular injury in shock and multiple organ failure. Prog Clin Biol Res 299:181–191
95. Webb LX, Winquist RA, Hansen ST (1986) Intramedullary nailing and reaming for delayed union or nonunion of the femoral shaft. A report of 105 consecutive cases. Clin Orthop 212:133–141
96. Weiland JE, Davis WB, Holter JF, Mohammed JR, Dorinsky PM, Gadek JE (1986) Lung neutrophils in the adult respiratory distress syndrome. Clinical and pathophysiologic significance. Am Rev Respir Dis 133:218–225
97. Wenda K, Runkel M, Degreif J, Ritter G (1993) Pathogenesis and clinical relevance of bone marrow embolism in medullary nailing – demonstrated by intraoperative echocardiography. Injury 24(suppl 3):73–81
98. Williams JJ, Moalli R, Calista C, Herndon JH (1990) Pulmonary endothelial injury and altered fibrinolysis after femur fracture in rabbits. J Orthop Trauma 4:303–308
99. Wozasek GE, Simon P, Redl H, Schlag G (1994) Intramedullary pressure changes and fat intravasation during intramedullary nailing: an experimental study in sheep. J Trauma 36:202–207
100. Wu CC, Shih CH, Chen WJ, Tai CL (1999) Effect of reaming bone grafting on treating femoral shaft aseptic nonunion after plating. Arch Orthop Trauma Surg 119:303–307
101. Wudel JH, Morris JA Jr, Yates K, Wilson A, Bass SM (1991) Massive transfusion: outcome in blunt trauma patients. J Trauma 31:1–7

CHAPTER 5

Biomechanics of Locked Intramedullary Fixation of Fractures

D. Dagrenat and I. Kempf

Introduction

There are many biomechanical advantages in using an intramedullary implant to fix a long bone fracture. First of all, placing a nail in the medullary canal provides a strong fixation with the lowest "shield effect" on the bone in comparison, for example, with a plate fixation. From a mechanical point of view, this low stress-shielding effect is explained by the nail being within the neutral fibre of the bone and therefore acting like a central tutor, which allows a harmonious share of the load along the bone [6]. The nail has mainly to support the stress in compression and rotation, while the stress in flexion, proportional to the distance between the implant and the axis of the bone, are minimized (Fig. 5.1 a, b).

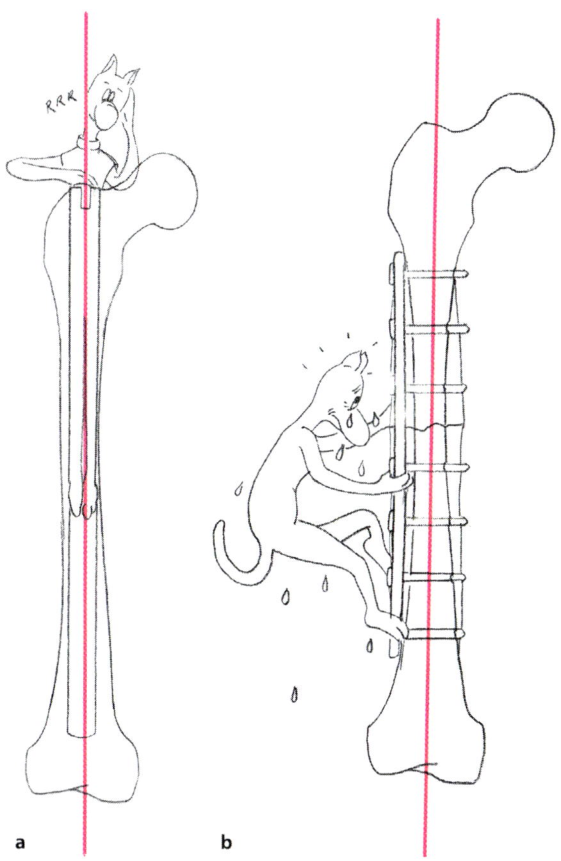

Fig. 5.1 a, b. The difference in stress-shielding between (**a**) a nail and (**b**) a plate

From a biological point of view, Rhinelander [27] has effectively demonstrated that placing a nail in the medullary canal impairs the medullary vascularization for only 3 weeks when the nail is implanted without reaming, and for 6 weeks when it is implanted after a reaming procedure. It has been shown by the same author that the endosteal mechanism of fracture healing was restored after this period of time. Furthermore, with the new developments in closed techniques, using the fracture table for the reduction and fluoroscopy for checking reduction and operation, it is not necessary to open the fracture site: it should even be avoided. The periosteal environment is therefore totally preserved, and we know how important it is to protect it, to allow for the spontaneous process of fracture healing via callus formation [9, 18, 25].

Design Principles

Curvature

The use of intramedullary nailing and the safe technique of nailing were developed by Küntscher [22]. In the 1940s, he presented his design of the implant with mechanical arguments and surgical technique. The hollow cylinder, more resistant in flexion than a full cylinder, the clover-leaf section and the posterior slot were chosen, as they provided the maximal stiffness in bending and allowed what Küntscher called "transverse elastic jamming" (Fig. 5.2), which was intended to control rotation. The reaming procedure efficiently provides the medullary canal with a consistent, homogeneous diameter, particularly within the fracture site. Reaming makes the nailing procedure safer by re-

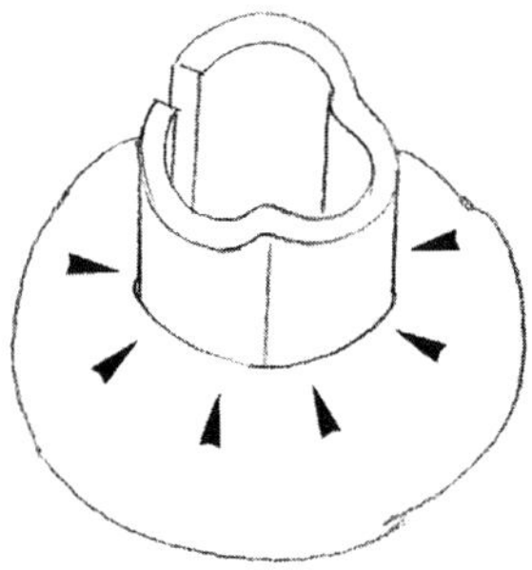

Fig. 5.2 The "clover leaf" section of the Küntscher nail, which is responsible for the transverse elastic jamming and resembles the carpenter's nail

ducing the risk of nail blockage. It also allows for the use of larger nails, which are more resistant to pressure: the stiffness of the nail rises to the fourth power in proportion to its diameter [4].

However, when this concept of transverse elastic jamming was verified, by cutting transverse sections of a nailed femur every 2 cm, it appeared that a satisfactory transverse tight fit was not achieved in any of the sections. In fact, it was later demonstrated that axial stability was also provided by other factors [16]. The original Küntscher nail was straight and, therefore, when it was implanted in a femur that had a normal sagittal curvature, a longitudinal 3- or 4-point jamming occurred in the sagittal plane, due to the difference in curvatures between the nail and the femur (Fig. 5.3). It is obvious that this longitudinal jamming is effective when there is a sufficient length of intact bone. The axial stability is also improved in vivo by the strength of the muscles around the fracture site and by the proper stability of the fracture fragments when they have been reduced and act as a stable gear. The last point is the anchorage of the tip of the nail in cancellous bone, especially in young patients.

The straight nail design impeded surgical technique causing a possible risk of splintering the bone fragments when introducing the nail. This is why all manufacturers provide a light sagittal curvature in the new femoral implants. For the tibial implant, the design has not varied from Küntscher's original nail. It is straight, with a proximal angle in the sagittal plane to avoid articular conflict on the knee.

The Locking Screws

The principle of locking by the use of screws was conceived to improve the stability of the fixation with intramedullary nail. This principle was in-

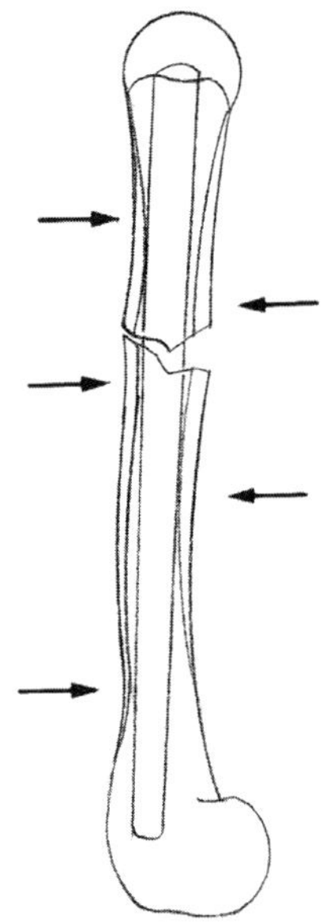

Fig. 5.3 The longitudinal 3-point jamming due to the difference in curvature between the nail and the femur

itiated by Küntscher [23] with his "Detensionsnagel" and developed by Klemm and Schellmann [21]. The impulse which caused the worldwide acceptance of the principle, came from the development of the Grosse and Kempf (GK) system [15], which provides a safe technique, particularly with the aiming device using fluoroscopy.

The locking palliate to some of the problems occasioned by Küntscher's nail:

- Rotational instability in the case of proximal or distal fractures, despite medullary reaming.
- Axial telescoping in comminuted fractures.

The Proximal Femoral Locking Screws

The purpose here is to obtain maximum stability, without impairing the stiffness of the proximal nail. The stresses on this region of the femur are particularly high, and the proximal part of the nail has been designed with the first 52 mm unslotted, in order to provide the best resistance to these stresses. Initially, the screw on the GK nail was placed through a thread on the proximal part of the nail, oblique at 130° (Fig. 5.4). This position provided a lock of the trochanteric area, the screw going from the greater to the lesser trochanter. It has been preferred to a transverse position, which needed to be lower on the nail and limited the indications for proximal fractures. The only disadvantage is the need for a double set of implants for left and right femurs. The screws are

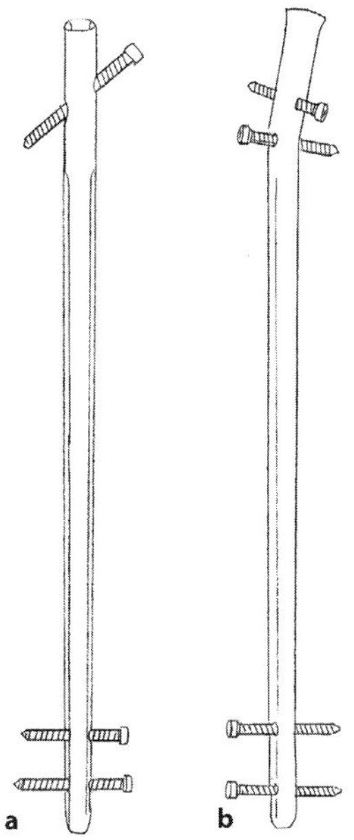

Fig. 5.4a, b. The locking screws in the GK nailing system: **a** femur; **b** tibia

self-tapping, fully threaded, with a diameter of 6.35 mm, which ensure their solidity and their grip in the bone. A precisely adapted ancillary system, fixed to the proximal tip of the nail, guides the screw through the nail after appropriate drilling.

Many designs are now available for proximal locking and include transverse locking screws and double oblique screws, to be utilized through the femoral neck. All these new designs broaden indications on proximal fractures and provide much-needed detection of points of weakness on the implant [20].

The Distal Femoral Locking Screws

On the GK nail, the distal part is pierced with two holes, each admitting a 6.22-mm-diameter screw (Fig. 5.4a). These screws are fully threaded and self-tapping, and they ensure a solid lock of the distal femur within the nail. The technique of distal locking requires the use of special ancillary equipment with fluoroscopy and aiming devices.

Many other systems can be used without a fluoroscope, using instead distal key bolts or pins emerging laterally, but these systems are much less resistant to compression and rotation than the screws and therefore have less control over impaction and axial stability [2, 12, 13].

The Proximal Tibial Screws

On the GK nail, the proximal locking is ensured by two screws, the proximal part of the nail being unslotted on its first 70 mm. It has one sagittal screw, placed obliquely upwards from the front to the back, and one transversal screw. This setting provides the best stability in all planes of the space for the proximal part of the tibia and facilitates the treatment of high metaphyseal fractures. The other configurations available generally use a proximal locking with two transverse screws but they assure less control of bending in the proximal tibia.

The Distal Tibial Locking Screws

This system is the same as in the femur with two distal locking screws. The diameter of both proximal and distal screws is 5 mm, sufficient for the tibia, and the screws are also fully threaded and self-tapping (Fig. 5.4b)

The Problem of Fatigue Failure of the Nail and Locking Screws

Many reports of fatigue failure emerge in literature the [5, 11, 29, 30]. Most of the reported fractures on the femoral GK nail happened on the proximal part of the nail, at the junction of the slotted and unslotted parts, making this a point of weakness as demonstrated by finite element analysis. Another point of weakness is within the distal holes in the nail, the ruptures being described almost exclusively on the upper one. These fractures were reported from the beginning of the clinical experience with the intramedullary locking nail, with a number of explanations.

The mode of manufacture was called into question because of the faulty welding at the junction of slotted and unslotted sections and was quickly discontinued. The nail is now built in one piece from a continuous tube, with no welding in any part. Clinical experience has also yielded another explanation: too much confidence in the implant, and perhaps a precipitate authorization of weight-bearing, has led to excessive stress on the nail, particularly for comminuted fractures. In addition, it should not be forgotten that errors are sometimes made in the early days of a new clinical technique.

More frequently, the risks of fracture or loosening of the locking screws have been reported, particularly with the implants of a diameter less than

6 mm for the femur and less than 5 mm for the tibia. Most of these screws of a small diameter are advocated with the use of thinner nails placed without reaming. From a biomechanical point of view, it is obvious that these implants are more fragile, that they are less fatigue resistant, and that using them without reaming compromises the fit of the nail in the medullary canal. The stability of the system is therefore seriously impaired, with a higher risk of secondary fracture displacement and a loosening of the implants. For these simple reasons, it seems dangerous to advocate:

- The common use of the unreamed nail for all indications.
- The use of only one distal lock when two locking screws can be used. Even if the rotational stability is almost the same with one screw, the load assumed by two screws in axial loading is much higher than with one screw.

Slotted or Unslotted Nails

The presence of a posterior slot on the nail has caused many clinical problems, including fatigue failure, relatively poor bending stiffness and low rotational stability, all of which lead to the phenomenon of induced axial torsion in clinical practice [28]. This induced torsion is due to the neutral fibre, or flexion axis of a slotted tube being displaced at the opposite side of the slot (Fig. 5.5). Therefore a flexion–compression loading produces a torque, in other words, when a bending load is placed on the slotted nail, it twists on itself. This problem has often been observed in clinical conditions. Sometimes the nail has twisted on introduction into the medullary canal, causing an additional difficulty for distal locking.

A few studies were performed to test unslotted nails [8, 17, 24]. As removing the slot increased the bending stiffness of the nail, the thickness of the unslotted nail was reduced to 1.35 mm instead of 1.7 mm for the slotted nail. Nevertheless, this decrease in thickness leads to a 25% increase in bending stiffness. At the flexion compression test, the ultimate strength was 50% higher for the unslotted nail. The maximal gain was obtained on tests of torsional rigidity, which was 20 times higher for an unslotted nail than for a slotted nail of the same diameter. And, of course, the fatigue tests showed the superior fatigue resistance of the unslotted nail.

Despite this improved mechanical performance in laboratory tests, the clinical use of the unslotted nail revealed a number of complications,

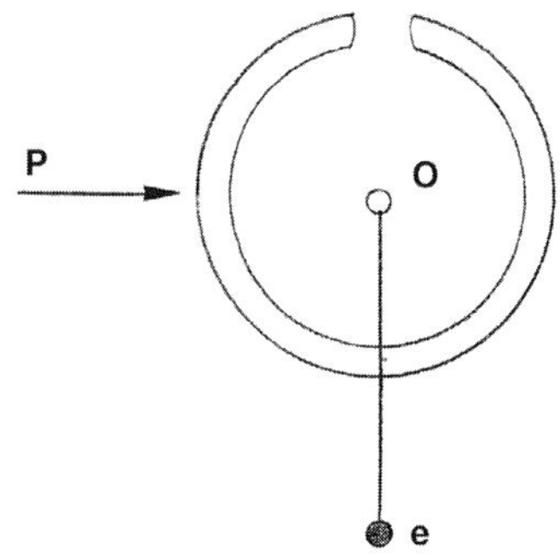

Fig. 5.5. Induced torsion. The displacement of the neutral fibre (*o* to *e*) of the nail, due to the slot, causes an adverse effect of torsion when applying a bending force

the greatest risk being a jamming or bursting of the medullary canal at the introduction of the nail [17]. The use of these nails requires more substantial reaming: 2–2.5 mm more than the diameter of the applied unslotted nail. Moreover, as the unslotted nail is stiffer, fitting to the shape of the medullary canal is no longer possible (transverse elastic jamming). Therefore, the introduction technique and especially the entry point, as well as the reduction achieved on the fracture table, must all be perfect. For these reasons, the authors [17, 24] recommend careful planning before using an unslotted nail, which should be reserved for very comminuted shaft fractures, pathological fractures on metastastic or very porotic bone and tumoral resections with massive allografts. The unslotted femoral nail is now replaced by the unslotted long Gamma nail with its extended indications. Small unslotted femoral and tibial nails are advocated for small tibiae or femurs whose medullary canal cannot admit the smallest slotted nail or for unreamed nailing in open fractures in patients with a normal canal diameter.

Dynamic/Static Fixation – Controversies on Dynamization

The initial authors [15] of the current clinical use of interlocked nailing have developed a few definitions, after a period of clinical experience:

- Dynamic locked nailing means that the nail is locked either proximally or distally. This system was advocated for stable simple fractures, proximal or distal. For these fractures, full weight bearing was immediately authorized and even encouraged, the authors arguing that the early weight bearing could promote the process of healing of the fractured bone.
- Static locked nailing means that the nail is locked proximally and distally. This static sys-

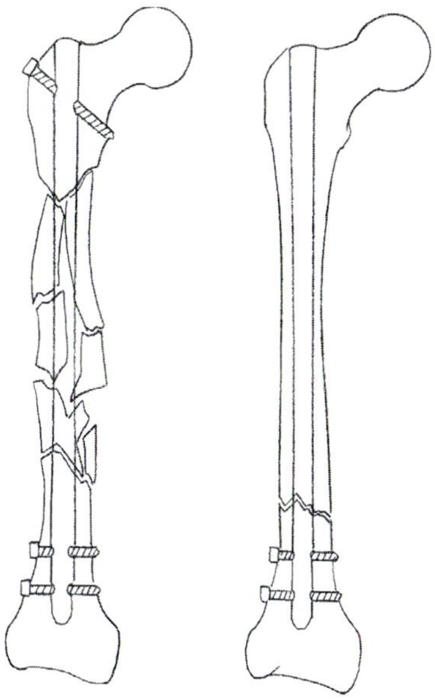

Fig. 5.6. Static and dynamic locking systems

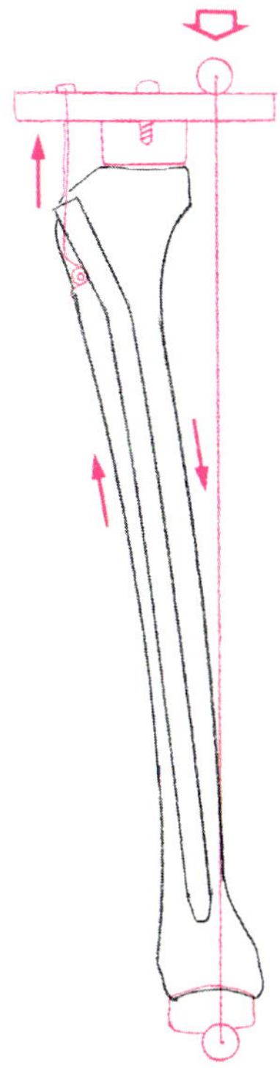

Fig. 5.7. In vitro testing of locked IM nailing

tem was advocated for unstable fractures, either in rotation or with a high risk of telescoping, and the corollary discharge of the limb for a certain period of time.

- Dynamization of the static system was advocated after a few weeks, before authorizing full weight bearing, by removing one of the locks, either proximal or distal, to change the static system to a dynamic one. This procedure of dynamization was intended to accelerate the process of healing (Fig. 5.6). These definitions have been confusing from a biomechanical point of view, and the aim of experiments has been to clarify the concepts.

In Vitro Testing

On a simple model, reproducing the physiologic load on a sheep tibia [7], the strains were measured via electric strain gauges both on the nail and the anterior aspect of the bone. The system was tested for various situations, including intact bone, single transverse osteotomy and resection of a segment, with two different fixations, either static or dynamic nailing (Fig. 5.7) [9, 10].

There is low stress shielding in flexion due to the nailing, either locked or unlocked (less than 20%). Neither dynamic or static locking interferes with the shield effect in flexion. The nail assumes nearly half of the stress in flexion, with a simple osteotomy with no difference between static or dynamic locked nailing. This also means that half of the load is assumed by the bone, and with that particular model there was no difference between the so-called dynamic and static systems. When bone loss was present, the static locked nail assumed most of the stress and the rupture was caused by nail buckling or cortical jamming. The test could not be performed with a nail alone or with a nail with a dynamic locking system.

From this simple experiment, we can deduce that intramedullary nailing is a load-sharing system rather then a stress-shielding one. We can also deduce that there is no difference in vitro between the static and dynamic systems, in terms of assuming the charge in bending.

In particular, the concept of dynamization was studied in an in vivo experiment in the AO laboratories [9]. The experiment compared the healing of an unstable fracture model on the sheep tibia, which was fixed initially with a static interlocking system. Two series of animals were used, one dynamized at 5 weeks and one with unchanged static systems. Both series had the same weight-bearing protocol, maintaining the sheep in hammocks until the 5th week with radiological tests every 7 days. After 11 weeks, the bones were tested mechanically, histologically, and on macroradiographs. All fractures healed uneventfully, via a strong external callus. At the end, there was no

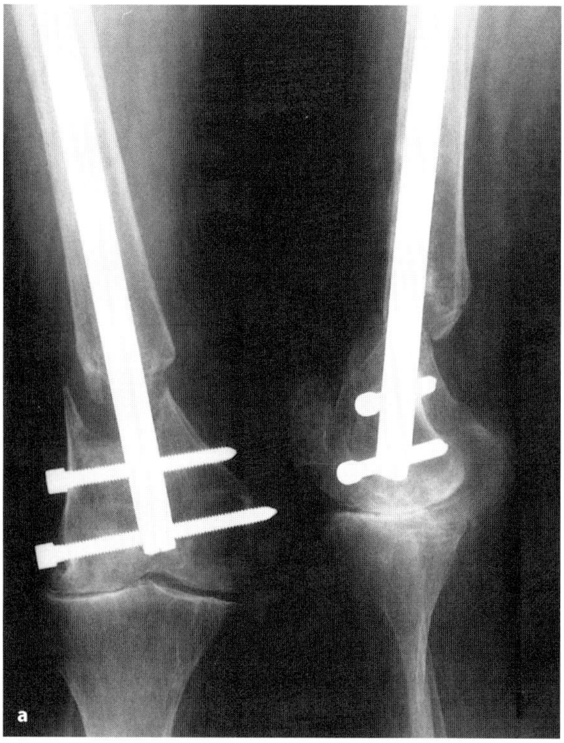

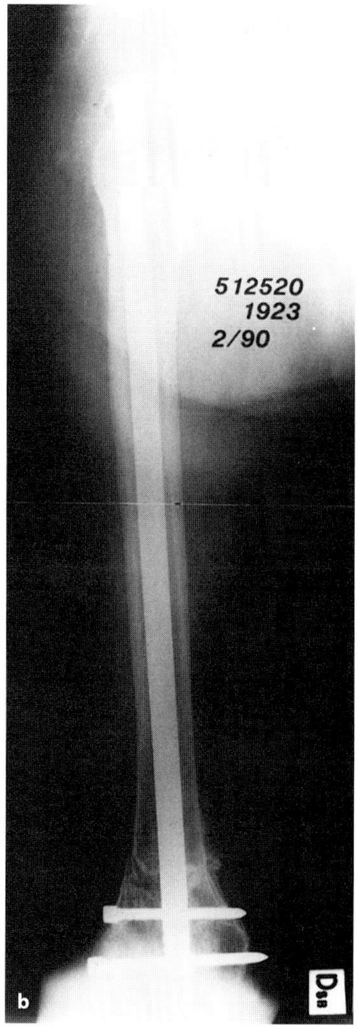

Fig. 5.8. a Remaining gap on a distal fracture treated by static locked nailing. Risk of progression to a non-union. **b** Dynamization: impaction of the fracture site, consolidation

difference between the two series in terms of the quality of healing and it could not be proved that the procedure of dynamization accelerated the healing process of healing. However, on two-thirds of the dynamized animals, a slight but visible impaction of the bone fragments was observed after dynamization; this closure of the fracture gap was accompanied by a centripetal closure of the external callus.

The clinical relevance of this experiment is that sound healing is not jeopardized by a static fixation, which is corroborated by many clinical series [3, 29, 30] and therefore, in the absence of a fracture gap between the bone fragments, early reoperation for screw removal can be avoided. Most complex fractures treated with the static interlocking nail follow this progression of healing. However, when a fracture gap remains as a result of static interlocking, with a risk of progressing to a pseudarthrosis or fatigue failure of the nail or locking screws, dynamization would be helpful or even necessary to bring the fracture fragments into contact (Fig. 5.8).

The dynamization procedure raises the point of when there is a gap remaining between the fracture fragments because of static locking. In this case, removing the proximal lock provides an impaction of the fracture site, as shown by the proximal tip of the nail coming out and subsequent consolidation.

Conclusion

It is generally agreed, from a biomechanical point of view, that locked medullary nailing represents a reference system, particularly adapted to the treatment of diaphyseal fractures of the lower limb. The medullary nail is a load-sharing system which helps natural healing via a strong external callus, and the locking makes its use safer even for complex fractures. However, one must not forget that the technique is demanding. The correct use of the ancillary systems must be learned in order to achieve correct implantation. This includes the use of the fracture table for fracture reduction, the optimal procedure for reaming and the use of fluoroscopy with the aiming devices for locking.

References

1. Aro HT, Chao EYS (1990) Effect of delayed dynamisation on healing of unstable experimental fractures in the canine tibia. Proceedings of the 36th annual meeting of the Orthopaedic Reasearch Society, New Orleans, LA, 5–8 Feb
2. Brooker AF, Brumback RJ (1988) Brooker-Wills nails in the treatment of infra-isthmal injuries of the femur. J Trauma 28:688–691
3. Brumback RJ, Uwagie-Ero S, Lakatos RP, Poka A, Bathon GH, Burgess AR (1988) Intramedullary nailing of femoral shaft fractures. Part II: Fracture healing with static interlocking fixation. J Bone Joint Surg Am 70:1453–1462
4. Bucholz RW (1987) Dilemmas and controversies in intramedullary nailing. In: Browner BO, Edwards CC (eds) The science and practice of intramedullary reaming. Lea and Febiger, Philadelphia, pp 85–89
5. Bucholz RW, Ross SE, Lawrence KL (1987) Fatigue fracture of the interlocking nail in the treatment of fractures of the distal part of the femoral shaft. J Bone Joint Surg Am 69:1391–1399
6. Chao EYS, Aro HT, Lewallen DG, Kelly PJ (1989) The effect of rigidity on fracture healing in external fixation. Clin Orthop 241:24–35
7. Cordey J, Schnetzer M, Brenwald J, Regazzoni P, Perren SM (1980) Direct in vivo measurements of torque and bending in sheep tibiae. In: Uhthoff HK (ed) Current concepts of internal fixation of fractures. Springer, Heidelberg Berlin New York
8. Covey DC, Saha S, Lipka JM, Albright JA (1990) Biomechanical comparison of slotted and non-slotted interlocking nails in distal femoral shaft fractures. Clin Orthop 252:246–251
9. Dagrenat D, Moncade N, Cordey J, Rahn BA, Kempf I, Perren SM (1993) An experimental study of dynamization following static medullary nailing in comminuted diaphyseal fracture. Unfallchirurgie, Heft 229, M. Brner/E. Soldner, Springer, Heidelberg Berlin New York
10. Dagrenat D, Moncade N, Cordey J, Rahn BA, Kempf I, Perren SM (1998) Effets de la dynamisation d'un enclouage verrouillé statique. Rev Chir Orthop [Suppl 2]:100–104
11. Franklin JL, Winquist RA, Benirschke SK, Hansen ST (1998) Broken intramedullary nails. J Bone Joint Surg Am 70:1463–1482
12. Hajek PD, Bicknell Jr HR, Bronson WO, Albright JA, Saha S (1993) The use of 1 compared with 2 distal screws in the treatment of femoral shaft fractures with interlocking intramedullary nailing. A clinical and biomechanical analysis. J Bone Joint Surg Am 75:519–525
13. Johnson KD, Tencer A, Blumenthal AA, Johnston DWC (1986) Biomechanical performance of locked intramedullary nail systems in comminuted femoral shaft fractures. Clin Orthop 206:151–161
14. Kempf I (1990) Enclouage centro-médullaire, Cahiers d'enseignement de la SOFCOT, no. 39, Expansion Scientifique Francaise, Paris
15. Kempf I, Grosse A, Beck G (1985) Closed locked intramedullary nailing. Its application to comminuted fractures of the femur. J Bone Joint Surg Am 67:709–720
16. Kempf I, Jaeger JH, Clavert JM, Mochel D, Glaesener R (1978) L'enclouage centro-médullaire avec alésage: Critique théorique et expérimentale des principes de Küntscher. Rev Chir Orthop 64:629–634
17. Kempf I, Karger C, Willinger R (1985) Locked intramedullary nailing: improvement of mechanical properties. In: Perren SM, Schneider E (eds) Biomechanics: current interdisciplinary research. Martines Nijhoff, Boston, pp 487–492
18. Kempf I, Meyrueis JP, Perren S (1983) La fixation d'une fracture: doit-elle être rigide ou élastique? Rev Chir Orthop [Suppl] 69:335–380
19. Kessler SB, Halfeldt KK, Peren SM, Schweiberer L (1986) The effect of reaming and intramedullary nailing on fracture healing. Clin Orthop 212:18–zz
20. Kinast C, Wyder H, Frirr R, Perren SM (1987) Biomechanical investigations of the proximal screw of interlocking nails. Orthop Trans 11:295
21. Klemm K, Schellmann WD (1972) Dynamische und statische Veriegelung des Marknagel. Monatsschr Unfallheilkd 75:568–575
22. Küntscher G (1962) Praxis der Marknagelung. Friedrich Karl Schattauer Verlag, Stuttgart
23. Küntscher G (1964) Die Nagelung des Defekttummersbruch. Chirurg 35:277
24. Laforest P, Karger C, Bouslama F, Taglang G, Grosse A, Kempf I (1994) Performances mécaniques des clous de tibia de Grosse et Kempf non fendus de faible diamètre. Rev Chir Orthop 80:36–43
25. MacKibbin B (1980) Radiologic and histologic characteristics of conservatively and operatively managed fractures. In: Uthoff HK (ed) Current concepts of internal fixation of fractures. Springer, Heidelberg Berlin New York
26. Olerud S (1987) The effects of intramedullary reaming. In: Browner BO, Edwards CC (eds) The science and practice of intramedullary reaming. Lea and Febiger, Philadelphia, pp 61–66
27. Rhinelander RR, Nelson CL (1973) The vascular and histologic response of diaphyseal cortex to experimental medullary nailing and reaming. J. Bone Joint Surg Am 55:1767
28. Schaeffer C, Willinger R, Renault D, Kempf I, Jaeger JH (1986) Theory of induced torsion and intramedullary nailing. In: Saha (ed) Biomechanical engineering V: recent developments. Pergamon, New York, pp 367
29. Winquist RA, Hansen ST, Clawson OK (1984) Closed intramedullary nailing of femoral fractures. J Bone Joint Surg Am 66:529–539
30. Wiss DA, Fleming CH, Matta JM, Clark D (1986) Comminuted and rotationally unstable fractures of the femur, treated with an interlocking nail. Clin Orthop 212:35–47

CHAPTER 6

Intramedullary Nail Systems

A. Speitling

Introduction

Intramedullary osteosynthesis is a well-established method for the treatment of fractured long bones. The first intramedullary shaft implantations were reported by Bircher as early as 1886 [1] and by Hey Grooves in 1912 [2]. Both failed due to selection of inadequate implant material, i.e. ivory and nickel coated mild steel, respectively. Today's intramedullary nail designs are based on Küntscher's nail presented in 1940 [3], Modney's locking nail in 1953 [4], and Küntscher's detensor in 1968 [5].

Since then, a huge variety of intramedullary implants have been designed, evaluated and presented in the literature. Only for internal fixation of the proximal femur, an amazing 79 different implants are listed [6] and this compilation is far from complete. Thus, it cannot be the objective of this chapter to provide a full survey on intramedullary nail systems commercially produced and clinically used today, but to give a synopsis of trends and representative implants.

Materials Used for Intramedullary Nails

Stainless steel was of outstanding importance for the clinical success of the intramedullary nail systems. Due to a lack of alternative materials, probably more than 95% of all nails ever implanted were made out of stainless steel; the focus here, therefore, will be mainly on stainless steel.

Of course, metallic intramedullary nails of commercial importance are also made out of titanium and its alloys. Both TiAl6V4 (TAV) and TiAl6Nb7 (TAN) have gained a market share of about 12% worldwide and up to 30% in specific markets during the past 5 years. The reader will find a full survey on the properties of these materials elsewhere [7].

Chemical Composition

A new epoch of implant material was marked by the introduction of the first corrosion-resistant steel in 1909 [8], an alloy of iron and about 12% chromium. All modern implant steels, as compared in Table 6.1, are based on the iron, chromium, and nickel alloy V2A, introduced by Krupp in 1920. This combination of the alloying elements significantly improved the strength, ductility, and corrosion resistance. In 1939, the first Küntscher nail was also made out of V2A.

Continuous improvements of the thermomechanical processing as well as the mechanical and chemical properties of implant steels can be related to changes in chemical composition. Based on improvements in melting technology, a lower carbon content (316L) and fewer nonmetallic inclusions with vacuum melting were possible (316LVM). Once again, ductility and corrosion resistance were improved. When introduced in 1976, the Grosse & Kempf nail was made out of this grade as it still is today. The alloy can be regarded as the gold standard for implant steels.

In parallel, a new class of nitrogen-alloyed steels has been developed since 1978 [9] and was first introduced by Howmedica under the brand name Orthinox to intramedullary nails in 1989, when the Gamma Nail was launched. In this steel, nitrogen is very effective for corrosion resistance, tensile strength, fatigue strength and it further stabilises the austenitic structure. Manganese partly replaces nickel and provides better strength. In the USA, the corresponding grade

Table 6.1. Stainless steel implant alloys

Implant alloy	Chemical elements (weight %)							
	C	Mn	Ni	Cr	Mo	N	Nb	Fe
Orthinox	0.03	4.0	9.0	20.5	2.2	0.4	0.3	Bal
22-13-5	0.02	5.0	12.7	21.4	2.3	0.3	0.2	Bal
316 LVM	0.02	1.2	13.5	18.0	2.8	–	–	Bal

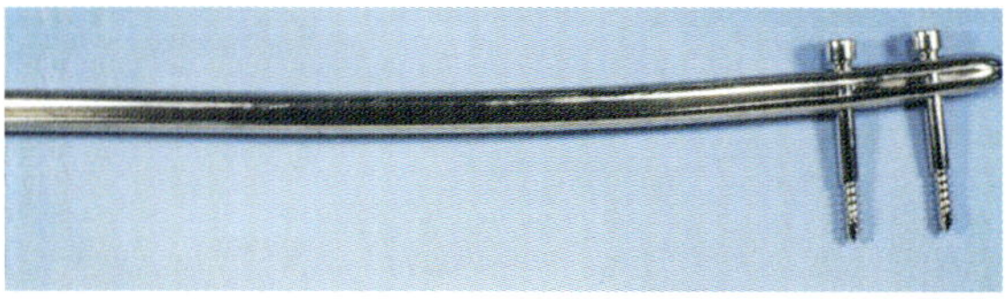

Fig. 6.1. Plastic deformation of an intramedullary nail in the frontal plane due to static overload by bending

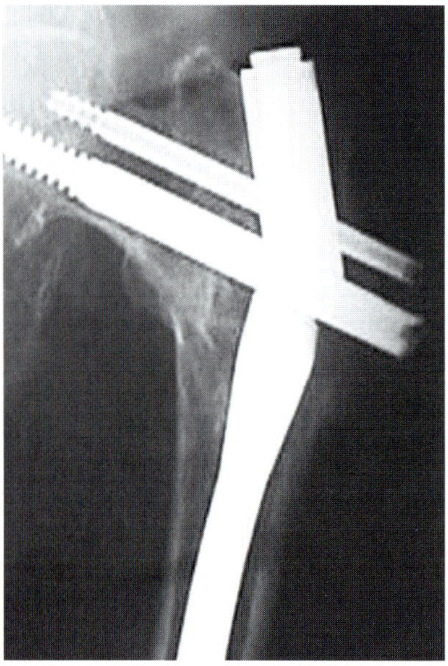

Fig. 6.2. Fatigue fracture of a proximal femoral nail via the proximal screw hole

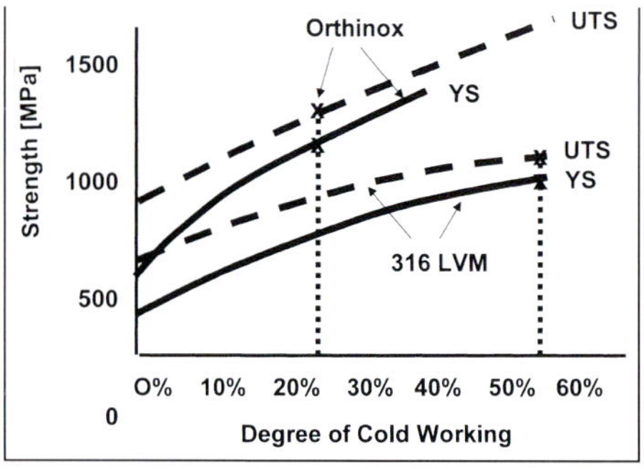

Fig. 6.3. Strength of stainless steels as a function of degree of cold working

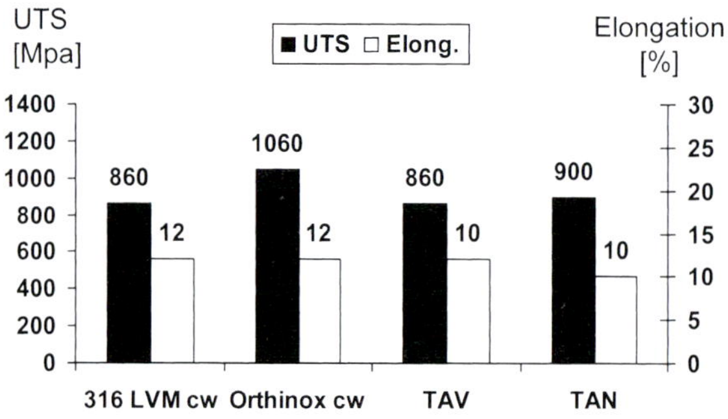

Fig. 6.4. Comparison of minimum requirements on tensile strength and elongation according to relating material standards

22-13-5 is considered as an alternative. However, this steel is only used in the USA and is not internationally standardised as implant material.

Mechanical Properties

The loads on implants are of static or dynamic nature. The term "static load" describes a one-time loading, e.g. one-time weight lifting. Static overload leads to nonreversible plastic deformation of the implant (Fig. 6.1).

The term "dynamic load" is used for repeated cyclic loading and unloading, e.g. implant loading during walking. Dynamic overloading leads to material fracture after a certain number of load cycles without plastic deformation of the material (Fig. 6.2). This is called fatigue fracture of the implant.

Behaviour Under Static Load

The static material properties are described by yield strength (YS), ultimate tensile strength (UTS), elongation, and modulus of elasticity. Yield strength represents the load level where plastic deformation of the material starts. Ultimate tensile strength gives the maximum bearable load until fracture of the material. Elongation is a value of the material's capacity for plastic deformation and the modulus of elasticity (Young's modulus) is a measure of the material's intrinsic rigidity.

The implant steels can be used in annealed and in cold worked conditions. Annealed steel provides low strength and a very high potential for plastic deformation. By cold working during or prior to manufacturing, the material strength can be increased (Fig. 6.3).

For steel implants, which have to be contoured during surgery like some bone plates, annealed steel would be used. For intramedullary nails only cold worked material is used. Typically, Orthinox is used in 20% cold-worked conditions and 316 LVM in 40%–50% cold-worked conditions.

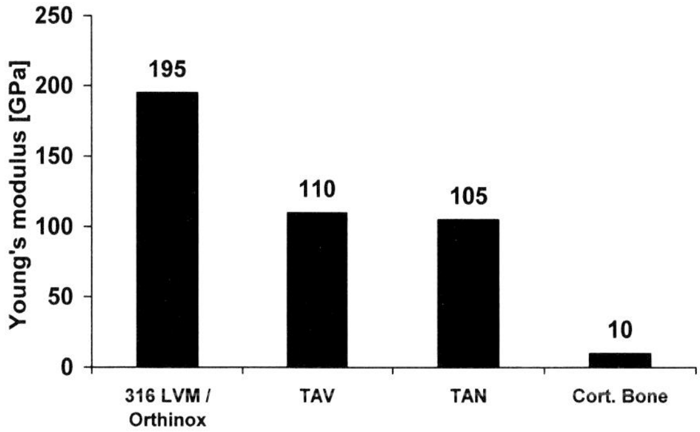

Fig. 6.5. Young's modulus for different materials

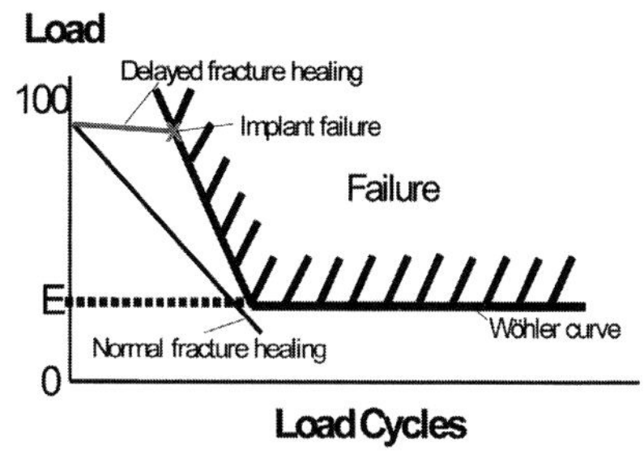

Fig. 6.6. Wöhler curve and relations to implant failure

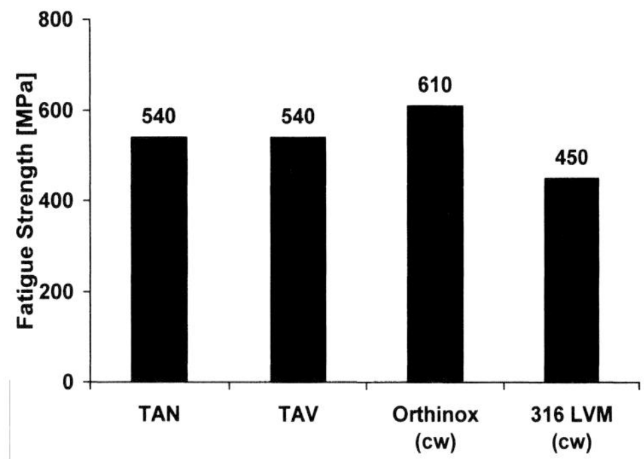

Fig. 6.7. Fatigue strength of different materials

Figure 6.4 shows a comparison of the minimum requirements on tensile strength and elongation according to the standards ISO 5832-1,3,9,11 for the different implant materials. The tensile strength and the elongation of TAV, TAN, and cold-worked 316 LVM are on one level. The highest strength is given for cold-worked Orthinox.

Young's modulus for the different materials is shown in Fig. 6.5. In comparison, cortical bone has the lowest Young's modulus, i.e. the least intrinsic rigidity. Young's modulus of TAN and TAV is approximately ten times higher than that of cortical bone; for 316 LVM and Orthinox, it is about 20 times higher.

Behaviour Under Dynamic Load

Fatigue is the most common cause of metallic implant failure (>99%). The material's behaviour under dynamic load is described by the Wöhler curve in Fig. 6.6. When a material is cyclically loaded by a load lower than the load E in Fig. 6.6, the material can withstand an infinite number of load cycles without failure. When the load is higher than E, material failure will occur after a certain number of load cycles. The higher the load the smaller the number of bearable load cycles to failure.

Implants for osteosynthesis are designed for load sharing with the bone, i.e. for the performance of the implant it is essential that the biomechanical load is continuously released during the implantation period. Directly after implantation, full weight bearing is expected, with a following load reduction on account of normal fracture healing (compare Fig. 6.6). Implant failure can occur when a delayed fracture healing is present and the implant is constantly loaded at a high load level (Fig. 6.6).

The fatigue strength of a material represents the load level E marked in Fig. 6.6 and is defined as the maximum load level where all tested material specimens reach 10^7 cycles without failure. Figure 6.7 gives the fatigue strength for different materials. The values were determined for smooth material specimens.

Orthinox made in a cold-worked condition provides the highest fatigue strength compared to all other generally used trauma implant materials.

The data given in Fig. 6.7 are valid only for smooth surfaces. When the material surface is notched by a thread, a locking hole, or by a scratch, the fatigue strength will be reduced by a factor of up to 5 depending on the notch geometry.

Biocompatibility

The described implant materials are all standardised in the ISO 5832 standards series for metallic implant materials. As an introduction to the ISO 5832 standards, the following statement is given:

> No known surgical implant material has ever been shown to cause absolutely no adverse reaction in the human body. However, long-term clinical experience of the use of the material referred to in this part of ISO 5832 has shown that an acceptable level of biological response can be expected when the material is used in appropriate applications.

There is not much to add. Although no implant material can be characterised as totally inert, complications related to the material are rare. If present at all, the body's reaction to the described materials for intramedullary nails is moderate and can generally be tolerated.

General Aspects of Intramedullary Nails

There is common agreement that the purpose of any osteosynthesis is to transmit the biomechanical forces and moments via the fracture line and to stabilise a fractured bone until the fracture is healed. There is less agreement on how the ideal intramedullary nail should look to achieve these objectives. Depending on multiple factors, e.g. bone, fracture type and reposition, gender, age, body weight, ethnic group, surgical technique, and postoperative mobilisation, the requirements vary. To meet these requirements, solid, cannulated, partially slotted, and fully slotted nails are available with star, cloverleaf, rectangular, circular, oval, and other cross sections.

The relative strength of the different principal nail cross sections is given in Table 6.2 [10], with the cannulated nail set at 100%. This demonstrates that independent of the material and diameter used, the strength can already be altered by a factor of 14. A slot has a moderate effect in bending and axial load but a severe effect in torsional strength. A typical absolute value for the bending strength of an 11-mm cannulated nail would be 70 Nm in 4-point bending, the torsional strength would be 58 Nm, and the axial strength 30 kN to plastic deformation. These data reflect the ability of a nail to transmit the biomechanical loads in a static situation. Under dynamic loads these strength values would have to be reduced by 50%–60%, depending on the load case and implant finish.

Fracture stabilisation, the second purpose here, is affected by the rigidity of the assembly of nail, locking screws, and bone. The bending stiffness of a nail is first of all proportional to its diameter [10, 11], of course with marked differences between nails with different wall thicknesses and different materials. However, stronger effects are seen on torsional rigidity, where open cross sections (slotted nails) differ more than one order of magnitude from closed cross sections (Table 6.3). Extremely flexible nails are marked by the design of Marchetti [12], with a torsional rigidity of only 0.03 Nmdeg^{-1}, determined in the author's own lab testing.

High bending and torsional rigidity effect higher insertion forces of a nail, due to the geometric

Table 6.2. Comparison of different cross sections of nails with the same 11-mm outer diameter and 8-mm inner diameter for cannulated and slotted nails, respectively, under axial compression, bending and torsion (relative units)

Profile	Axial strength	Bending strength	Torsional strength
Solid	150	130	140
Cannulated	100	100	100
Slotted	90	90	10

Table 6.3. Torsional rigidity of closed (cl) and slotted (sl) Grosse & Kempf nails according to ASTM F383 [10]

Diameter (mm)	10	11	12	13	14
Profile	cl	cl	sl	sl	sl
Rigidity (Nmdeg^{-1})	1.48	1.92	0.13	0.19	0.22

mismatch between nail and bone [11]. In extreme cases this may even cause femoral bursting [13]. However, the torsional and bending stiffness of the nail–bone system reaches only 10% (torsion) and 80% (bending) of the intact bone [14].

This is certainly important with regard to the third purpose, i.e., to enable fracture healing. Clinical practice has shown that the demand for absolute stabilisation of the fracture, as postulated by the Arbeitsgemeinschaft Osteosynthese (AO) in the 1970s and produced in very rigid plate designs, would generate atrophic bone [15]. It is accepted that callus-free healing, even after dynamic compression plating, is not the rule [16]. In other words, healing is normally based on callus formation. Even after perfect reduction, there are incongruities at the fracture site that will result in gaps [17]. In this case a very stiff implant will suppress the callus formation [17] due to stress shielding. On the other hand, a very flexible nail will cause excessive motion, which may result in a hypertrophic nonunion. Both complications – either of atrophic or hypertrophic origin – are rare in intramedullary nailing [11, 18].

Although the mechanisms of fracture healing are not fully understood, it seems that the bone is able to cope with the flexibility of the majority of nails used today. As an additional option, the stiffness of the whole construct can be modified by several features. It can be enhanced by means of a compression screw, especially in torsion [19] and can be reduced by dynamisation of the nail either by removal of the locking screws or by use of oblong locking holes. In an external fixation model this has been shown to create significantly more callus [20, 21] than the rigid fixation.

Femur Nails

The femur is probably the ideal bone for intramedullary fixation. Access to the medullary cavity is possible by both orthograde and retrograde techniques. It has a nearly continuous bend in antecurvation, a quite round medullary cavity, and the biggest cortical wall thickness of all long bones [22]. Corresponding to this the biomechanical loads and requirements on implant strength – especially on the proximal femur – are higher than in other long bones. This is ideally addressed by an intramedullary nail. Due to its central positioning, the bending moment generated by the hip force is much smaller if compared with a laterally positioned plate [23]. Thus most actual trends in intramedullary fixation devices and the differentiation of indications for these devices are first seen on this bone.

Maximum nail sizes were up to 18 mm in the 1960s. Parallel to improvements in material strength, the average nail sizes were reduced from typically 15 mm to 12 mm on the femur [24], with the minimum marked at 8.5 mm. This permits minimal or even unreamed techniques, reflecting the actual trend to minimally invasive surgery.

As an example, a representative intramedullary portfolio for the femur of just one manufacturer, Stryker Trauma, is given in Fig. 6.8.

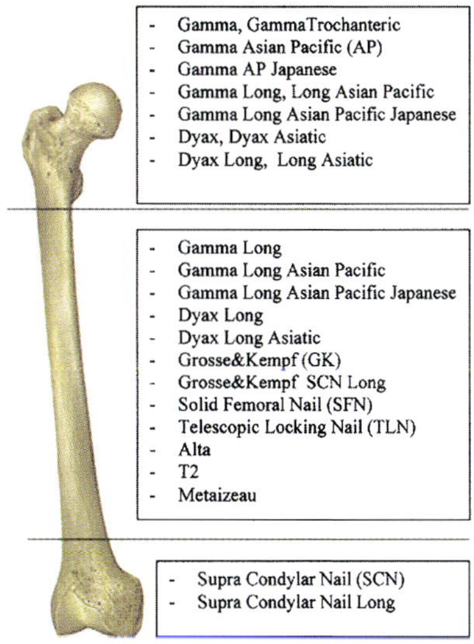

Fig. 6.8. Nailing systems for the proximal, diaphyseal, and distal femur

On stable and unstable shaft fractures, the Grosse & Kempf nail could be regarded as the original design, with all others derived from it. As material for the various intramedullary nails, stainless steels and Ti6Al4V are used, the latter reflecting the need for nickel-free and MRI-compatible materials. All, except the SFN, are cannulated. The range of diameters is from 8.5 mm up to 16 mm, the length between 260 mm and 500 mm.

The SFN addresses fractures with significant soft tissue injury, polytrauma, or thorax trauma patients. Here, a solid nail, used in the unreamed technique, has been considered advantageous, although this is still subject to controversy [25, 26].

Three nails, the TLN, IC, and T2, can be used to apply compression on the fragments and to dynamise by means of a sleeve or an oblong hole. As shown above, this stimulates callus formation and permits fine tuning of the torsional rigidity.

As for the present, the latest innovation implants for retrograde nailing were designed to treat diaphyseal and distal fractures, especially in obese patients and in cases of hip arthroplasty. The only system comprising all features, i.e. ortho- and retrograde nails, small diameters, titanium, and compression, is the T2 nail, which is built on a common screw and instrument platform.

For the proximal femur and its higher biomechanical loads, stronger implants were designed. Gamma (Orthinox) or Dyax (TAV) nails are listed (Fig. 6.8), both in several ethnic versions and with comparable features as shaft nails. All have a proximal diameter of 17 mm, the distal diameter is between 10 mm (Long Asian) and 14 mm (Standard). Alternative designs are shown in Fig. 6.9. Indications are stable and unstable intertrochanteric, pertrochanteric, and high subtrochanteric fractures for the short nails. The long nails are the missing link to shaft nails, indicated for combined shaft and subtrochanteric fractures, pathologic fractures, malunions, and revision procedures.

Analogous to the proximal femur, and with increasing acceptance of the retrograde access, specialised short and long implants for the distal femur were designed. The diameter is 11 mm, the length ranges from 170 mm to 320 mm. Indications are stable and unstable supracondylar and distal femoral fractures. To improve fragment fixation in the very distal metaphyseal area, a specific design of locking screws is exigent (Fig. 6.10). Supracondylar nails can be used with most knee prostheses and all hip endoprostheses.

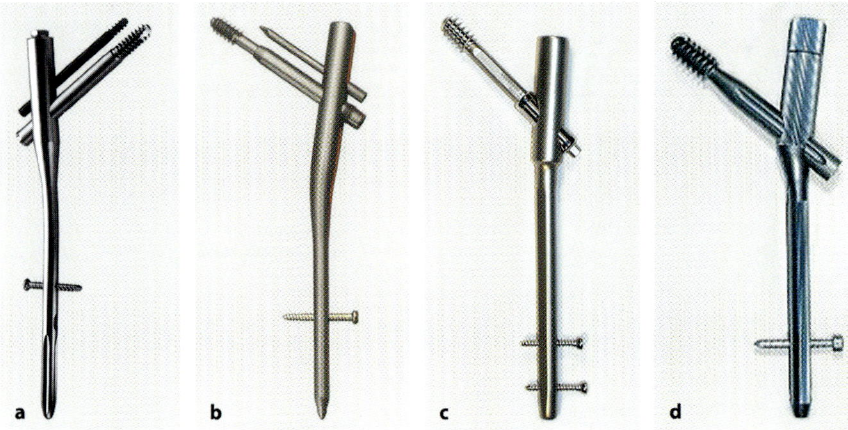

Fig. 6.9. Intramedullary nails for the proximal femur (**a** Switzerland, **b** Germany, **c** USA, **d** Japan) based on Gamma Nail design

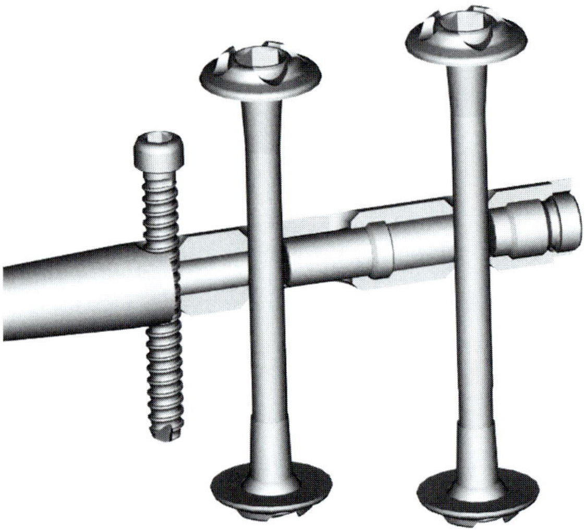

Fig. 6.10. Standard and condylar locking screws in SCN

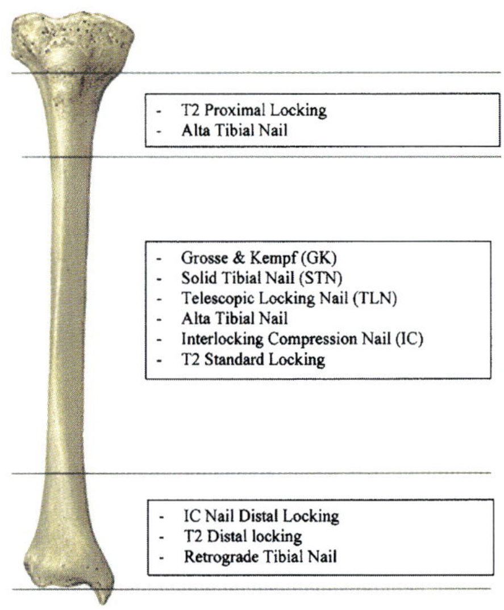

Fig. 6.11. Nailing systems for the proximal, diaphyseal, and distal tibia

Tibia and Fibula Nails

The tibia has a triangular cross section which is per se less suitable to stabilisation with a circular nail. Only by using a locking nail with proximal and distal locking screws can sufficient axial and rotational stability be provided. Typical diameters of tibia locking nails have always been smaller than those given for femur nails. This is in accordance with the lower biomechanical loads, compared with the femur. Today the average nail is 11 mm, with an extreme marked at 7.5 mm.

A representative survey, the Stryker Trauma portfolio of nails used for the tibia, is given in Fig. 6.11, a typical set of instruments in Fig. 6.12.

The locking nails are provided in lengths ranging from 240 mm to 485 mm, the diameter from 7.5 mm to 15 mm. All nails except one are straight in their middle part, with the typical Herzog bend proximally (Fig. 6.13) and a smaller distal bend for ease of insertion. The only fully straight nail is the TLN, where the insertion point requires a more dorsal choice.

Other features of tibial nails – steel and titanium, slotted, nonslotted, and solid designs, compression features – have the same background and indications as for femoral nails.

Although one could imagine the same specialisation and thus the same variety of intramedullary implants as in the femur, anatomy and the difficulty of retrograde nailing have been regarded as an obstacle. The Retrograde Tibial Nail is intended to expand the experience. However, few cases of retrograde nailing have been reported so

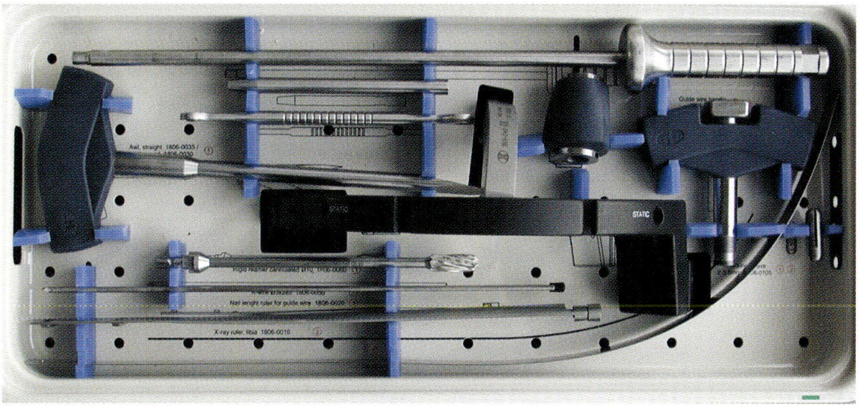

Fig. 6.12. Instrument tray for tibial nails

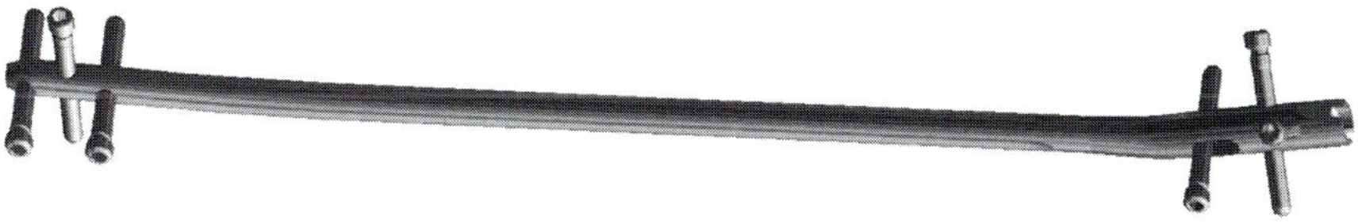

Fig. 6.13. The T2 Standard Tibia Nail

far [27]. In the meantime, Alta and T2 nails for the proximal tibia as well as IC and T2 nails for distal tibia indications offer the most dedicated design.

Only a few instruments need to be dedicated to the tibia nail alone, in case of the STN it is the target device and a smaller drill for locking screws. Most are for general purposes and can be used for both the femur and tibia, e.g. a nail holding screw, depth gauge, wrench, socket wrench, drill guide sleeve, awl, and countersink, the latter with innovative Elastosil handles for improved grip.

The anatomy of the fibula and the frequency of fractures in the distal fibula led to the development of retrograde fibula nails, as presented in 1993 [28]. Typical shaft size is either 3.5 mm or 4.5 mm, the length is 150 mm. Locking can only be done in the distal end of the nail, providing a certain degree of stabilisation, but no rotational control. Although certain problems with the standard treatments (plate, rush pin) have been reported, nailing of the fibula is not very common.

Humerus Nails

Like the tibia, the humerus has an irregular medullary cavity, with a very oval cross section distally, opening like a trumpet at its proximal end. Since the biomechanical loads [29] are much below those of the lower extremity, smaller implants are sufficient.

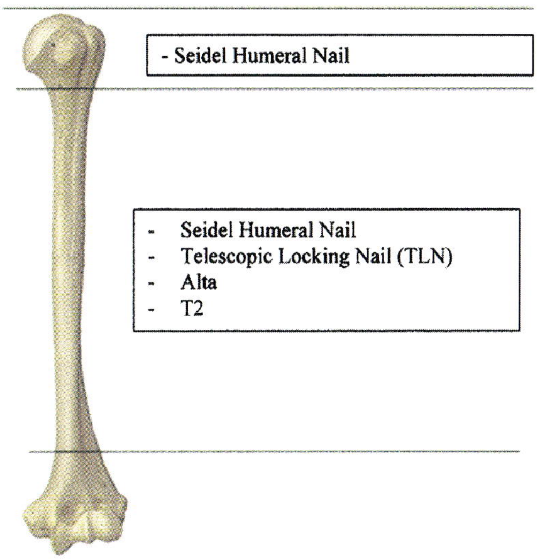

Fig. 6.14. Locking nail systems for the humerus

A survey of nail systems is shown in Fig. 6.14. Typical nail shaft sizes are 6–9 mm in diameter and a length of 140–320 mm. Both ortho- (Seidel, TLN, Alta, T2) and retrograde nailing (Alta, T2) are common. Materials are implant steel and titanium alloy. Due to the smaller diameters, all nails are nonslotted, but mostly cannulated.

For proximal humerus fractures, the Seidel nail offers a lateral cap washer as a specific feature. In addition, this nail has a distal locking mechanism based on spreading metal flanges, which follows the minimally invasive concept but has a limited stability if compared to distal locking screws.

Ulna and Radius Nails

The ulna and radius, like the fibula, have a small medullary cavity and are curved in several planes. This requires small and flexible, probably malleable implants. Access to the medullary canal is possible via orthograde (ulna) and retrograde (radius) techniques.

Nailing systems are offered, for example, by Biomet, AOS, and Stryker, either dedicated nails in the diameter range 3.5–5 mm, all offering locking features, Metaizeau pins in the size 2–4 mm, or Rush pins. In addition, the Stryker ulna nail offers compression and distraction features. The length is between 180 mm and 260 mm.

Indications are diaphyseal fractures and correction osteotomy. Although results are encouraging [30, 31], the method is not commonly used.

Summary

Early intramedullary nails failed due to the inadequate implant materials. Biocompatibility and strength issues have been successfully addressed by stainless steel and titanium alloys. In addition, the biological concept of fracture healing after intramedullary fixation had to be postulated and experienced. The introduction of reaming in order to prepare the medullary canal for insertion of large nails and the invention of locking screws to stabilise fractures after repositioning were important milestones to fully establishing the intramedullary concept.

Today, intramedullary locking nail systems for all long bones are available and in clinical use. Stronger, sometimes solid nails allow using smaller diameters and thus minimally or even nonreamed techniques.

Orthograde as well as retrograde nail insertion is customary. Indications are extended to the metaphyseal areas. As first seen on the femur, this led to the development of several specific implants. It is expected that the other long bones will be segmented in a similar way and that the method of intramedullary nailing still has potential for innovations.

References

1. Bircher, H (1886) Eine neue Methode unmittelbarer Retention bei Frakturen der langen Röhrenknochen. Langenbecks Arch Chir 34:410–422
2. Hey Grooves EW (1912) Some clinical and experimental observations on the operative treatment of fractures, with especial reference to the use of intramedullary pegs. BMJ 2:1102–1105
3. Küntscher G (1940) Die Marknagelung von Knochenbrüchen. Langenbecks Arch Klin Chir 200:443–455
4. Modney MT, Bambara J (1953) The perforated cruciate intramedullary nail: preliminary report of it's use in geriatric patients. J Am Geriatr Soc 11:579–588
5. Küntscher G (1968) Die Marknagelung des Trümmerbruchs. Langenbecks Arch Klin Chir 322:1063–1968
6. Calandruccio RA et al. Internal fixation devices for fractures of the proximal femur. AAOS Committee on the history of orthopaedic surgery
7. Kramer K-H (2000) Implants for surgery – a survey on metallic materials. In: Stallforth H, Revell P (eds) Materials for medical engineering. Wiley-VCH, Weinheim, pp 9–29
8. Schuster J (1975) Die Metallose. Enke Verlag, Stuttgart
9. Truman JE (1978) An austenitic stainless steel of improved strength and corrosion resistance. Stainless Steel Industry 6:21–32
10. Harder HE, Speitling A (1995) Stabilität von Marknägeln unter Belastung. In: Gahr RH, Hein W, Seidel H (eds) Dynamische Osteosynthese, Springer, Berlin, pp 24–33
11. Johnson KD, Tencer A (1990) Mechanics of intramedullary nails for femoral fractures. Unfallchirurgie 93:506–511
12. Hargreaves DG, Warren PJ, Pereira JA, Hollingdale JP (1996) Complications following the use of the Marchetti flexible intramedullary nail. Injury 27:735–738
13. Johnson KD, Tencer AF, Sherman MC (1987) Biomechanical factors affecting fracture stability and femoral bursting in closed intramedullary nailing of femoral shaft fractures, with illustrative case presentations. J Orth Trauma 1:1–11
14. Tencer AF, Johnson KD, Johnston DWC, Gill K (1984) A biomechanical comparison of various methods of stabilization of subtrochanteric fractures of the femur. J Orthop Res 2:297–305
15. Kreusch-Brinker R (1995) Biomechanik nach operativ versorgter Femurfraktur. In: Gahr RH, Hein W, Seidel H (eds) Dynamische Osteosynthese, Springer, Berlin pp 62–65
16. Schwyzer HK, Cordey J, Brun S, Matter P Perren SM (1984) Bone loss after internal fixation using plates, dermination in humans using computed tomography. In: Perren SM, Schneider E (eds) Biomechanics. Current interdisciplinary research. Martinus Nijhoff, Dordrecht, pp 191–195
17. Chao EYS, Aro HT (1997) Biomechanics of fracture fixation. In: Mow VC, Hayes WC (eds) Basic orthopaedic biomechanics, Lippincott-Raven, Philadelphia, pp 317–351
18. Gelis T, Jakob M (1995) Vergleichende klinische Ergebnisse nach Femurnagelung und Verplattung. In: Gahn RH, Hein W, Seidel H (eds) Dynamische Osteosynthese. Springer, Berlin, pp 86–88
19. Bühren V (2000) Intramedullary compression osteosynthesis. Unfallchirurgie 103:708–720
20. Jiun-Jer W, Shyr HS, Chao EY, Kelly PJ (1984) Comparison of osteotomy healing under external fixation devices with different stiffness characteristics. J Bone Joint Surg Am 66:1258–1264
21. Reikeras O, Reigstadt A (1985) Healing of stable and unstable osteotomies in rats. Arch Orthop Trauma Surg 104:161–163
22. Donald GD, Pope MH (1985) Design of intramedullary nails. In: Seligson D (ed) Concepts of intramedullary nailing, Grune & Stratton, Olrando, pp 69–90
23. Haynes RC, Pöll RG, Miles AW, Weston RB (1997) An experimental study of the failure modes of the Gamma Locking Nail and AO Dynamic Hip Screw under static loading: a cadaveric study. Med Eng Phys 19:446–453

24. Wenda K, Runkel M, Rudig L (1995) Oberschenkelmarknagelung ohne Aufbohren. In: Gahr RH, Hein W, Seidel H (eds) Dynamische Osteosynthese. Springer, Berlin, pp 98–106
25. Cole AS, Hill GA, Theologis TN, Gibbons CLMH, Willett K (2000) Femoral nailing for metastatic disease of the femur: a comparison of reamed and unreamed femoral nailing. Injury 31:25–31
26. Bosse MJ, McKenzie EJ, Riemer BL, Brumback RJ, McCarthy ML, Burgess AR, Gens DR, Yasui Y (1997) Adult respiratory distress syndrome, pneumonia, and mortality following thoracic injury and a femoral fracture treated either with intramedullary nailing with reaming or with a plate. J Bone Joint Surg Am 79:799–809
27. Hofmann GO, Gonschorek O, Bühren V (1999) Retrograde tibial nailing: anatomical considerations and first clinical experience. Osteo Intl 7:162–169
28. Wu YS, Zhang FB (1993) The treatment of tibial and fibular fractures with a rectangle-shaped intramedullary nail. Contemp Orthop 26:279–288
29. Brand D, Knopf U, Seidel H, Schneider E (1996) Stabilisierung von Humerusschaftfrakturen – vergleichende biomechanische Untersuchungen. Osteo Int 4:235–245
30. Lefèvre C, Poureyron Y, LeNen D (1995) Intramedullary locking nail of the ulna – implant, device, indications. Proceedings of the 3rd Trauma Course AIOD Formation, Strasbourg, pp 12–13
31. Lefèvre C, Poureyron Y, LeNen D (1995) Intramedullary locking nail of the radius. Proceedings of the 3rd Trauma Course AIOD Formation, Strasbourg, pp 14–15

CHAPTER 7

Time of Radiation Exposure During Intramedullary Nailing Procedures

J.-C. Dosch and M.G. Dupuis

Introduction

Intraoperative radiation exposure during intramedullary nailing procedures is still of current interest. What is the mean exposure time and how is it distributed intraoperatively? Is there a time–dose relationship? When does it begin to become biologically noxious to the patient and to the operating room personnel? In this chapter, our objective is to give some elements of answer, mainly through the analysis of X-ray exposure times.

Materials and Methods

When the new Centre de Traumatologie et d'Orthopédie was opened in Strasbourg in 1975, it was decided to keep a record of all exposure times and the names of surgeons performing under image intensifier control. Our 4773 measurements have been progressively fine-tuned to allow a better control over the distribution of X-ray exposure. Series no. 1 (1976–1983) only gives information about overall exposure time during femoral and tibial intramedullary nailings. Series no. 2 (1984–1990) also includes distal interlocking time, using the Lafforgue and Grosse targeting technique. Series no. 3 (1991–1995) provides full data on reduction and guide rod insertion time, nail insertion time, and distal interlocking time.

Philips image intensifiers have been used in all cases. These are exclusively handled by electroradiology technicians, a permanent team of seven or eight people who are qualified to deal with the specific problems of radiation protection and radiation exposure to the operating room personnel. From 1976 to 1984, we used BV 22 X-ray imagers. Between 1984 and 1991, we gradually renewed our equipment and replaced our BV 22 units with fibre optic BV 25 imagers. The milliamp scale (mA) is legally limited to 3 mA for fluoroscopic use. The kilovolt scale (kV) is graduated from 40 kV to 100 kV in 10-kV increments. Current doses vary according to region and projection. The mA range is from 0.2 to 2.8, and kV from 45 to 80 (Table 7.1). Accuracy of exposure time is 5 s.

Table 7.1. Settings of voltage (in kilovolts, kV) and current (in milli-amperes, mA)

Area	Projection	kV	mA
Hip	Frontal	65–75	1.5–2.7
Hip	Profile	70–80	2.7–2.8
Knee	Frontal/profile	55–55	0.3–1
Ankle	Frontal/profile	45–50	0.2–0.3
Shoulder	Frontal	55	1–1.5

All surgical operations were performed on orthopaedic tables. Reduction of the fracture site was assessed using the image intensifier, while diaphyseal axes where checked on full-size X-rays intraoperatively. We do believe this is indispensable, owing to the peripheral distortion of the image on the monitor. The nailing technique itself was initiated provided that the X-ray was satisfactory.

Systematic use of a 0.5-mm-thick lead apron provided protection from ionizing radiation. Lead gloves were indispensable for reduction manoeuvres. Exposure to the operating room personnel was monitored on portable dosimeters, for collection and monthly analysis by industrial medicine.

Results

Overall Exposure Time – Series No. 1 (1976–1983)

A total of 1423 measurements were taken during intramedullary nailing procedures: 705 involved the femur, 452 of which were locked (IMLN) and 253 were not (IMN); 718 involved the tibia, 459 of which were locked (IMLN) and 259 were not (IMN).

A quick decrease in exposure times (Tables 7.2, 7.3) can be noted in both femoral (from 520 to 240 s) and tibial (from 591 to 185 s) nailings. Also, the standard deviation significantly de-

Table 7.2. Femoral nailing: average irradiation time (series no. 1)

Femur	1976	1977	1978	1979	1980	1981	1982	1983
IMLN								
m	520	482	320	272	240	242	222	210
SD	317	256	210	143	141	168	130	130
n	44	40	50	65	79	61	54	60
IMUN								
m	335	369	232	188	168	182	153	120
SD	235	225	98	95	75	80	132	71
n	39	60	33	29	16	25	25	26

IMLN, intramedullary locked nail (452 cases); IMUN, intramedullary unlocked nail (253 cases); m, mean value; SD, standard deviation.

Table 7.3. Tibial nailing: average irradiation time (series no. 1)

Tibia	1976	1977	1978	1979	1980	1981	1982	1983
IMLN								
m	591	492	273	250	212	200	182	185
SD	260	297	183	148	146	102	98	141
n	40	34	51	51	86	76	66	55
IMUN								
m	310	249	183	182	90	106	130	90
SD	160	103	126	170	45	63	66	48
n	47	81	34	30	16	16	23	12

IMLN, intramedullary locked nail (459 cases); IMUN, intramedullary unlocked nail (259 cases); m, mean value; SD standard deviation.

creases, which suggests that series no. 1 is still within the training phase of the nailing technique. The discrepancy between IMN and IMLN exposure times corresponds to distal interlocking time. A fine analysis (using the Mann-Whitney *U* test) shows that this discrepancy is significant in the tibia. This is due to the fact that simple nailing of the tibia is specifically used to treat simple midshaft fractures, which are technically easy to manage.

Overall Exposure Time – Series No. 2 (1984–1990)

During this period, fibre optic image intensifiers were gradually introduced. This new technology facilitates a reduction in the necessary X-ray exposure by 60% for an equal period of time. In this series, an intramedullary locking nail was used in 997 cases (femur 515, tibia 482). The average exposure time (Table 7.4) was 218 s for the femur and 178 s for the tibia, including all indications. The average distal interlocking time (Table 7.4) is the same for the femur and tibia (57 and 58 s, respectively), but it varied according to the type of fracture (Tables 7.5, 7.6). The fractures requiring a more extensive fluoroscopic control are,

Table 7.4. Average values of nailing and locking irradiation times for femur and tibia (series no. 2)

	No. of cases	Locking time	Total time
Femur	$n=515$	57	218
Tibia	$n=482$	58	178

Table 7.5. Femoral nailing and locking irradiation times (mean and range values) versus type of fracture (series no. 2)

Femur	Locking time	Total time
Comminuted (n=71)	53 (5–120)	235 (60–660)
Segmental (n=16)	54 (10–120)	230 (120–360)
Proximal (n=50)	40 (10–90)	190 (60–360)

Table 7.6. Tibial nailing and locking irradiation times (mean and range values) versus type of fracture (series no. 2)

Tibia	Locking time	Total time
Comminuted (n=26)	42 (25–70)	170 (120–300)
Segmental (n=27)	58 (5–120)	230 (120–480)
Spiral (n=87)	61 (15–180)	185 (60–360)

for the femur: comminuted fractures (235 s) and segmental fractures (230 s), and for the tibia: segmental fractures (230 s) and spiral fractures (185 s).

Overall Exposure Time – Series No. 3 (1990–1995)

This is the most complete series: 207 humeral nails, 441 femoral nails, 458 tibial nails, and 1247 Gamma nails (Table 7.7).

Humerus. The average overall exposure time was 57 s, going up to 92 s for segmental fractures and to 83 s for comminuted fractures (Table 7.8). The average reduction time was 30 s (ranging from 81 s for comminuted fractures to 17 s for fractures with a third fragment). The average nail insertion time was much more consistent, ranging from 27 s for segmental fractures to 49 s for fractures with a third fragment. The longest time (460 s) was recorded during the treatment of an old pseudarthrosis, where insertion of the guide rod was particularly difficult.

Femur. The average overall exposure time (Table 7.9) was 160 s, including all indications (126 s for pseudarthroses, 156 s for osteotomies, 165 s for fractures). The longest time (600 s) was recorded during osteotomy of a malunion, using an endo-

Table 7.7. Irradiation times (mean and range values) versus kind of nailing (2353 cases) (series no. 3)

Type of Nails	Reduction	Nailing	Locking	Total time
Humerus (*n*=207)	30 (5–460)	39 (5–240)	–	57 (5–485)
Femur (*n*=441)	56 (5–250)	67 (5–550)	46 (10–195)	160 (5–600)
Tibia (*n*=458)	38 (5–290)	50 (5–345)	48 (10–230)	133 (25–430)
G-Nail (1247)	15 (0–180)	49 (5–540)	–	64 (10–610)

Table 7.8. Humeral nailing and reduction times (average and range values) versus type of fractures (167 cases) (series no. 3)

Humerus	Reduction	Nailing	Total time
Comminuted (*n*=12)	81 (5–440)	36 (10–90)	83 (15–485)
Segmental (*n*=3)	65 (15–120)	27 (15–35)	92 (50–150)
Spiral (*n*=40)	23 (5–100)	40 (5–240)	54 (10–240)
Transversal (*n*=71)	34 (5–460)	39 (5–240)	59 (10–470)
Oblique (*n*=22)	27 (5–135)	44 (5–110)	58 (25–175)
Third Fragment (*n*=19)	17 (5–50)	49 (10–170)	59 (10–170)

Table 7.9. Femoral and tibial irradiation nailing times (mean and range values) versus indication of nailing (899 cases) (series no. 3)

	Fracture	Pseudarthrosis	Osteotomy
Femur			
Mean value	165	126	156
Range	5–490	45–320	55–600
Number of cases	376	36	29
Tibia			
Mean value	134	122	122
Range	25–430	25–380	50–285
Number of cases	399	40	19

medullary saw. The average reduction time was 56 s, with a maximum of 250 s for loss of reduction, due to the breakage of a part of the orthopaedic table intraoperatively. The average nail insertion time was 67 s, ranging from 58 s for oblique fractures to 94 s for segmental fractures. The average locking time was about 46 s and remained unchanged irrespective of the type of fracture (Table 7.10).

Tibia. In all indications (Table 7.7), the average overall exposure time was 133 s (122 s for pseudarthroses and osteotomies, 134 s for fractures). The average overall reduction time for fractures was 38 s, with a maximum of 290 s for a refracture, underneath the callus of an old fracture originally treated with external fixation. The average nail insertion time was 50 s, ranging from 44 s for oblique fractures to 68 s for segmental fractures. The average locking time was about 48 s and was steady (Table 7.11).

Gamma Nail. A gamma nail is indicated for the treatment of fractures of the proximal end of the femur. The average overall exposure time was 64 s, with a maximum of 610 s for a staged fracture (neck plus severely comminuted shaft fracture, treated with a long gamma nail). A thorough

Table 7.10. Femoral reduction, nailing and locking irradiation times (mean and range values) versus type of fractures (364 cases) (series no. 3)

Femur	Reduction	Nailing	Locking	Total time
Comminuted (*n*=48)	77 (5–250)	73 (20–225)	48 (20–190)	197 (60–380)
Segmental (*n*=14)	75 (30–170)	94 (20–210)	37 (15–70)	204 (120–330)
Spiral (*n*=51)	51 (5–140)	62 (20–190)	52 (20–195)	163 (70–490)
Transversal (*n*=127)	58 (5–230)	65 (5–250)	43 (15–130)	152 (10–450)
Oblique (*n*=51)	55 (5–180)	58 (20–160)	48 (10–180)	156 (45–360)
Third fragment (*n*=73)	55 (5–190)	71 (5–230)	48 (15–130)	171 (50–390)

Table 7.11. Tibial reduction, nailing and locking irradiation times (mean and range values) versus type of fractures (433 cases) (series no. 3)

Tibia	Reduction	Nailing	Locking	Total time
Comminuted (*n*=28)	50 (5–290)	51 (5–140)	53 (20–185)	151 (35–420)
Segmental (*n*=29)	44 (5–150)	68 (15–140)	46 (25–100)	155 (75–320)
Spiral (*n*=124)	36 (5–180)	51 (10–300)	45 (10–210)	132 (45–420)
Transversal (*n*=90)	39 (5–255)	49 (10–345)	45 (10–230)	123 (25–430)
Oblique (*n*=52)	40 (5–140)	44 (5–140)	45 (10–120)	122 (50–260)
Third fragment (*n*=100)	36 (5–115)	54 (5–210)	52 (10–150)	142 (50–330)

Table 7.12. Reduction and nailing times (mean and range values) for 1054 Gamma nails on the basis of the Ender classification (series no. 3)

Gamma nails	Reduction	Nailing	Total time
Type I/II (n=444)	11 (2–90)	35 (5–280)	45 (10–280)
Type III/IV (n=352)	13 (4–105)	40 (5–150)	53 (10–190)
Type V/VI (n=94)	19 (5–165)	53 (10–230)	72 (15–290)
Type VII/VIII (n=164)	19 (5–90)	67 (10–295)	87 (15–330)

analysis of pertrochanteric fractures using the Ender classification (Table 7.12) shows that the average reduction time was about 15±4 s and was steady. On the other hand, the average nailing time increased in proportion to the type (35 s for types I and II, 40 s for types III and IV, 53 s for types V and VI, and 67 s for types VII and VIII).

Discussion

Image intensifiers are currently being used more and more in operating rooms [2, 6, 8]. Compared to X-rays, they are indeed a significant improvement in terms of comfort and time savings. This technological advance has given rise to a new type of surgery: closed procedures. Of course, the dark side of the picture is, up to a point, the ionizing radiation hazard, but it can be controlled and monitored. Combating radiation involves having a better appreciation of the hazard and providing more information to make the operating room personnel aware of it. For this reason, we felt it necessary to record all exposure times during our radiosurgical procedures.

The average overall nailing time (AONT) is the summation of average overall times relating to reduction (AORT), nail insertion (AOIT), and distal interlocking (AOLT). The downward trend reflects the efficacy of the fight against radiation. Series no. 1 is within the training phase of the nailing technique. In fact, a quick decrease in AONT can be noted between 1976 and 1983, where the times drop from 520 s to 210 s for the femur, and from 591 s to 185 s for the tibia. Knowing intermediate times (AORT, AOIT, AOLT) allowed us to consolidate and then improve AONT. The decrease in AONT was confirmed in series no. 2 and no. 3, from 218 s to 160 s for the femur and from 178 s to 133 s for the tibia.

The average overall AOLT varied according to the radiographer's experience. Between series no. 2 and series no. 3, this time decreased from 57 s to 46 s for the femur and from 58 s to 48 s for the tibia. A fine analysis of AOLT shows that this time is actually unrelated to the site of distal interlocking (femur or tibia) and to the type of fracture. This demonstrates the reliability of the Lafforgue and Grosse targeting device and, above all, the necessity of a homogeneous team of experienced radiographers who have been specifically trained in intraoperative fluoroscopy.

AORT and AOIT depend on the surgeon's skill. These times are still rather high. This is mainly due to the Centre de Traumatologie et d'Orthopédie (CTO) in Strasbourg currently being a training centre that welcomes new young surgeons who are willing to learn the nailing technique; such sessions take place every 6 months. A number of other reasons are to be taken into consideration, such as investigation of borderline indications by the most experienced surgeons.

Direct and Scattered X-rays. The summation of AORT and AOIT is the overall time of X-ray exposure to the surgeon, while AONT is exposure to the radiographer. This is because we always use the targeting device, which allows the surgeon to stand away from the direct radiation field, as delimited by the tube-intensifier virtual cone (maximum 11° taper angle at its top). The surgeon also stands away from scattered radiation, which is minimal, particularly because of a double collimation (diaphragm) and Cu and Al filtration at the tube outlet. This eliminates soft rays which spoil the quality of the fluoroscopic image and have a negligible toxicity (due to very low energy) that is absorbed by a few millimetres of soft tissue (skin).

One must bear in mind that reduction in these two types of radiation is proportional to the square of the distance in room air. Under normal conditions, scattered X-rays are hardly recordable with ionic dosimeters beyond 40 cm and for 300 s. Therefore, it is almost impossible for a surgeon who uses the Lafforgue and Grosse targeting device to be in contact with this radiation field.

Radiation Dose-Exposure Time Relationship. In diagnostic radiology, this relationship is *directly proportional* (mA fluoroscopy 3 mA and kV 105 kV), when exposure is *discontinuous.* The same holds true for the dose–biological effects relationship, although this is a much more complex problem, mainly due to a varying tissue sensitivity (the most sensitive tissues are the stroma of the gonad, the thyroid gland tissue, and the lens) [1, 3–5, 7, 9].

Two factors may influence this relationship, with severe biological effects, compared to radiation exposure:

- Massive (body area) and intense exposure
- Continuous exposure preventing tissue recovery (cell debt or non-amortization of the life span of cells).

In practice, these two conditions never meet.

Legislation Regarding X-ray Exposure. Over all these years, the standards set by industrial medicine for film badges have never been exceeded because we take care that the operating room personnel actually wear a film badge (57% to 89%).

Maximum permissible dose (MPD) has been replaced by effective dose equivalent, only applying to external exposure. Limits are as follows:

	Cumulative result (12 months)	Cumulative result (3 months)
Whole body	50 mSv	30 mSv
Skin	500 mSv	300 mSv
Lens	150 mSv	90 mSv
Hands, fore-arms, feet and ankles	500 mSv	300 mSv
Women in the reproductive years		12.5 mSv
Pregnancy from declaration to delivery		10 mSv (9 months)

The new mSv unit (milliSievert)-old mRad ratio is 1 to 100.

1 Sv=100 Rad.

For guidance:

- X-ray of the pelvis = 1–2.8 mSv = 1 week skiing at 2000 m (cosmic radiation)
- Teleradiograph of the spine – AP and lateral views = 4 mSv
- EDE (or MPD) = 20–50 AP X-rays of the pelvis – homogeneous distribution over 1 year
- Natural telluric radiation is 2 mSv per year in Lozère, compared to 1 mSv at the seaside

Legislation:

- Decree no. 86-1103 of 2 October 1986, modified by decree no. 91-963 of 19 September 1991
- Circular letter DH/8D no. 200 of 3 August 1987, issued by the Department of Health and Human Services
- Order of 19 April 1968 has been extended by the order of September 30, 1987, specifying the "conditions of use for personnel working with dosimeters"
- Order of 28 August 1991: recommendations to factory doctors (abrogates order of 23 April 1968)
- Decree no. 88-521 of 18 April 1988, specifying the limits for persons exposed occupationally to radiation
- Decree no. 94-604 of 19 July 1994 regarding general principles applying to ionizing radiation protection.

References

1. Auboiroux B (1986) La radioprotection dans le domaine médical. Etude de dosimétrie des extrémités. Mémoire ingénieur C.N.A.M. 8 July 1986
2. Barry TP (1984) Radiation exposure to an orthopedic surgeon. Clin Orthop 182:160–164
3. Bross IDJ, Ball M, Falens S (1979) A dosage response curve for the one-rad range: adult risks from diagnostic radiation. Am J Public Health 69:130–136
4. Chanteur J (1988) Radioprotection: le decrét du 2 octobre 1986. Arch Mal Prof 49:269–275
5. Germanaud J, Sabattier R, Baurrier B (1992) La radioprotection en milieu hospitalier. Arch Mal Prof 53:245–255
6. Giachino A, Cheng M (1980) Irradiation to the surgeon during pinning of femoral fractures. J Bone Joint Surg Br 62:227–229
7. Merriam GR, Focht EF (1957) A clinical study of radiation cataracts and the relationship to dose. Am J Roentgenol 5:759–785
8. Miller ME, Davis ML, MacClean CR, Davis JG, Smith BL, Humphries JR (1983) Radiation exposure and associated risks to operating-room personnel during use of fluoroscopic guidance for selected orthopaedic surgical procedures. J Bone Joint Surg Am 65:1–4
9. National Council on Radiation Protection and Measurements (1975) Review of current state of radiation protection philosophy, report no. 43, Washington, D.C. National Council on Radiation Protection 1975

CHAPTER 8

Distal Targeting in Locking Nails

G. TAGLANG

Introduction

Since the first findings of G. Küntscher [4] with his "Detensionsnagel," which was in fact a prototype of the locking nail, everybody agrees that the best system to lock a nail to the bone is a screw system. Some authors have described various systems with fins [1] or pins, but the results have shown a greater instability of the locking system, especially in comminuted fractures, distal fractures and fractures in the elderly (with a high grade of osteoporosis). On the other hand, many problems have occurred during the removal of the devices [2]. For all these reasons, the majority of the locking nails currently on the market are locked with screws.

It seems that the main problem is to find the holes in order to perform an adequate locking at the distal part of the nail. Historically, the first system in use by Küntscher, and later by Klemm and Schellmann, was a free-hand system. We used this system for 2 years, but our impression was of a certain overload of irradiation to the surgeon's hands. For these reasons, Lafforgue and Grosse (in collaboration with Dudey – a fluoroscopy technician) developed a target device mounted on the image intensifier. This technique has proved to be the most effective way of dealing with irradiation for all the surgical team. Pennig and Brug [5] later worked on a new free-hand target device and added modifications and improvements to that technique.

Prerequisites

The supine position facilitates the use of the image intensifier and thus the distal targeting technique. We are also convinced that this position is best for reducing a femoral fracture, especially in a polytrauma situation.

The first step in every technique is to position the image intensifier so that the distal hole in the nail appears perfectly round on the screen. In fact, this is the most difficult step of all, and the X-ray assistant must be well trained for it (Fig. 8.1).

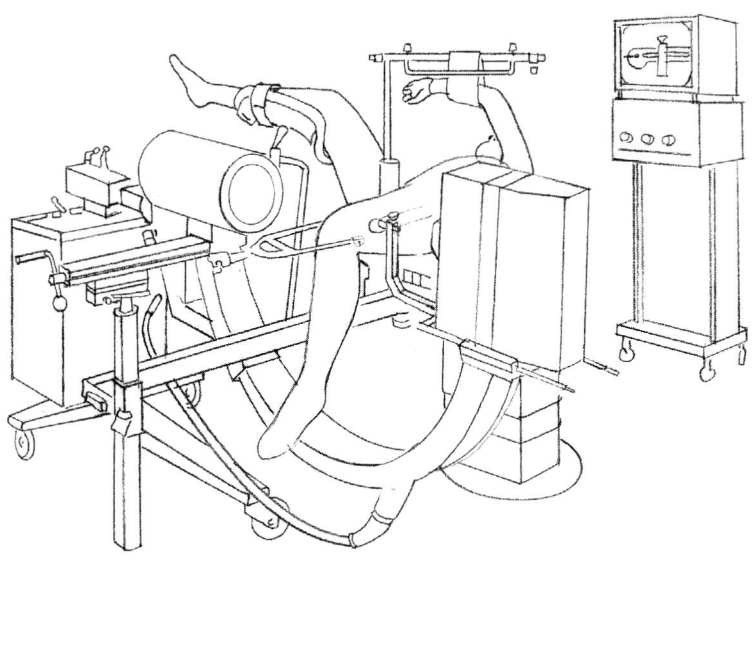

Fig. 8.1. Optimal positioning of the patient on the fracture table and positioning of the image intensifier for the distal locking

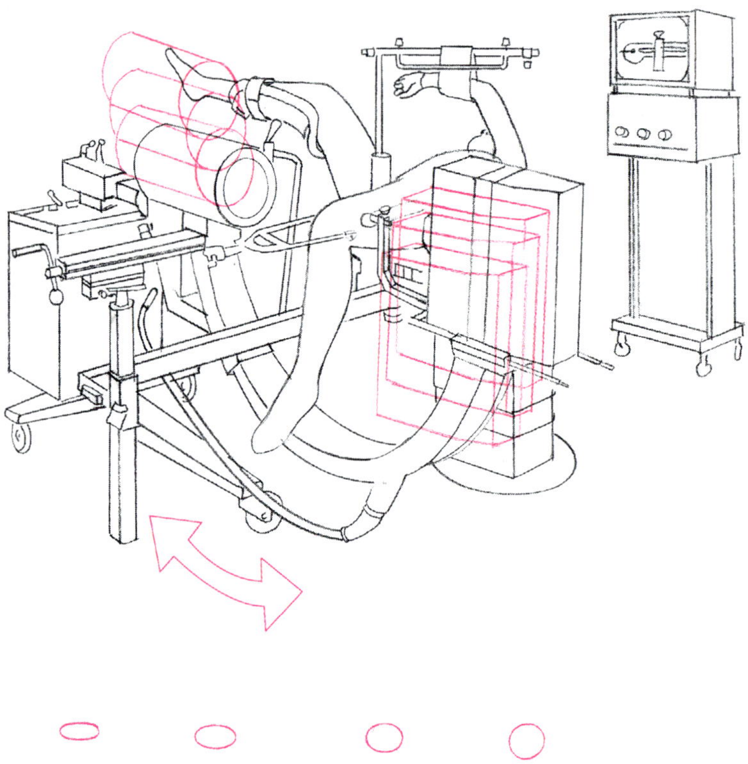

Fig. 8.2. Basic principle of distal targeting to correct an elliptical horizontal hole image, by rotating the C-frame in the vertical plane

General Rules

The most important rule is to correct one plane at a time. In fact, the hole is never perfectly round at the first control; it appears to be elliptical most of the time. The X-ray assistant must correct this by adjusting the position of the C-frame.

The hole on the screen may be elliptical and horizontal due to faulty positioning of the image intensifier in the vertical plane. The correction must be done in this plane. One must bear in mind that the C-frame can move in the vertical plane from 0° to 90° in one direction and only 10° in the other direction (if you consider the neutral position as the neutral position of the tube). This means that the position of the nail in the medullary canal is also very important, a point which will be discussed later in this chapter (Fig. 8.2).

The same elliptical and horizontal hole on the screen may also be caused by faulty positioning of the image intensifier in the horizontal plane. In fact, the image intensifier is not really perpendicular to the medullary canal (and therefore to the nail). The X-ray technician must move the image intensifier in the horizontal plane (Fig. 8.3).

We have frequently observed a combination of both maladjustments, and it is very important to correct the position in one plane at a time, first in the horizontal plane and later in the vertical plane, to obtain perfect alignment between the X-ray beam and the centre of the hole.

The Particular Case of the Femur

As the distal part of the femur is locked from lateral to medial, the image intensifier is positioned with the X-ray tube on the lateral side and the amplifier in contact with the thigh. As the distal targeting imposes in the vertical plane an optimal positioning, and the degree of flexibility in this plane cannot be more than 10° in one direction, it is preferable that the nail is put in place in a light external rotation, otherwise the C-arm will have to pass above the thigh, and this is not easily done.

The Particular Case of the Tibia

The tibia is installed neither in a vertical plane nor in a horizontal plane. This can increase the difficulty of the distal targeting, because displacements of the C-arm are made in an oblique plane. The distal part of the tibia is locked from medial

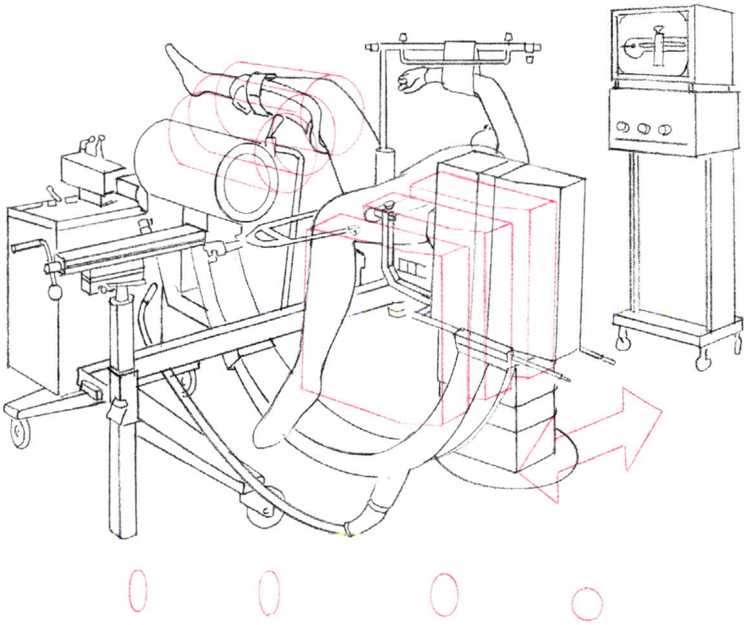

Fig. 8.3. Basic principle of distal targeting to correct an elliptical vertical hole image, by moving the C-frame in the horizontal plane

to lateral, which means that the tube must be placed at the medial part of the tibia.

Precautions

One has to remember that the nail can become deformed during the nailing essentially in the A-P plane (as a result of bending) rather than in the frontal plane (rotation). This explains the problems with the nail-mounted target devices, even with very rigid nails. However, these deformities are now very rare because the nails are less pliable than they were in the beginning. This is especially true of the small diameter nails without slots. On the other hand, we ream routinely 1.5–2 mm over the nail diameter.

One other important precaution is to perfectly centralise the drill before drilling, avoiding the sideslip of the drill. This can be observed at the distal part of the femur, where the natural tendency is a posterior sideslip. This problem is easy to solve by using a pointed awl (or a Steinmann pin with the free-hand technique) to pierce the first cortex (lateral for the femur or medial for the tibia).

Various Techniques

Grosse-Lafforgue Device (Image-Intensifier-Mounted Target Device) [3]

Use of this targeting method minimises radiation exposure to the surgeon, as it is mounted on the X-ray tube side of the image intensifier, and can be manoeuvred remotely by the X-ray technician. With this technique there is no direct or diffused radiation to the hands of the surgeon.

After the X-ray beam is aligned to produce a perfectly round hole on the monitor screen, the target device is folded down in line with the beam and manoeuvred against the patient's thigh. The concentricity of the circles made by the targeting device and the distal hole is verified, making adjustments as necessary. A skin incision is made, the pointed awl is introduced through the barrel of the sighting device and its tip is used to pierce the lateral cortex (Fig. 8.4).

The Femur

A 5-mm drill guide sleeve is passed through the sighting device and both cortices are drilled, using the 5-mm drill. The current devices for the femur are now colour-coded, and the standard colour code for the femur is black.

The drill and guide sleeve are removed and a depth gauge inserted through the sighting device

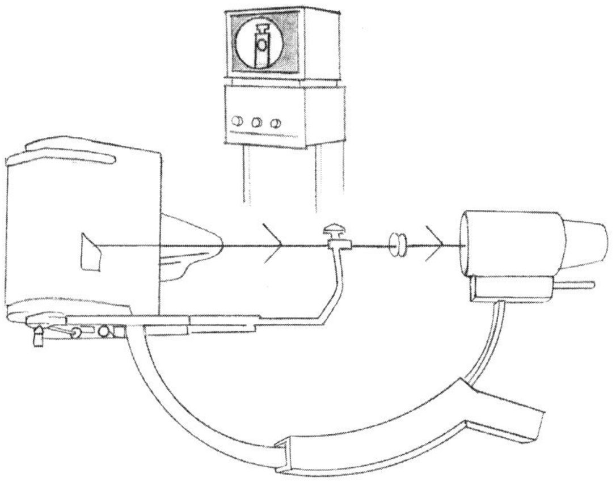

Fig. 8.4. The principle of the Grosse-Lafforgue target device mounted on the image intensifier

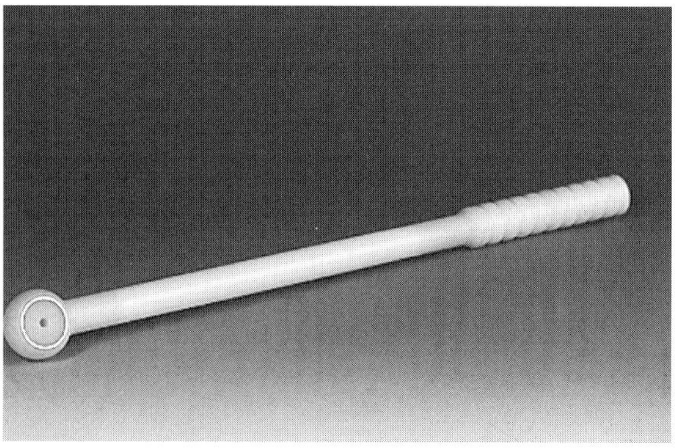

Fig. 8.5. Pennig's free-hand target device

to determine the required screw length; the barrel of the measuring gauge acts as a substitute for the normal guide, being brought into contact with the bone.

Using the screwdriver, a 6.28-mm fully-threaded screw is placed through the sighting barrel and driven through both cortices. The second screw is then targeted and placed in a similar manner. Due to the potential deformity of the distal part of the nail, it is not possible to directly target the second hole without using the C-frame again.

The Tibia

The same technique is used, but both cortices are drilled with a 3.7-mm drill (colour code: yellow). The size of the self-tapping fully threaded screw is 4.6 mm.

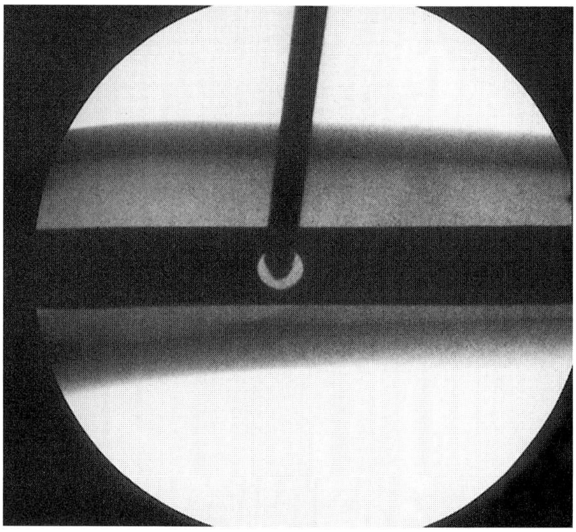

Fig. 8.6. The Steinmann pin in the centre of the image of the distal hole

Free-Hand Technique

This technique has been modified and developed from Küntscher's original technique by Pennig and Brug [5] in Münster, Germany. The device used in this technique is a radiolucent polyethylene handle with two metallic rings at the distal part (Fig. 8.5).

The essential first step in using this device is to align the image intensifier with the most distal screw hole of the nail until a perfect circle is seen. A 4-mm Steinmann pin is passed through the free-hand device and, using the image intensifier, placed against the soft tissue to indicate the stab wound incision site.

After the incision is made and with the image intensifier on, the free-hand device is used to place the Steinmann pin in the exact centre of the visualised hole. The point of the pin is firmly held against the proximal cortex (Fig. 8.6).

With the pin stationary, the device is moved until both alignment rings appear as one and the pin appears to be a dot in the centre of the single ring. The mallet is then used to tap the pin through the near cortex and into the screw hole in the nail, up to but not into the far cortex (Fig. 8.7).

The pin is kept in place and the targeting device is removed. The special drill guide is then introduced over the pin and up to the near cortex. The Steinmann pin is removed, using pliers or the Jacob's chuck. The drill guide is firmly held while the pin is removed.

The 5-mm drill bit is used to drill through both cortices. The drill guide and drill are then

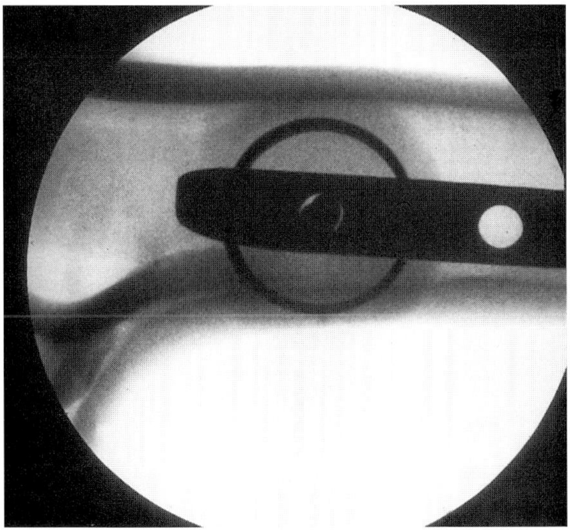

Fig. 8.7. The Pennig target device with the concentric rings and the Steinmann pin in the middle of the hole

removed. The measurement is performed using the depth gauge, which has an integral sleeve that should contact the near cortex to give the correct distance. A screw of appropriate length is placed in a free-hand fashion. The same steps are repeated to target the second hole.

Nail-Mounted Device

The basic idea with a nail-mounted device is to perform the distal targeting without the use of irradiation. This device is not very reliable. The potential problem of the rotation and/or bending of the nail makes it particularly unsuitable for young patients with hard cortices. We used a prototype for 2 years, but experienced difficulties in aligning the image of the holes and the image of the barrel, even when using adjustment knobs.

References

1. Brooker Jr AF, Brumback RJ (1998) Brooker-Wills nails in treatment of infra-isthmal injuries of the femur. J Trauma 28:688–691
2. Ebraheim NA, Milem CA, Jackson WT (1993) Compli cated removal of the distal locking device of Brooker-Wills. Clin Orthop 290:275–278
3. Kempf I, Grosse A, Lafforgue D (1978) L'apport du verrouillage dans l'enclouage centro-médullaire des os longs. Rev Chir Orthop Reparatrice Appar Mot 64:635–651
4. Küntscher G (1964) Die Nagelung des Defekttrümmerbruchs. Chirurg 35: 277
5. Pennig D, Brug E, Kronholz HL (1988) A new distal aiming device for locking nail fixation. Orthopedics 11:1725–1727

CHAPTER 9

Femoral Fractures

K.S. Leung and A. Grosse

Introduction

The femur is surrounded by a very vascular muscular envelope, and the fracture fragments are well perfused even if there are comminutions. Healing of femoral fractures is uneventful most of the time, provided the fracture fragments are not devitalised. It is true that many femoral fractures may be treated by non-operative means that include skeletal traction or functional bracing. However, the disadvantages of prolonged hospitalisation in traction and complications such as shortening and rotational deformities make these non-operative methods unpopular. Operative treatment helps to prevent these complications and facilitate early rehabilitation after injury. While open reduction and internal fixation is definitely one form of treatment [47] with predictable outcome, closed reduction and intramedullary fixation is much preferred. With this modern concept of fracture treatment, the ultimate goals are minimal trauma to soft tissues and the preservation of fracture haematoma to facilitate fracture healing [5, 48, 55, 61].

Diaphyseal fracture of the femur is the best indication for closed intramedullary fixation. In fact, one of the earliest applications of intramedullary fixation of fractures started with femoral fractures. However, intramedullary fixation of long bone fractures according to Küntscher's design and method can only treat fractures in midshaft with minimal comminution. With the increasing incidence of high-energy trauma, femoral fractures are frequently associated with comminutions and involve more proximal and distal segments. Simple intramedullary nailing [7, 61] cannot control the rotational and the shortening deformities of these unstable fractures [56]. The use of locked intramedullary nailing widens the applications of this closed technique into the treatment of all unstable and stable femoral shaft fractures [1, 2, 4, 6, 8, 11, 15, 18, 19, 23, 25, 30, 31, 34, 39, 46, 50, 52, 53, 63].

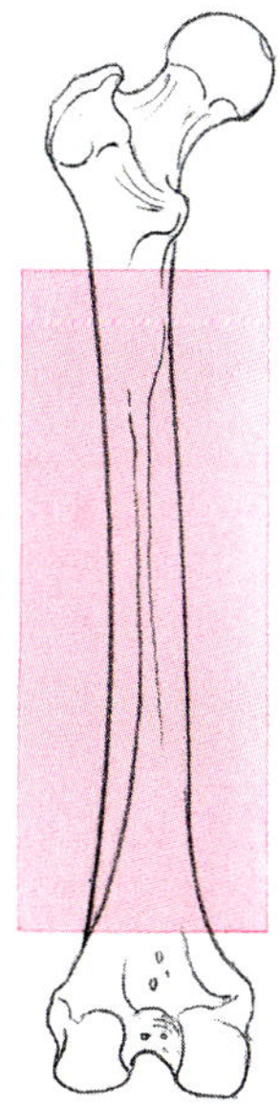

Fig. 9.1. The locked nail extends the indication of intramedullary nail fixation for femoral fractures. Fractures from subtrochanteric to supracondylar regions can be treated with locked intramedullary nails

Indications

The intramedullary locked nail is indicated in all unstable fractures occurring from the subtrochanteric [56, 61] to supracondylar regions of the femur (Fig. 9.1). Fractures with third fragments, long spiral fractures, segmental fractures [60], and comminuted fractures [39, 57], with or without bone loss, are the best indications for intramedullary locked nailing. Extended indications may include proximal and distal fractures (see other volume), open fractures, delayed union and non-union, lengthening and shortening osteotomies [35, 56], and reconstructive limb salvage surgery after tumour resections.

Preoperative Preparation

Evaluation

Patients with femoral fractures are usually the victims of high-energy trauma where associated injuries are not uncommonly found. These life-threatening conditions must be treated and the patient stabilised before the fracture is fixed. Radiological examination with good quality film should be done to exclude pelvic injuries as well as ipsilateral hip and knee fractures [9]. In the case of comminutions and bone loss, it is essential to take an X-ray measurement of the contralateral femur to determine the length and the size of the nail to be inserted.

Temporary Skeletal Stabilisation

While the patient is waiting for surgery, temporary skeletal stabilisation is necessary to control pain and facilitate the subsequent nailing procedure. Skeletal traction should be applied by either distal femoral, or proximal tibial Steinmann pin insertion. If the nailing procedure is expected to be carried out within 48 h, distal femoral pin traction should be done as it is a much more efficient skeletal traction system than proximal tibial pin traction. Distal femoral pin traction is also used if there is concomitant ligamental injuries of the knee. However, if it is anticipated that the nailing procedure cannot be performed within 48 h, proximal tibial pin traction is a safer method of preventing potential pin tract infection around the femoral pin sites, which may increase the risk of infection after the nailing procedure.

It is recommended to have slight over-traction at the fracture sites by applying a traction force of 10–15 kg, in order to facilitate proper closed reduction of the fractures during operation.

Timing of Surgery

Fixation of the fractures should be done as soon as the patient's other life-threatening conditions are stabilised. Early fixation of the fractures decreases mortality and morbidity; it also facilitates nursing care and speeds rehabilitation.

Operative Technique

Anaesthesia and Positioning

The operation can be performed under spinal and general anaesthesia. If the distal femoral pin has not been inserted, it should be inserted before the patient is positioned on a fracture traction table. It is strongly recommended that traction through the distal femoral pin should be used, in order to provide efficient traction and reduction manoeuvre. Proximal tibial traction or foot piece traction should only be used in very special situations.

The patient is placed supine on the traction table (Fig. 9.2). This position simplifies the achievement of anatomical reduction [41] and the use of a C-arm in distal locking. It also has physiological advantages for patients with poly-trauma and multiple fractures. However, in an extremely obese patient, the lateral decubitus position may be helpful for access to the entry point in the greater trochanter.

The injured limb is attached to the traction table directly, with the distal femoral pin through an adjustable stirrup (Fig. 9.3). Care should also be taken to prevent placing the leg and the foot in a dependent position. The contralateral lower limb is positioned by flexing, abducting and externally rotating the hip and flexing the knee (Fig. 9.3). This will make it easier to manoeuvre the image intensifier.

The upper trunk should be flexed laterally towards the opposite side. A restrainer should be attached to keep the trunk in position during the reduction manoeuvre, and throughout the whole operation (Fig. 9.4) [16]. Care must be taken that there is no pressure on the arm or the wall of the chest.

Image Intensifier

The image intensifier should be positioned on the medial side of the fractured limb, with the intensifier end on the medial side of the injured limb, when taking lateral imaging (Fig. 9.2). This will facilitate an unobstructed distal targeting procedure and avoid the phenomenon of magnification. The manoeuvre of the C-arm should be tested before draping, so that the whole femur can be properly imaged in two planes without the interference of the contralateral limb and the traction bars of the orthopaedic table.

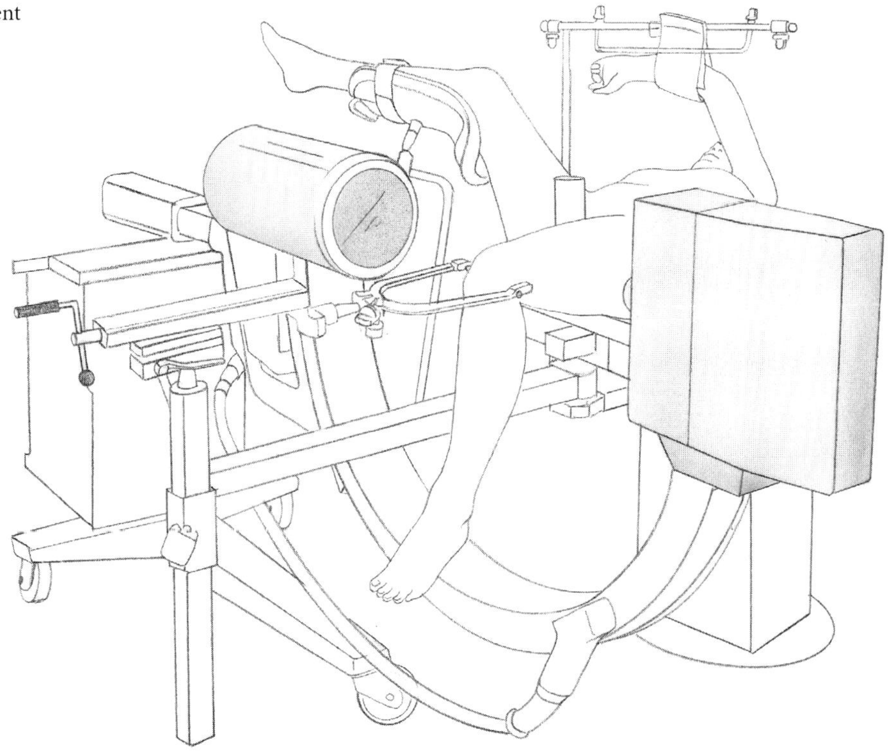

Fig. 9.2. Position of the patient on a traction table

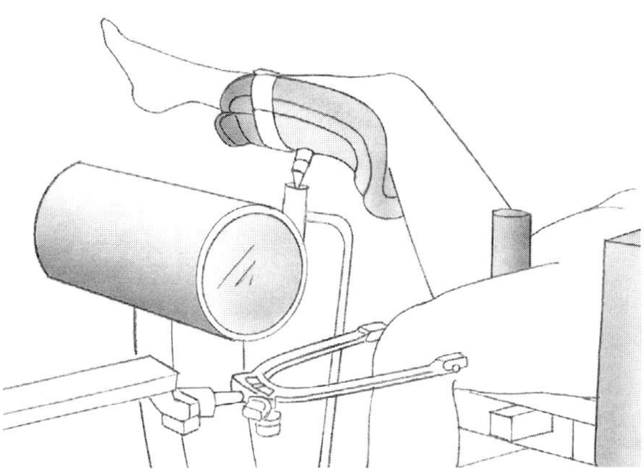

Fig. 9.3. One of the designs of the stirrups for skeletal traction through the distal femur. Note the position of the contralateral lower limb

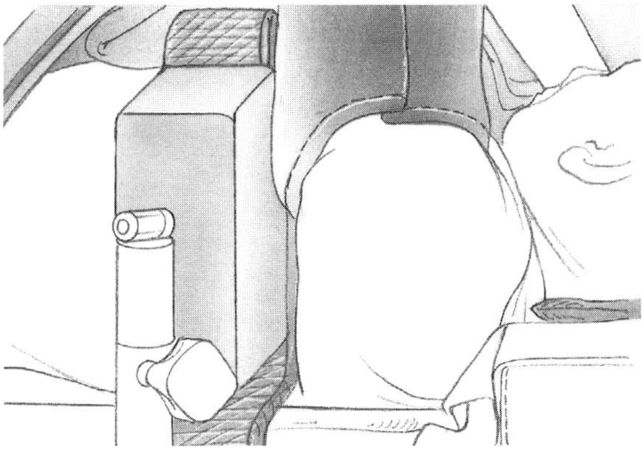

Fig. 9.4. Positioning of a restrainer to keep the upper trunk laterally flexed

Closed Reduction

The fracture should be reduced as *anatomically* as possible before surgical incision is made.

With the distal femoral traction pin attached to the traction table by an adjustable stirrup, longitudinal traction is applied while adducting the thigh. The length of the femur can be restored without difficulty. Varus and vulgus deformities can be corrected by adducting and abducting the distal segment. The more proximal the fracture, the more vulgus the proximal segment. Fine adjustment can be made through the stirrup. Reduction of the fracture in the frontal plane can be achieved with this manoeuvre

Rotational deformity can be corrected by matching the cortical thickness of the proximal and distal segments. External rotation of the proximal segment is a very common configuration, due to the action of relatively unopposed ex-

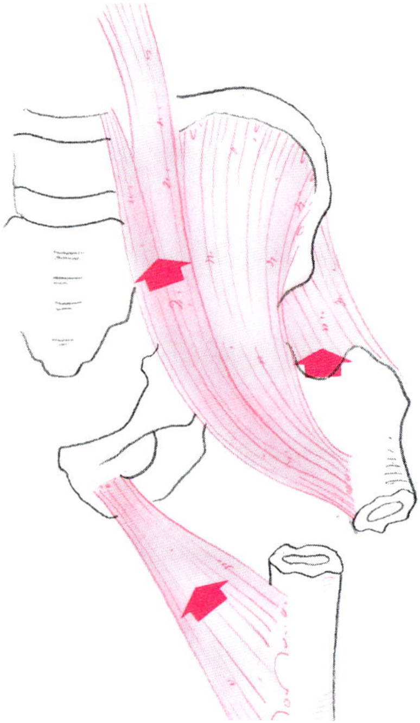

Fig. 9.5. Different muscles acting on the proximal segment in a subtrochanteric fracture which is flexed, rotated externally, and abducted

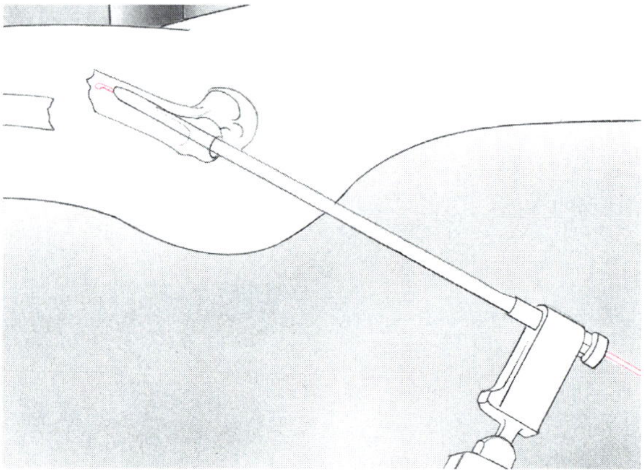

Fig. 9.6. The use of a repositioning guide in assisting the reduction of a subtrochanteric fracture. The use of a small Küntscher nail (9 mm) serves the same purpose

ternal rotational forces. The more proximal the fracture, the more external is the proximal segment rotation.

By carefully performed reduction in the frontal plane, satisfactory alignment on the lateral plane can be obtained in most cases.

Subtrochanteric Fractures

The marked deformities associated with this fracture are due to the actions of unopposed proximal muscles (Fig. 9.5): these include the short rotators of the hips together with the strong psoas causing external rotation, hip abductors causing abduction of the proximal segment, and the strong psoas causing flexion deformity. As a result of these actions, anatomical reduction by the closed method is difficult. In order to reduce the fracture, excessive adduction of the lower limb should be avoided and reduction should be controlled with one plane first if possible. The fracture can then be reduced during operation by using a nail of a smaller diameter: the technique proposed by Küntscher – after the intramedullary canal is entered, the medullary canal of the proximal segment is reamed to 9–9.5 mm. (The entry point on the tip of the greater trochanter must be carefully identified due to the commonly associated deformities. Also see below for the entry site for the intramedullary canal.) A short, 9-mm nail containing the reamer guide, is then inserted; it can then be used to control the proximal segment to reduce the fracture. The reamer guide can then be passed after the fracture is reduced and aligned. The specially designed repositioning guide may simplify the procedure by reducing the proximal fragment (Fig. 9.6).

Supracondylar Fractures

The fractured limb should be adducted with extension at the knee joint, to obtain anatomical reduction.

Comminuted Fractures

Reduction of comminuted fractures is usually not difficult. To control the length, the contralateral limb serves as the reference. To control rotational deformity, a good imaging of the lesser trochanter should be obtained to determine the degree of external rotation, so that the distal segment can be aligned accordingly.

Draping and Sterilisation

The region from the iliac crest to the whole thigh down to the knee is cleansed and disinfected. Surgical drapes are placed, allowing exposure of the thigh from the iliac crest to the distal femoral traction pin.

Incision and Entry Point

A 5-cm, horizontal incision is made from the greater trochanter towards the iliac crest (Fig. 9.7). After incising the deep fascia, the abductor muscle is split along the muscle fibre and retracted with a self-retaining retractor. The entire superior surface of the tip of the greater trochanter can be palpated. With this surface divided into three equal segments, the entry point is between the anterior third and the middle third (Fig. 9.8). In many incidences, this point is represented by a small depression which one can always feel if careful palpation is done. The posterior one-third of the greater trochanter does not align with the medullary canal of the femur and should not be taken into consideration in determining the entry point.

We recommend that the entry point for the femoral medullary canal should be on the tip of the greater trochanter instead of the piriformis fossa for the following reasons:

a) There is much less chance of injuring the ascending cervical arteries, hence the possibility of avascular necrosis of the femoral head can be minimised.
b) Biomechanically, the entry point in the piriformis fossa weakens the femoral neck in respect to the bending forces acting on the femoral head. It thus increases the possibility of iatrogenic fractures in the femoral neck during nailing procedure and after the operation [27, 33, 40, 43, 49].
c) In extremely overweight patients, the entry point on the greater trochanter is better placed for insertion [44].

The lateralised incision has the potential risk of impingement of the tip of the nail into the medial cortex and may lead to iatrogenic fracture of the medial cortex in the proximal femur (see "Nail Insertion").

An accurate entry point can be located by using a sharp fine awl, which perforates the greater trochanter at the determined entry point. The entry hole is then enlarged by reciprocating movements with a pointed curve awl. The direction of the entry of the awl should follow the gentle curvature from the tip of the greater trochanter into the medullary canal. If required, the entry of the awl can be monitored with an image intensifier. The newly designed awl consists of two parts (Fig. 9.9). The central pointed awl perforates the cortex in the entry point. The conical part maintains the position for the insertion of the reamer guide.

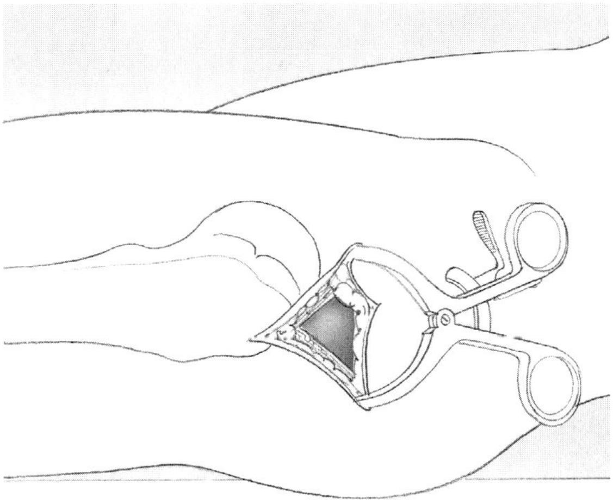

Fig. 9.7. The incision in the trochanteric area

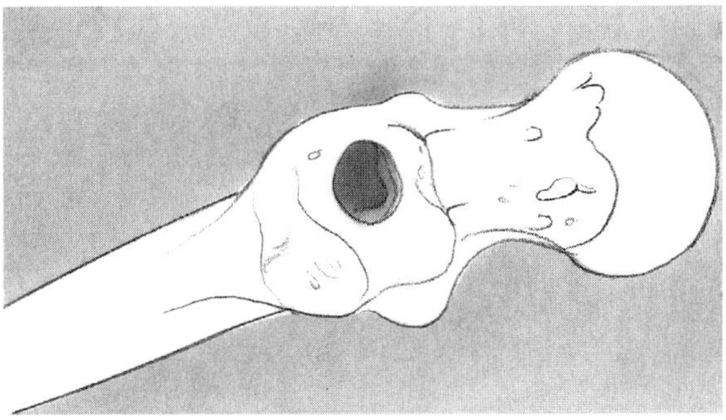

Fig. 9.8. The entry point between the anterior third and the middle third on the greater trochanter

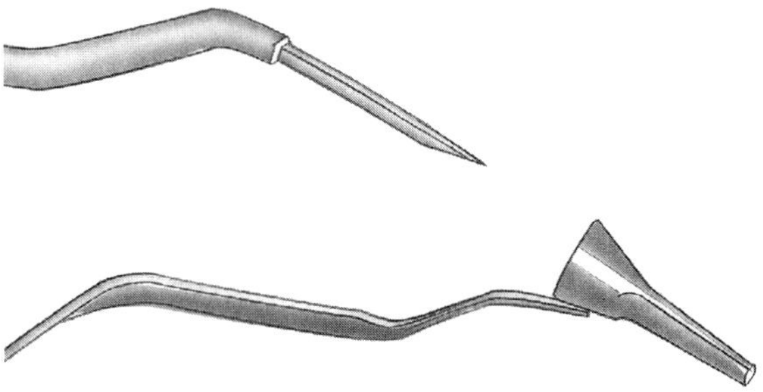

Fig. 9.9. The pointed awl in two parts. A central sharp awl for perforating the cortex at the tip of the greater trochanter. The outer conical part maintains the passage for the reamer guide

Reamer Guide Rod

A pre-curved olive-tip reamer guide held by a Jacob's chuck is inserted along the same curved tract to the medullary canal (Fig. 9.10). Again, care must be taken so that it will not impinge on the medial cortex of the femur. The pre-curved tip facilitates its passage through individual frac-

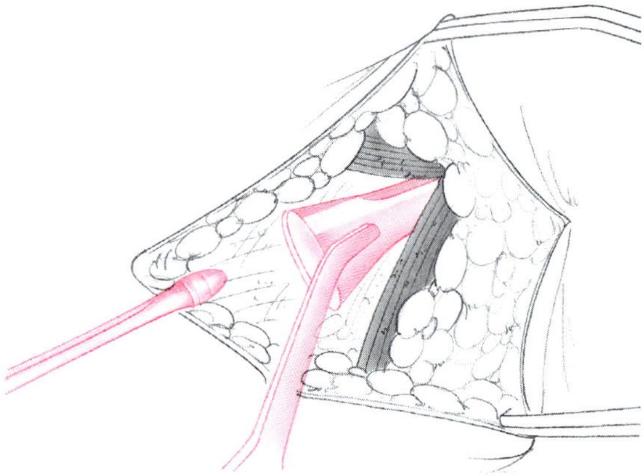

Fig. 9.10. A pre-curved olive-tip reamer guide is inserted into the femoral canal through the conical part of the awl

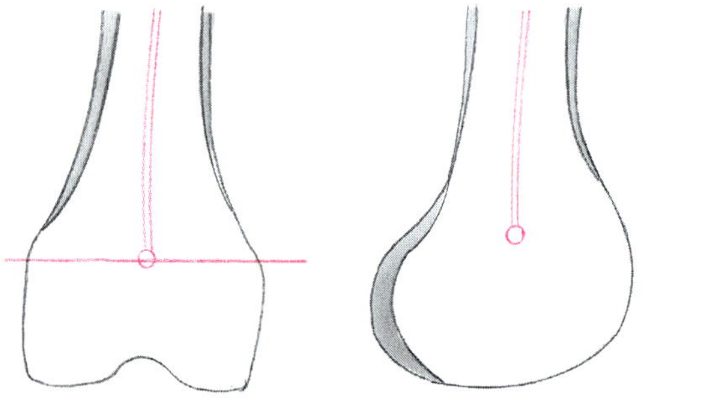

Fig. 9.11. The tip of the reamer guide should be centralised in the distal part of the femur

ture fragments and enables the reduction of translational displacements of major fragments. The passage of the reamer guide rod is monitored with the image intensifier in both the frontal and lateral planes. The feeling of the contact of the tip with the inner cortex of the femur ensures good positioning of the guide and helps to limit X-ray exposure by reducing the need for frequent screening with the image intensifier [17, 18, 38, 40]. After passing through the fracture site, the tip of the reamer guide is centralised in the subchondral area of the distal femur in both the frontal and sagittal planes (Fig. 9.11). Eccentric placement of the reamer guide may lead to uneven reaming and possible misalignment of the fracture fragments.

At this stage, the length of the nail to be inserted is determined by placing the calibrated nail guide beside the reamer guide, with its tip at the entry point. The correct length of the nail can then be determined by subtracting the protruding reamer guide length from the graduated nail guide.

Reaming

Reaming usually begins with a 9-mm flexible reamer. A tissue protector may be used to prevent frictional injury to the surrounding soft tissue. The reamer should only be switched on after the reamer head has been completely inserted into the medullary cavity. The initial resistance is usually in the entry point as well as in the trochanteric region. The isthmus is the other region that has resistance to reaming. Repeated reaming with a reamer head of the same diameter should be done whenever resistance is felt. Reaming in 0.5-mm increments should be continued until 1.5–2 mm larger than the chosen nail diameter. Reaming should be carried out with the minimum of pushing and without excessive force. Care should be taken to make sure that the reamer guide rod is in the correct position each time the reamer head is redrawn for exchange.

Comminuted Fractures and Bone Loss [29]

When reaming through an area of comminuted fractures, the reaming machine should be switched off and the reamer advanced by a gentle push. Reaming should only be resumed in the intact femoral diaphysis.

Segmental Fractures

The reaming of the segmental fracture has the potential hazard of causing the segment to rotate with the reamer. In femur, the chance of rotation is minimal, due to the strong attachment of the linea Aspera. However, extra caution should be taken, with gentle reaming and frequent monitoring with the image intensifier.

Nail Insertion

The nail cannot pass over the curved olive-tipped reamer guide rod; it must be exchanged for a straight nail guide rod. A Teflon tube is passed over the reamer guide rod to the distal femur (Fig. 9.12). The reamer guide rod is then removed and the nail guide inserted. The Teflon tube is then removed and the position of the nail guide should be checked with the image intensifier.

The nail of the selected diameter and length is mounted on the driving device, with the nail-holding bolt which must be firmly tightened with the socket wrench. The nail is then introduced

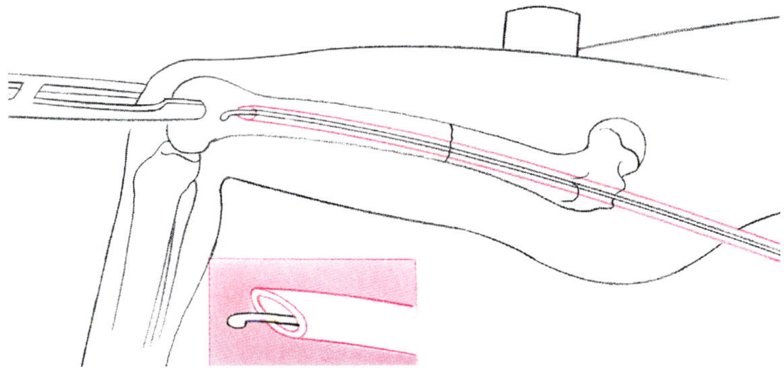

Fig. 9.12. The Teflon tube is passed over the reamer guide

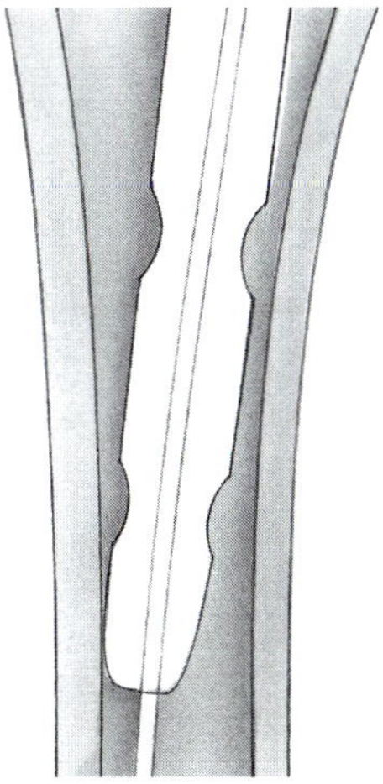

Fig. 9.13. The tip of the nail is monitored with the C-arm in order to avoid impinging onto the medial cortex of the proximal femur during insertion

over the nail guide rod. The nail is pushed in manually as far as possible and then impacted gently with the mallet to its final position in the medullary canal. The tip of the nail should be monitored constantly with the image intensifier, in order to avoid impinging on the medial cortex (Fig. 9.13). Pushing the nail towards the patient may be helpful at this stage. As the nail is impacted with the mallet, it is necessary to ensure that the nail stays in contact with the driving device, by constantly checking that the nail-holding screw is firmly tightened and the nail guide rod does not back out.

Over-traction of the fracture site should be corrected, by releasing the traction when the tip of the nail passes the fracture site into the distal segment, before it is completely inserted to allow final impaction.

When the nail is impacted to its final position, the nail guide can then be removed.

Proximal Locking

Proximal locking is indicated in all unstable diaphyseal fractures and fractures in the proximal metaphysis/diaphysis which are rotatory unstable. Proximal locking can be done with various screw configurations. The use of the diagonal locked screw has the advantages of a further increase in the working length of the nail and the maximum purchase on the bone by the screw. With this design, a very proximal fracture with an intact lesser trochanter can be treated satisfactorily.

Before proximal locking, the nail-holding bolt must be firmly tightened, using the socket wrench to ensure the nail is in contact with the driving/targeting device (Fig. 9.14). The tissue protector and the obturator assembly is passed through the target device and is brought into contact with the lateral cortex of the greater trochanter, through an incision wound penetrating the skin and the fascia lata. The tissue protector is secured in position by tightening the thumb screw. After the obturator has been removed, a pointed awl is introduced through the tissue protector and pierces the lateral cortex with the aid of a mallet. The guide sleeve for a 5-mm drill is inserted into the tissue protector, and both cortices are drilled, using the 5-mm drill bit (colour code: black) (Fig. 9.15). The drill sleeve is removed and the length of the proximal locking screw is determined with the depth gauge (Fig. 9.16). A 6.28-mm self-tapping screw of the correct length is then positioned through the tissue protector without malalignment and driven into both the cortices (Fig. 9.17).

The proximal targeting device can be removed. A proximal plug may be placed in the end of the nail, to prevent bone in-growth and facilitate subsequent removal. The wound is temporarily packed with a saline gauge, before closure at the end of the operation.

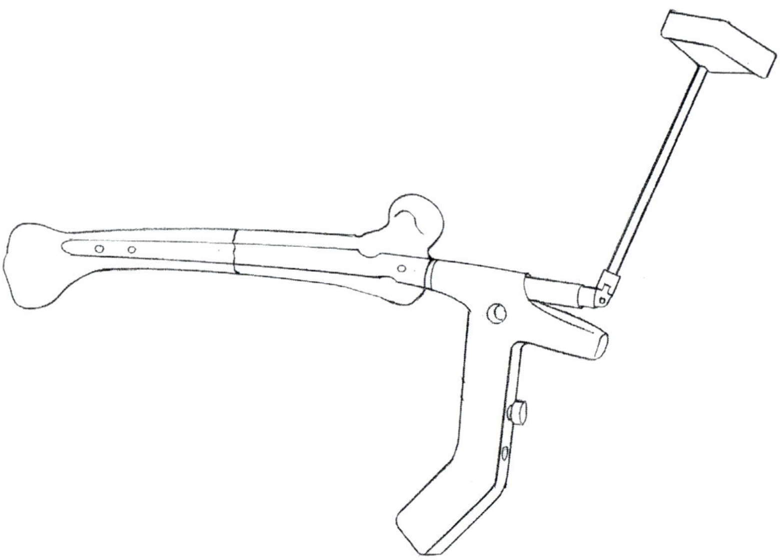

Fig. 9.14. The nail holding bolt must be tightened before proximal locking procedures

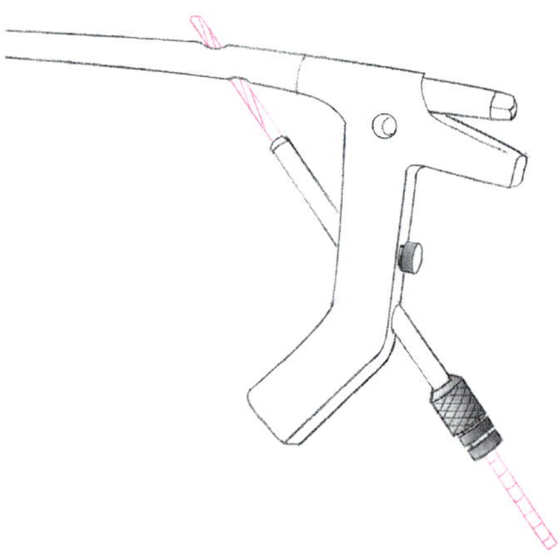

Fig. 9.15. Both cortices must be drilled with a 5.0-mm drill bit

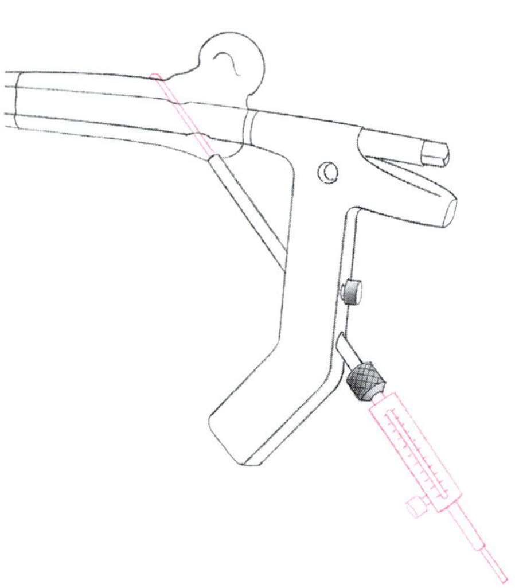

Fig. 9.16. The length of the screw inserted is measured with a depth gauge. The inner drill sleeve is removed before measuring

Distal Locking

Distal locking (see Chap. 8, this volume) is indicated in all unstable diaphyseal fractures and fractures in the distal diaphyseal/metaphyseal with rotatory instability [21]. The screws are inserted from the lateral side of the thigh. Two fully threaded 6.28-mm screws are needed to ensure maximal stability [22]. In bones of poor quality, Vécsei screws may be used with advantage (Fig. 9.21a, b).

Closure

The wound is closed in layers, after copious irrigation of the proximal incision wound to wash away the reamed material, which may be a potential source of ectopic calcification [12, 32, 42]. A suction drainage is inserted, but not too near the entry point of the medullary cavity. The distal incision wounds can be closed with skin sutures only. The distal femoral traction pin can then be removed with an aseptic technique. A light pressure bandaging is applied to the whole lower limb to control the post-operative swelling. It is recommended that the bandage should be kept for at least 1 week after the operation to prevent recollection of haematoma around the fracture site.

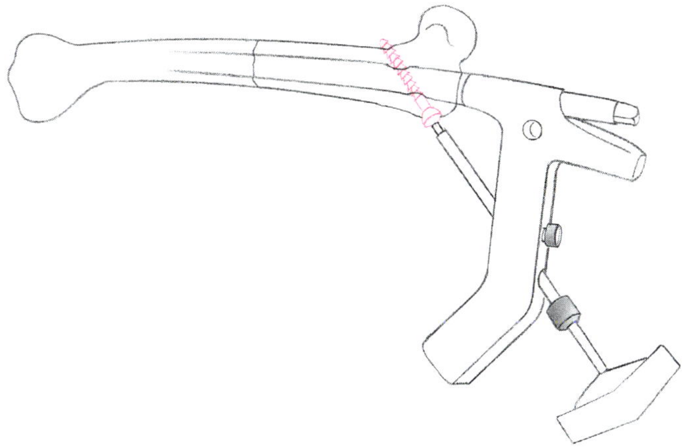

Fig. 9.17. A 6.28-mm self-tapping screw is inserted through two cortices

Post-operative Management

The lower limb is elevated on a Braun's frame with the hip and knee flexed to 90°. This is important because it allows drainage and decreases swelling. It also allows maximal stretching of the quadriceps muscle, which is usually injured with the fracture. The position will prevent contracture of the quadriceps during healing. The use of a continuous passive motion (CPM) machine prevents adhesions and fibrous contracture of the quadriceps.

Radiographs are taken to ensure good reduction and stable fixation. Mobilisation of the limb should be initiated as soon as the patient's condition allows. Most patients can start to walk with graduated weight-bearing [26]. When there is significant comminution or bone loss, weight-bearing may be allowed if there is early callus formation. Full weight-bearing may be allowed if there is corticalisation of the callus. For dynamically locked fractures, walking with weight bearing can be started immediately. Muscle strengthening exercise should be commenced at the same time with an emphasis on the abductors of the hip.

Dynamisation: The Removal of Locked Screws During the Course of Fracture Healing

The practice of dynamisation has been mostly abandoned in femoral fractures fixed with slotted locked nails. This practice is supported by much clinical experience as well as by animal experiments [10, 13, 51, 61]. The slotted nail with a static locked configuration provides considerable axial flexibility for normal fracture healing [36]. However, dynamisation is indicated in fractures fixed with more rigid nails, such as the unslotted or solid nail. Furthermore, it may be practised in fracture with over-distraction and definite delayed union 3–4 months after fracture fixation.

Dynamisation is done by removing the locked screw(s) further away from the fracture site.

Removal of Implants

Removal of implants is indicated when there is constant irritation, which is not uncommonly encountered in the distal locked screws. Removal should only be considered after there is clinical and radiological union, with good corticalisation of callus. It is recommended that the removal should be carried out at least 2 years after operation.

The distal screws are removed through the old incisions. The proximal incision is made and the proximal screw is removed. The proximal nail end is approached and the proximal cap or bony overgrowth (if there is any) is removed. To assemble the extraction instrumentations, the adapter is screwed onto the small extraction shaft which is then attached into the nail with a 10-mm socket wrench. The adapter is removed and the long extraction shaft with a handle is attached to the small extraction shaft (Fig. 9.18). The nail can then be removed with the help of the sliding hammer.

Errors and Potential Hazards

Positioning

To guard against the trunk on the same side of the injured limb, the restrainer should be installed before traction is applied for reduction. Traction without this restrainer will cause the trunk to rotate around the perineal counter traction pole. There have been reports of patients falling off the

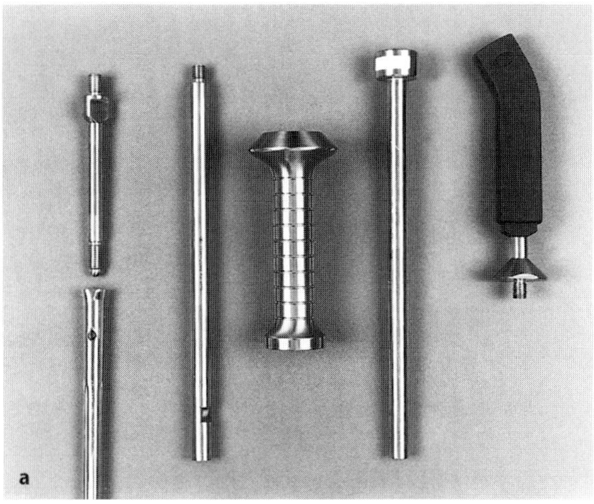

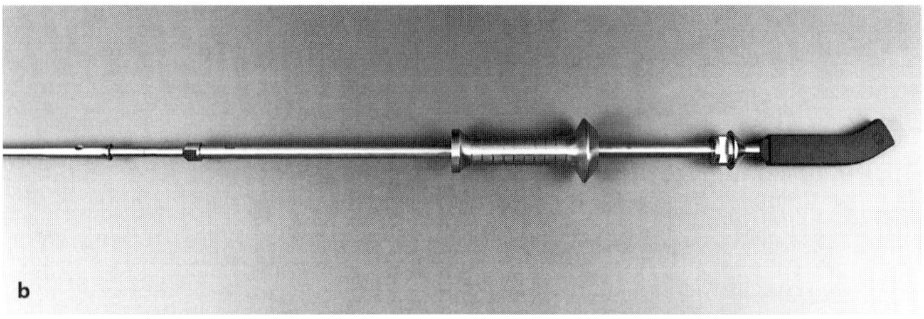

Fig. 9.18 a, b. The extraction device: **a** different parts, **b** assembly

operating table when traction that was too strong was applied without the restrainer [16]. Such strong traction should be avoided, as it may cause injury to the soft tissue around the perineum. Scrotal haematoma and pudendal nerve injury have been reported [14, 28, 46].

Entry Point

The recommended entry point is on the tip of the greater trochanter on the frontal plane. For more proximal fractures and subtrochanteric fractures, the entry point has to be medialised, so as to correct the common vulgus deformity.

Reaming

Reaming should always be gentle and gradual, in order to prevent an increase in intramedullary pressure, which may lead to marrow content embolisation. Although the exact role of these marrow emboli in causing complications in the trauma patient is still not clear, care should always be taken to minimise the embolisation (see Chap. 4, this volume).

The reamer head may sometimes become jammed. This can occur if the medullary canal is too tight, if the reamer head is not sharp, or if the reaming is done with too much force. The jammed reamer can only be removed by extracting it together with the reamer guide rod. The olive tip of the reamer guide rod serves as the extractor when it is retracted.

Nail Insertion

With the patient in a supine position and the entry point in the tip of the greater trochanter, there is a definite risk of the tip of the nail impinging on the medial cortex in the subtrochanteric area and causing iatrogenic fractures (Figs. 9.19). It is therefore necessary to keep the nail adducted during insertion.

Internal rotation of the nail during insertion is a common complication and should be avoided by controlling the handle of the driving device carefully during insertion.

Torsional deformity of the distal part of the nail is usually due to a relatively narrow [61] medullary canal compared to the diameter of the nail and to forceful impaction with the mallet.

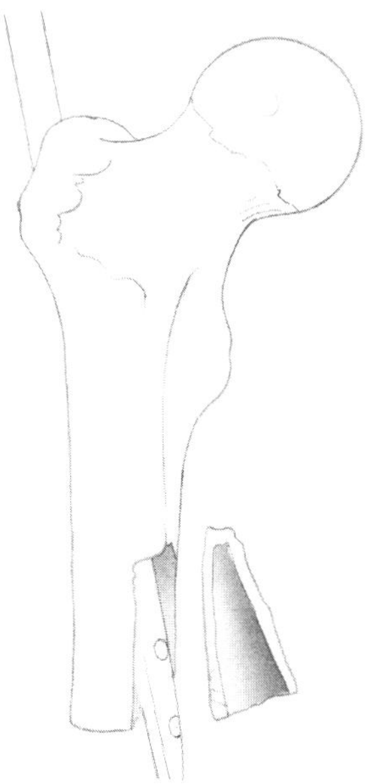

Fig. 9.19. Iatrogenic fracture of the medial cortex due to nail insertion. The nail should be maximally adducted during insertion

This is more common with the use of the slotted nail in fixing femoral fractures with an intact isthmus. Over-reaming of the isthmus to 1.5–2.0 mm is recommended in such situations.

If jamming of the nail occurs or repositioning of the nail is needed, the nail is retracted by using the repositioning adaptor, which fits into the hole in the targeting device (Fig. 9.20) and the extraction shaft with the sliding hammer.

Locking Screws

The most common mode of screw failure is loosening. The cause may be one of the following:

a) The use of screws that are too short.
b) If the fracture has extended to the screw hole or new fracture has developed during screw hole preparation.
c) Osteoporotic bone where the standard screw may not be able to purchase well into the far cortex. The use of Vécsei spreading screws (Fig. 9.21) may help to increase the purchase, by increasing the anchorage of the screw into the screw hole of the nail. This will prevent the backing out of the screws and help to maintain fixation.

Unslotted Nails

Unslotted nails have a smaller diameter than slotted nails. The torsional rigidity is almost 20 times that of the slotted nail, which ensures that the mechanical properties are comparable even though the diameter is smaller [37]. Owing to their rigidity and smaller diameter, the difficulty of insertion and distal targeting is increased. Over-reaming to at least 2 mm is recommended. Extra caution must be taken in preventing iatrogenic fractures during insertion, as the nail is less yielding [3]. Proximal locking is done with the same drill (colour code: black) and the same screw as with the slotted nail while in distal lock-

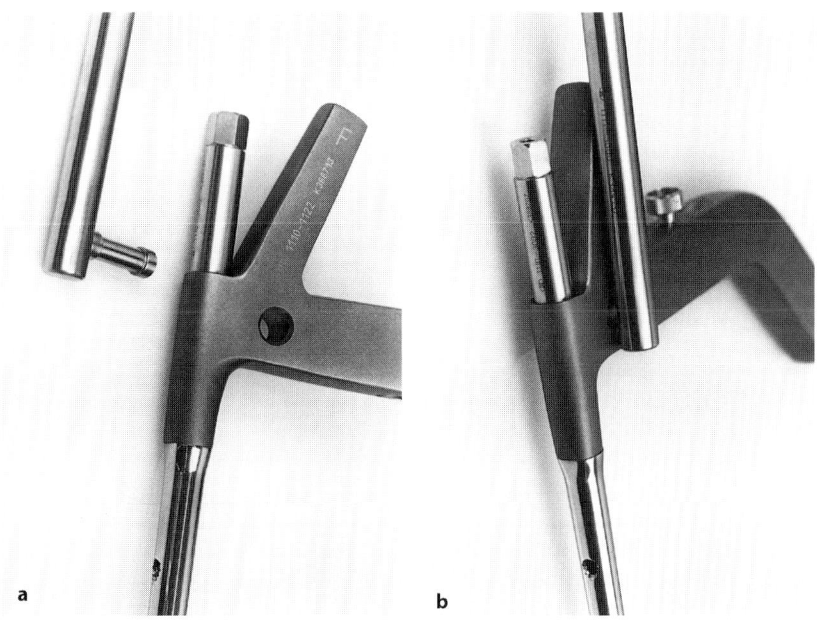

a b

Fig. 9.20 a, b. The use of the repositioning adaptor hooked **a** onto the proximal targeting device **b** for retraction of nail during insertion of the nail

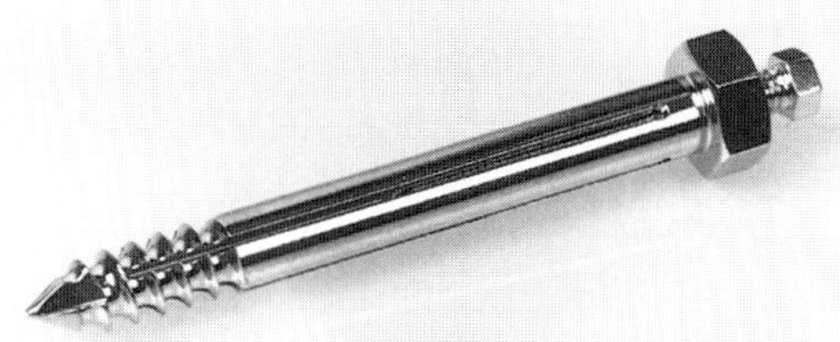

a

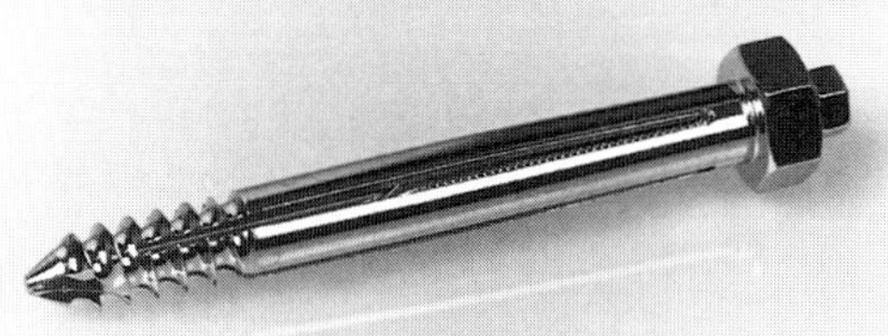

b

Fig. 9.21 a, b. The Vécsei spreading screws **a** for osteoporotic bone fixation and **b** spread

ing. A smaller drill bit (3.7 mm) (colour code: yellow) and smaller screws (4.6 mm) are used.

Unslotted nails are indicated in patients with a smaller medullary canal. They also provide additional advantages in open fractures, where they can be inserted with or without reaming in patients with a normal canal diameter. Bearing the weight while walking is not recommended prior to good callus formation. Dynamisation may be indicated in fractures fixed with unslotted nails.

Open Fractures

All grades of open fractures in the femur can be safely treated with intramedullary locked nails, which provide excellent skeletal stability for the early management of soft tissue injuries [11, 20]. The very vascular muscular envelope provides an excellent environment for controlling infection and fracture healing. All nails should be *static locked* and the principles of management for open fracture should always be strictly followed.

Post-nailing Infection

To maintain the fracture, stability is vital to combat infection in the medullary cavity. Infection should be treated energetically with intravenous antibiotic(s), to which the bacteria are sensitive. Collection of infected discharge should be drained surgically. The intramedullary locked nail should not be removed. If the infection cannot be controlled with conservative means, exchange nailing after thorough intramedullary debridement should be performed. Again, the *static locked* configuration is recommended (see Chap. 14, this volume) [24, 45].

Nailing Abnormal Femoral Canal

In patients with previous pathologies in the femur, the medullary canal may be occluded. It is recommended that the medullary cavity should be carefully opened with a pointed guide, and then reaming should follow. The use of a long drill bit may be helpful in opening the medullary cavity. This will facilitate the passage of the reaming guide rod for proper reaming procedure.

References

1. Alho A, Stromsoe K, Ekeland A (1991) Locked intramedullary nailing of femoral shaft fractures. J Trauma 31:49–59
2. Alho A, Ekeland A, Stromsoe K (1992) Femoral shaft fractures in the elderly treated with Grosse-Kempf slotted locked intramedullary nail. Ann Chir Gynaecol 81:366–371
3. Alho A, Moen O, Husby T, Ronningen H, Skjeldal S (1992) Slotted versus non-slotted locked intramedullary nailing for femoral shaft fractures. Arch Orthop Trauma Surg 111:91–95
4. Beaty JH, Austin SM, Warner WC, Canale ST, Nichols L (1994) Interlocking intramedullary nailing of femoral-shaft fractures in adolescents: preliminary results and complications. J Pediatr Orthop 14:178–183
5. Bednar DA, Ali P (1993) Intramedullary nailing of femoral shaft fractures: reoperation and return to work. Can J Surg 36:464–466
6. Benirschke SK, Melder I, Henley MB, Routt ML, Smith DG, Chapman JR, Swiontkowski MF (1993) Closed interlocking nailing of femoral shaft fractures: assessment of technical complications and functional outcomes by comparison of a prospective database with retrospective review. J Orthop Trauma 7:118–122
7. Bråten M, Terjesen T, Rossvoll I (1993) Torsional deformity after intramedullary nailing of femoral shaft fractures. Measurement of anteversion angles in 110 patients. J Bone Joint Surg Br 75:799–803
8. Browner BD (1986) Pitfalls, errors, and complications in the use of locking Küntscher nails. Clin Orthop 212:192–208
9. Brumback RJ, Reilly JP, Poka A, Lakatos RP, Bathon GH, Burgess AR (1988) Intramedullary nailing of femoral shaft fractures. Part I: decision-making errors with interlocking fixation. J Bone Joint Surg Am 70:1441–1452

10. Brumback RJ, Uwagie-Ero S, Lakatos RP, Poka A, Bathon GH, Burgess AR (1988) Intramedullary nailing of femoral shaft fractures. Part II: Fracture-healing with static interlocking fixation. J Bone Joint Surg Am 70:1453–1462
11. Brumback RJ, Ellison Jr PS, Poka A, Lakatos R, Bathon GH, Burgess AR (1989) Intramedullary nailing of open fractures of the femoral shaft. J Bone Joint Surg Am 71:1324–1331
12. Brumback RJ, Wells JD, Lakatos R, Poka A, Bathon GH, Burgess AR (1990) Heterotopic ossification about the hip after intramedullary nailing for fractures of the femur. J Bone Joint Surg Br 72:1067–1073
13. Brumback RJ, Ellison TS, Poka A, Bathon GH, Burgess AR (1992) Intramedullary nailing of femoral shaft fractures. Part III: Long-term effects of static interlocking fixation. J Bone Joint Surg Am 74:106–112
14. Brumback RJ, Ellison TS, Molligan H, Molligan DJ, Mahaffet S, Schmidhauser C (1992) Pudendal nerve palsy complicating intramedullary nailing of the femur. J Bone Joint Surg Am 74:1450–1455
15. Cameron CD, Meek RN, Blachut PA, O'Brien PJ, Pate GC (1992) Intramedullary nailing of the femoral shaft: a prospective, randomized study. J Orthop Trauma 6:448–451
16. Christie J, Court-Brown C, Kinninmonth AW, Howie CR (1988) Intramedullary locking nails in the management of femoral shaft fractures. J Bone Joint Surg Br 70:206–210
17. Coetzee JC, van der Merwe EJ (1992) Exposure of surgeons-in-training to radiation during intramedullary fixation of femoral shaft fractures. S Afr Med J 81:312–314
18. Costa P, Carretti P, Giancecchi F, Pignedoli P, Rotini R, Tartaglia I (1988) The locked Grosse-Kempf intramedullary nail in the treatment of diaphyseal and metaphyseal fractures of the femur and tibia. Ital J Orthop Traumatol 14:475–482
19. Graham GP, Mackie IG (1988) Experience with the A.O. locking femoral nail. Injury 19:249–253
20. Grosse A, Christie J, Taglang G, Court-Brown C, McQueen M (1993) Open adult femoral shaft fracture treated by early intramedullary nailing. J Bone Joint Surg Br 75:562–565
21. Grover J, Wiss DA (1995) A prospective study of fractures of the femoral shaft treated with a static, intramedullary, interlocking nail comparing one versus two distal screws. Orthop Clin North Am 26:139–146
22. Hajek PD, Bicknell Jr HR, Bronson WE, Albright JA, Saha S (1993) The use of one compared with two distal screws in the treatment of femoral shaft fractures with interlocking intramedullary nailing. A clinical and biomechanical analysis. J Bone Joint Surg Am 75:519–525
23. Hanks GA, Foster WC, Cardea JA (1988) Treatment of femoral shaft fractures with the Brooker-Wills interlocking intramedullary nail. Clin Orthop 226:206–218
24. Jenny JY, Jenny G, Kempf I (1994) Infection after reamed intramedullary nailing of lower limb fractures. A review of 1,464 cases over 15 years. Acta Orthop Scand 65:94–96
25. Johnson KD, Johnston DW, Parker B (1984) Comminuted femoral-shaft fractures: treatment by roller traction, cerclage wires and an intramedullary nail, or an interlocking intramedullary nail. J Bone Joint Surg Am 66:1222–1235
26. Johnson KD, Tencer AF, Blumenthal S, August A, Johnston DW (1986) Biomechanical performance of locked intramedullary nail systems in comminuted femoral shaft fractures. Clin Orthop 206:151–161
27. Johnson KD, Tencer AF, Sherman MC (1987) Biomechanical factors affecting fracture stability and femoral bursting in closed intramedullary nailing of femoral shaft fractures, with illustrative case presentations. J Orthop Trauma 1:1–11
28. Kao JT, Burton D, Comstock C, McClellan RT, Carragee E (1993) Pudendal nerve palsy after femoral intramedullary nailing. J Orthop Trauma 7:58–63
29. Kempf I, Grosse A, Beck (1985) Closed locked intramedullary nailing. Its application to comminuted fractures of the femur. J Bone Joint Surg Am 67:709–720
30. Kempf I, Grosse A, Taglang G, Bernhard L, Moui Y (1991) Interlocking central medullary nailing of recent femoral and tibial fractures. Statistical study apropos of 835 cases. Chirurgie 117:5–6, 478–487
31. Keogh P, Maher M, EcElwain J (1991) Grosse-Kempf intramedullary nailing of femoral fractures. Ir Med J 84:59–61
32. Keret D, Harcke HT, Mendez AA, Bowen JR (1990) Heterotopic ossification in central nervous system-injured patients following closed nailing of femoral fractures. Clin Orthop 256:254–259
33. Khan FA, Ikram MA, Badr AA, al-Khawashki H (1995) Femoral neck fracture: a complication of femoral nailing. Injury 26:319–321
34. Klingler K, Käch K, Eberle H (1989) Indications and results of interlocking nailing of the femur. Helv Chir Acta 56:79–83
35. Kraemer WJ, Hearn TC, Powell JN, Mahomed N (1996) Fixation of segmental subtrochanteric fractures. A biomechanical study. Clin Orthop 332:71–79
36. Kyle RF, Schaffhausen JM, Bechtold JE (1991) Biomechanical characteristics of interlocking femoral nails in the treatment of complex femoral fractures. Clin Orthop 267:169–173
37. Laforest P, Karger C, Boudlama F, Taglang G, Grosse A, Kempf I (1995) Mechanical performance of non slotted small diameter nails of Gross and Kempf. Rev Chir Orthop Reparatrice Appar Mot 80:36–43
38. Levin PE, Schoen Jr RW, Browner BD (1987) Radiation exposure to the surgeon during closed interlocking intramedullary nailing. J Bone Joint Surg Am 69:761–766
39. Lowdon IM, Williamson DM, Nelson IW, Cockin J (1989) Technical considerations of the AO interlocking nail. Injury 20:222–225
40. Müller LP, Suffner J, Wenda K, Mohr W, Rudig L (1996) Radiation burden to the hands of surgeons in intramedullary nailing. Unfallchirurgie 22:253–259
41. Majkowski RS, Baker AS (1991) Interlocking nails for femoral fractures: an initial experience. Injury 22:93–96
42. Marks PH, Paley D, Kellam JF (1998) Heterotopic ossification around the hip with intramedullary nailing of the femur. J Trauma 28:1207–1213
43. Miller SD, Burkart B, Damson E, Shrive N, Bray RC (1993) The effect of the entry hole for an intramedullary nail on the strength of the proximal femur. J Bone Joint Surg Br 75:202–206
44. Ostrum RF (1996) A greater trochanteric insertion site for femoral intramedullary nailing in lipomatous patients. Orthopedics 19:337–340
45. Patzakis MJ, Wilkins J, Wiss DA (1986) Infection following intramedullary nailing of long bones. Diagnosis and management. Clin Orthop 212:182–191
46. Peyser A, Libergall M, Mosheiff R, Segal D (1991) Interlocked intramedullary nailing of the femoral shaft. Harefuah 121:511–515
47. Rüedi T (1990) Intramedullary nailing with interlocking. Arch Orthop Trauma Surg 109:317–320
48. Richards RR, Waddell JP, Sullivan TR, Ashworth MA, Rorabeck CH (1984) Infra-isthmal fractures of the femur: a review of 82 cases. J Trauma 24:735–741
49. Simonian PT, Chapman JR, Selznick HS, Benirschke SK, Claudi BF, Swiontkowski MF (1994) Iatrogenic fractures of the femoral neck during closed nailing of the femoral shaft. J Bone Joint Surg Br 76:293–296
50. Thoresen BO, Alho A, Ekeland A, Stromsoe K, Folleràs G, Haukebo A (1985) Interlocking intramedullary nailing in femoral shaft fractures. A report of forty-eight cases. J Bone Joint Surg Am 67:1313–1320

51. Vécsei V, Häupl J (1989) The value of dynamic adjustment in locking intramedullary nailing. Aktuel Traumatol 19:162–168
52. White GM, Healy WL, Brumback RJ, Burgess AR, Brooker AF (1986) The treatment of fractures of the femoral shaft with the Brooker-wills distal locking intramedullary nail. J Bone Joint Surg Am 68:865–876
53. Wilson-MacDonald J, Owen JW, Lowdon I, Fergusson CM (1987) Early experience with closed interlocking medullary nailing of the femur. Injury 18:390–395
54. Winquist RA, Hansen Jr ST (1980) Comminuted fractures of the femoral shaft treated by intramedullary nailing. Orthop Clin North Am 11:633–648
55. Winquist RA, Hansen Jr ST, Clawson DK (1984) Closed intramedullary nailing of femoral fractures. A report of five hundred and twenty cases. J Bone Joint Surg Am 66:529–539
56. Wiss DA, Brien WW (1992) Subtrochanteric fractures of the femur. Results of treatment by interlocking nailing. Clin Orthop 283:231–236
57. Wiss DA, Fleming CH, Matta JM, Clark D (1986) Comminuted and rotationally unstable fractures of the femur treated with an interlocking nail. Clin Orthop 212:35–47
58. Wiss DA, Brien WW, Stetson WB (1990) Interlocked nailing for treatment of segmental fractures of the femur. J Bone Joint Surg Am 72:724–728
59. Wolf H, Schauwecker F, Tittel K (1984) Malrotation following intramedullary nailing of the femur. Unfallchirurgie 10:133–136
60. Wu CC, Shih CH (1993) Effect of dynamization of a static interlocking nail on fracture healing. Can J Surg 36:302–306
61. Wu CC, Shih CH, Chen YJ (1989) Adult femoral shaft fracture treated with an intramedullary nail. Chang Keng I Hsueh 12:141–147
62. Wu CC, Shih CH, Lee ZL (1991) Subtrochanteric fractures treated with interlocking nailing. J Trauma 31:326–333
63. Zuckerman JD, Veith RG, Johnson KD, Bach AW, Hansen ST, Solvik S (1987) Treatment of unstable femoral shaft fractures with closed interlocking intramedullary nailing. J Orthop Trauma 1:209–218

CHAPTER 10

Tibial Fractures

K.S. Leung

Tibial fractures can be treated with cast, functional bracing and operative treatment. Operative treatment is indicated in unstable fractures, open fractures and tibial fractures in polytraumatised patients and patients with multiple fractures [1, 2, 7, 14]. With operative treatment, closed intramedullary nailing is the preferred method for most of the diaphyseal fractures as the soft tissue envelope of the tibia is not as forgiving as that in the femur. Conventional intramedullary fixation without locking in tibial fractures is indicated in the middle third of fractures with bony cortical contact, i.e. stable fractures [7, 9]. These include transverse fractures and short oblique fractures. The locked intramedullary nail is indicated in unstable fractures with comminution or long spiral fracture patterns. Fractures in more proximal or distal regions can also be treated with locked intramedullary nails. In open fractures, the locked intramedullary nail also provides better mechanical stability for early soft tissue handling. The introduction of locked intramedullary nails broadens the applications of closed intramedullary fixation for tibial fractures.

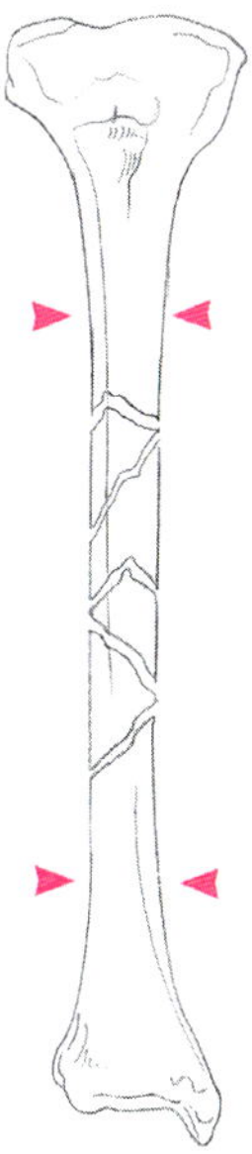

Fig. 10.1. The intramedullary locked nail is indicated in unstable fractures occurring in the middle 60% of the tibia. With slight modification of the technique, more distal fractures may also be treated with this technique

Indications

The intramedullary locked nail is indicated in unstable fracture occurring in the middle 60% of the tibia (Fig. 10.1). Fractures with butterfly fragments, long spiral fractures, metaphyseal fractures, pathological fractures, segmental fractures, comminuted fractures and fractures with bone loss are now best treated with locked intramedullary nailing. Extended indications for the use of intramedullary locked nails may include proximal and distal fractures, open fractures, delayed or non-union [2–4, 7, 13, 14].

Pre-operative Preparation

Evaluation

Patients suffering from acute trauma must be stabilised. Associated injuries, complications, particularly neurovascular damage, compartment syndrome and fat embolism, must be identified and managed accordingly with priority. The injured limb is splinted temporarily and elevated to decrease swelling while waiting for operation. Plain radiography of the injured limb is taken, including the joint proximally and distally. Proximal and distal propagation of the fracture lines must be looked for carefully with good quality films. In cases where there is significant shortening and deformity, a radiograph of the opposite leg is taken for accurate assessment of the length.

An open fracture requires early operative treatment according to the principles of open fracture management.

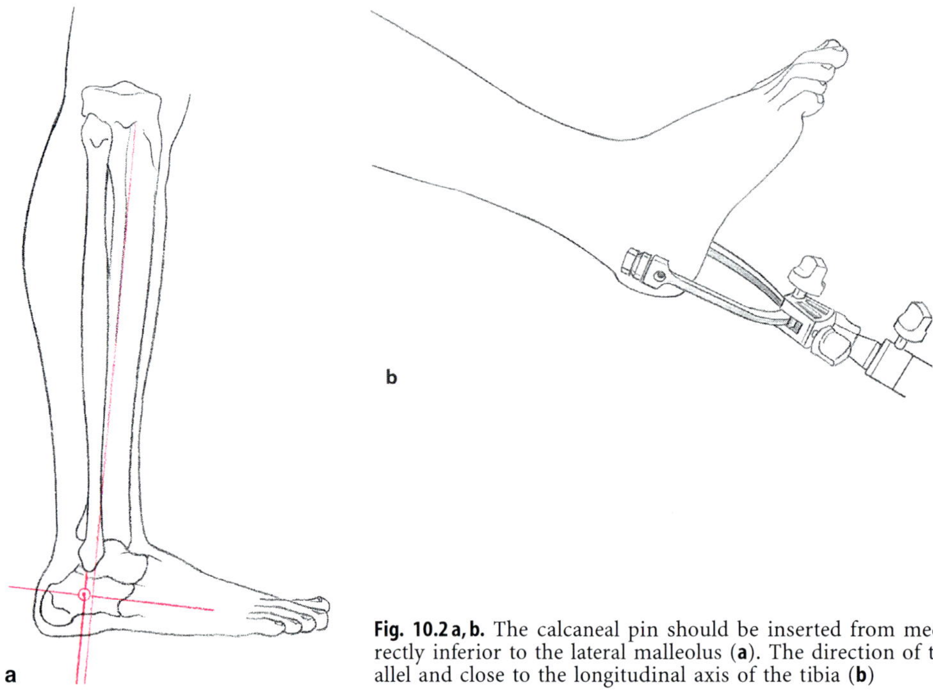

Fig. 10.2 a, b. The calcaneal pin should be inserted from medial to lateral, 2 cm directly inferior to the lateral malleolus (**a**). The direction of the traction will be parallel and close to the longitudinal axis of the tibia (**b**)

Timing

Timing of the operation depends on the general condition of the patient and the local soft tissue status. Although there is no absolute contra-indication for intramedullary fixation of fractures with significant soft tissue injury, other complications of soft tissue injury must be treated with priority. Early fixation decreases morbidity, decreases mortality, facilitates nursing care and speeds rehabilitation.

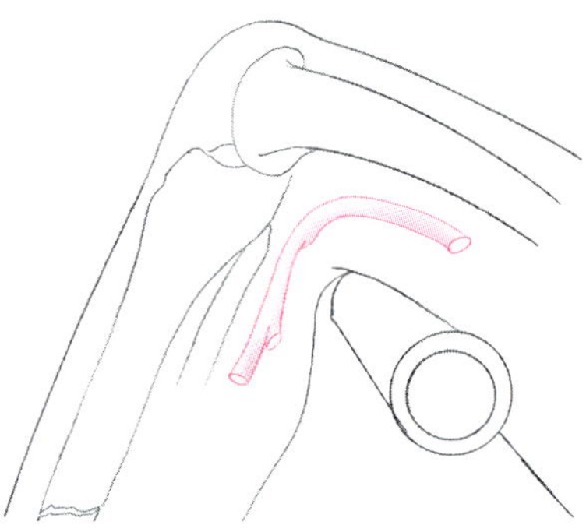

Fig. 10.3. The knee rest should be placed against the distal thigh to provide counter traction without creating pressure against the popliteal neurovascular bundle

Operative Technique

Positioning and Anaesthesia

The operation can be performed under either spinal or general anaesthesia. The patient is placed supine on an orthopaedic traction table. Skeletal traction on the injured limb is provided by a calcaneal pin inserted from the medial to the lateral direction after the patient is anaesthetised (Fig. 10.2). The calcaneal pin should be inserted 2 cm posterior and 2 cm inferior to the lateral malleolus to counteract the pull of the calf muscles. In cases where distal locking is not indicated, traction applied through the foot piece without skeletal traction may be sufficient to control the length and rotatory deformity. Proximally, the knee is supported by a well-padded knee rest placed against the distal part of the posterior thigh which provides counter traction (Figs. 10.3, 10.4). Care must be taken not to put the knee rest against the popliteal fossa, as this causes compression on the neurovascular bundle and displacing the proximal fragment anteriorly. It will also push the neurovascular bundle anteriorly and increase the risk of injury during drilling of the sagittal proximal locking screw [6]. The two knee guards are put against the femoral condyles to prevent rotation (Fig. 10.5). The knee is then flexed to about 90° and the calcaneal Steinmann pin attached to the traction system via an adaptive stirrup (Fig. 10.6). Inadequate flexion brings the inferior pole of patella into the operative field and

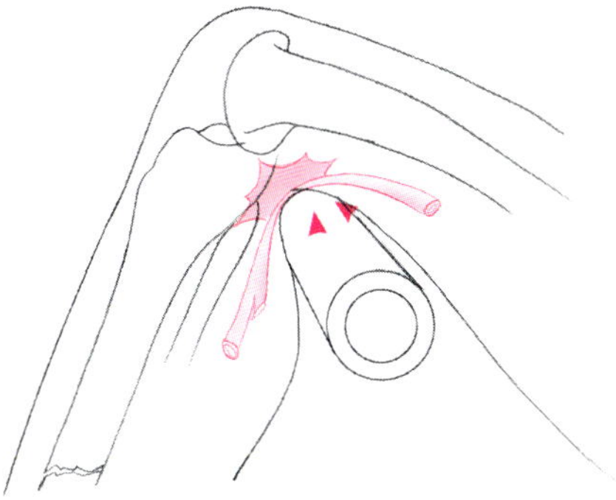

Fig. 10.4. Incorrectly placed knee rest against the popliteal fossa displaces and compresses the neurovascular bundle

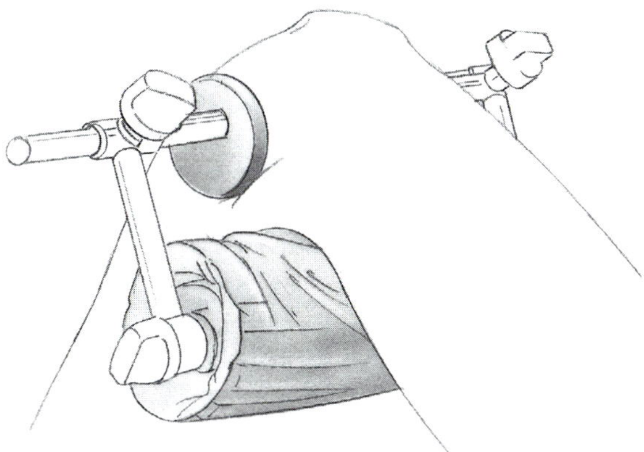

Fig. 10.5. The knee guards are placed against the femoral condyles to control rotation. They must not compress on the fibular neck causing peroneal nerve neuropraxia

makes it difficult to access the medullary cavity (Fig. 10.7 a). Increasing the knee flexion will facilitate instrumentation and nail insertion but makes imaging of the proximal tibia difficult (Fig. 10.7 b). A compromise in the degree of the knee flexion must be made and confirmed with the C-arm positioning.

The entry to the medullary cavity must be through the tibial tuberosity in the postero-inferior direction.

The contralateral limb is supported on a leg rest and kept out of the way by flexion, with abduction at the hip (Fig. 10.8).

Closed Reduction

Reduction is achieved by longitudinal traction through the calcaneal pin, with adjustment on rotational and varus/valgus forces. Coarse adjustment of the varus/valgus displacements can be made by adjusting the attachment hole on the

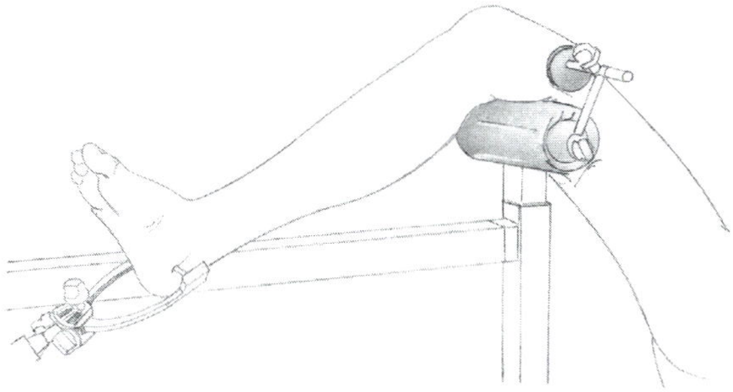

Fig. 10.6. The knee should be flexed to about 90° on the traction system

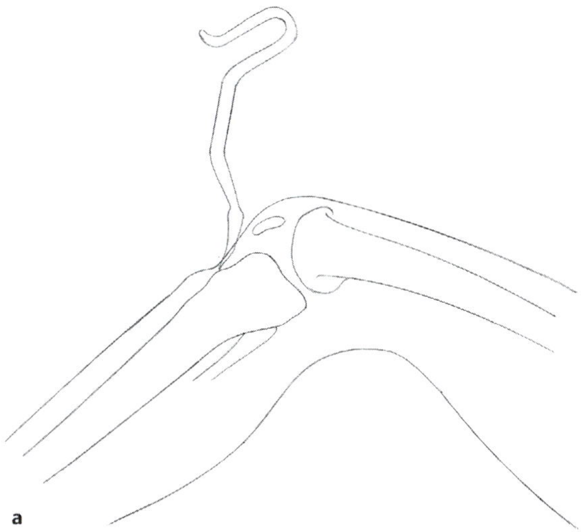

a

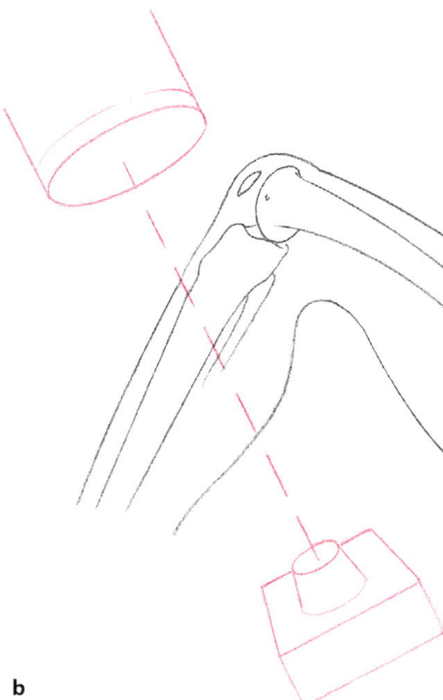

b

Fig. 10.7. a With inadequate flexion, the inferior pole of the patella will obscure the entry point. **b** With excessive flexion, a good anteroposterior X-ray of the proximal tibia cannot be obtained

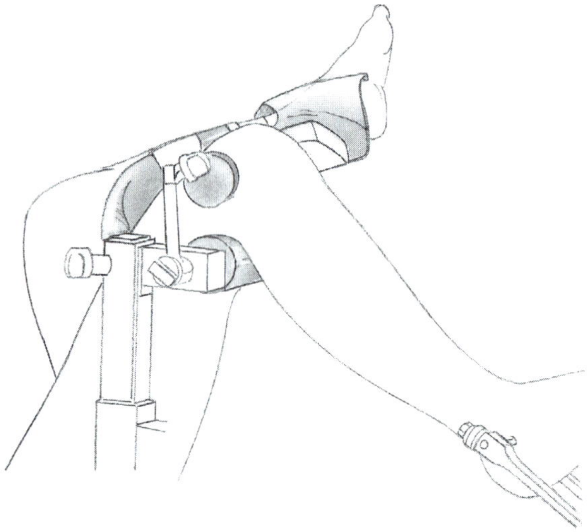

Fig. 10.8. The contralateral limb is positioned on a leg rest with hyperflexion and abduction at the hip

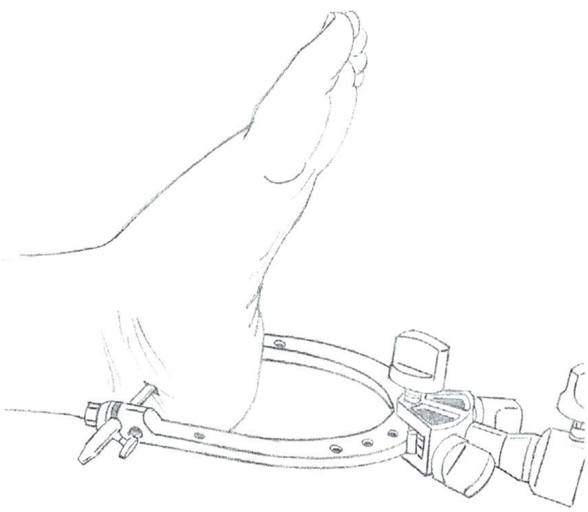

Fig. 10.9. Varus/valgus can be adjusted by changing the attachment position on the stirrup

stirrup (Fig. 10.9) and on traction forces by adjusting the traction device of the traction table. Fine adjustment of the varus and valgus displacement can be achieved with the two adjustment screws on each side of the traction device. As the anteromedial surface of the tibia is subcutaneous, palpation along the surface usually gives a good guide to the reduction. Aligning the second toe to the tibial tuberosity serves as a good guideline for correcting the rotational deformity.

As in all closed techniques, fracture reduction should be achieved as anatomically as possible.

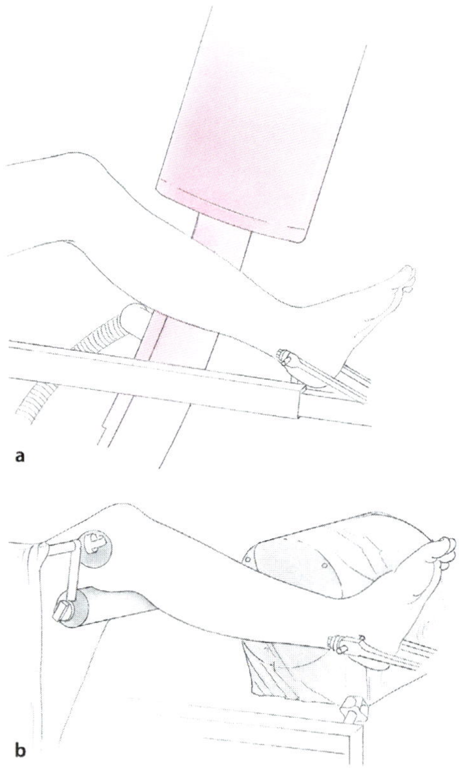

Fig. 10.10 a, b. Positioning the C-arm on the lateral side allows easy interchange between anteroposterior (**a**) and lateral (**b**) imaging

X-ray Control

Either one-plane or a two-plane image-intensified fluoroscopic units may be used. The C-arm should be positioned on the lateral side of the patient with the intensifier end on the lateral side for lateral views and on the upper end for anteroposterior views (Fig. 10.10 a, b). This should be checked before draping so that the whole tibia can be imaged in both planes without interference from either the contralateral limb or the traction bars. It should also be possible to swing the C-arm perpendicular to the leg to give true anteroposterior and true lateral images (see the section on positioning). Care should be taken to ensure the proximal tibia can be imaged properly.

Draping and Sterilisation

The whole tibia should be exposed and sterilised. The proximal drape wraps round the knee rest and knee guards, exposing the whole patella. The distal drape wraps round the calcaneal pin, giving access to distal tibia. Additional large side drapes

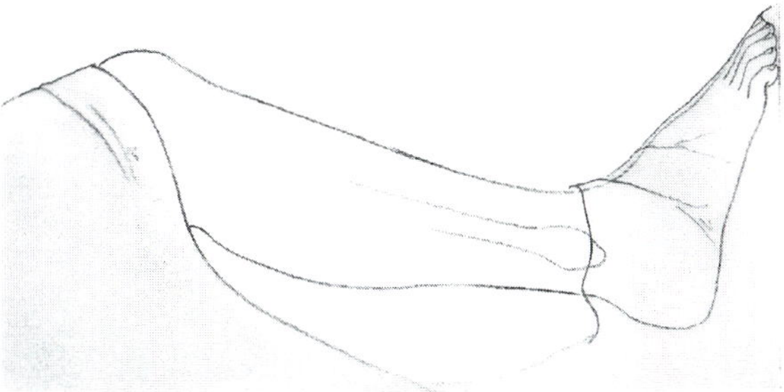

Fig. 10.11. The surgical field is draped to allow access to the entry point, proximal locking and distal locking sites. Additional large side drapes keep the C-arm covered during manipulation

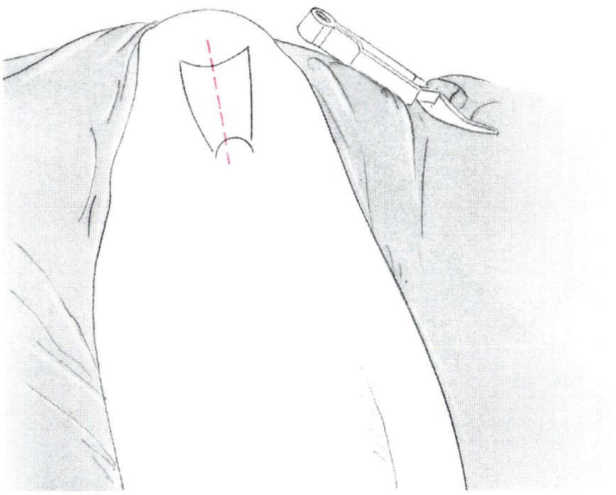

Fig. 10.12. Mid-line skin incision

are set up to keep the C-arm covered when it is positioned into the lateral position (Fig. 10.11).

Incision and Entry Point

A mid-line longitudinal incision is made over the patellar tendon (Fig. 10.12). It extends from the lower pole of the patella to just 10 mm distal to the tibial tuberosity. This gives a better exposure with easy extension proximally or distally where there is a need. A transverse incision midway between the knee joint line and tibial tuberosity may also be used with better cosmetic result.

The patellar tendon is split longitudinally between the lateral two-thirds and the medial one-third to expose the tibial tuberosity (Fig. 10.13). The anterior knee fat pad is gently displaced posteriorly. The insertion of the patellar tendon onto the tibial tuberosity is detached slightly from the midline with a sharp scalpel. The approach to the tibial medullary canal must be extra-articular [6].

An accurate entry point is important to ensure smooth introduction of the nail. The site of entry should be in line with the medullary cavity, which lies slightly medial to the tibial tuberosity (Fig. 10.14). It should not encroach on the tibial plateau [6].

The entry hole is created accurately with a sharp fine awl. It is then enlarged by a reciprocating movement with a pointed curved awl, which is introduced along its curvature so that its handle comes to lie parallel to the tibial shaft (Fig. 10.15). This avoids penetration of the posterior cortex and possible neurovascular damage (Fig. 10.16). This procedure may be facilitated by the use of the two-part curved awl with its conical sleeve designed for easy passage of the reamer guide (Fig. 10.17).

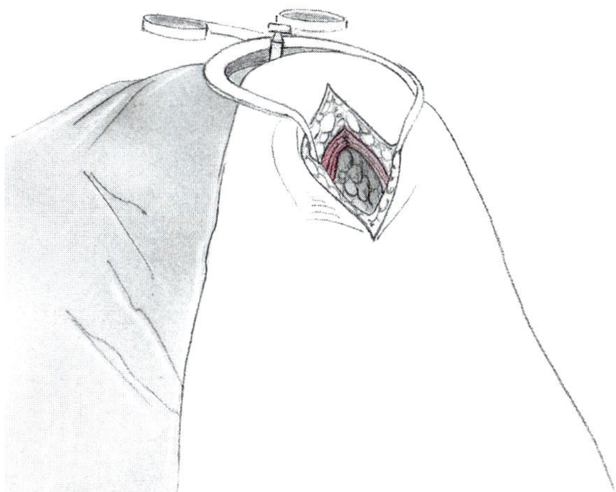

Fig. 10.13. Split patellar approach with partial stripping of the patellar tendon insertion

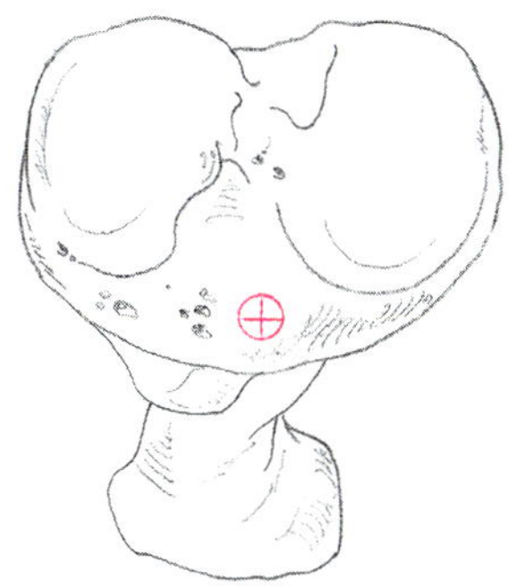

Fig. 10.14. The centre line of the medullary cavity lies slightly medial to the tibial tuberosity

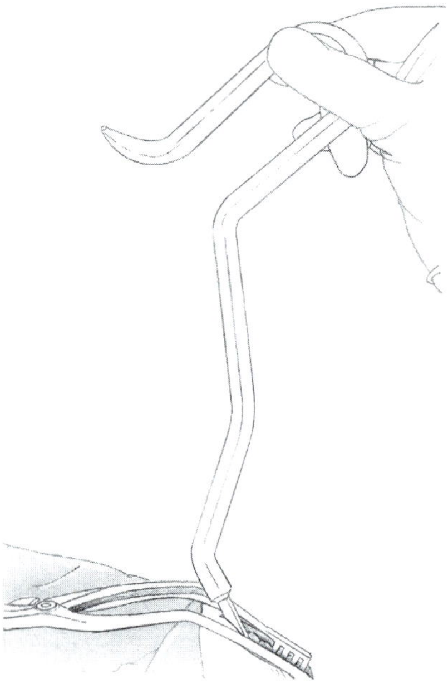

Fig. 10.15. Correct insertion of the curved awl along its curvature

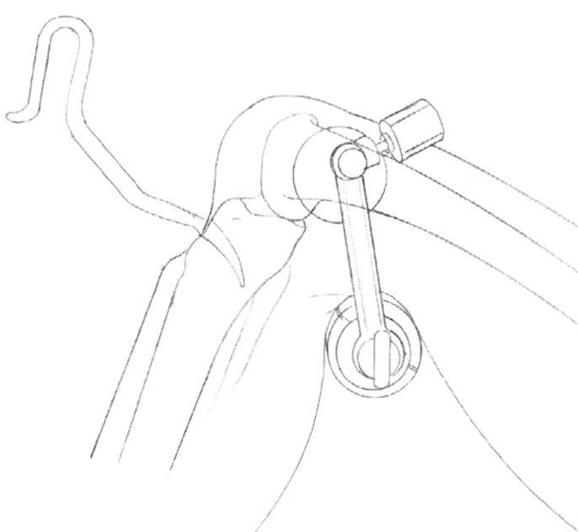

Fig. 10.16. An incorrectly inserted awl may penetrate the posterior cortex and the popliteal neurovascular bundle

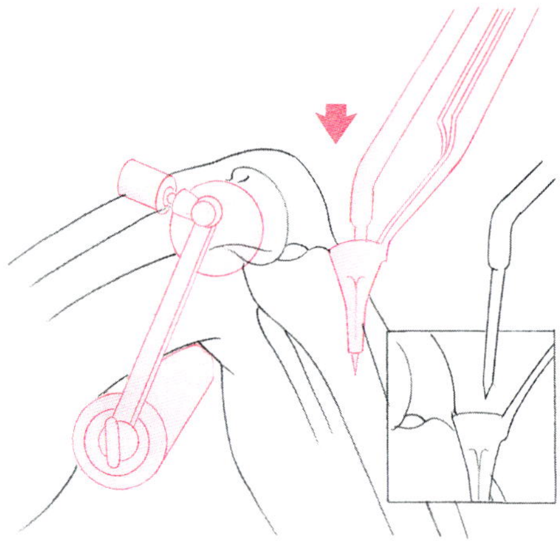

Fig. 10.17. The use of the two-part curved awl facilitates the passage of the reamer guide

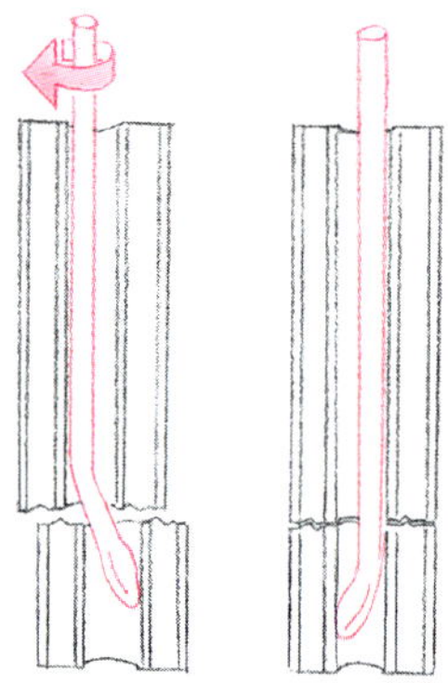

Fig. 10.18. The curved tip of the guide rod can be used to reduce the fragments by rotating the tip in the distal fragment and bringing the ends into alignment

Reamer Guide Rod

The olive-tipped reamer guide rod is introduced along the same curved tract in order to avoid penetrating the posterior cortex. The tip should be prebent to facilitate passage through individual fragments and enable reduction of any translational displacement. The rod is rotated under X-ray guidance to introduce its tip across the fracture site into the distal fragment. Once a secure length has been introduced, the rod is rotated again to achieve reduction (Fig. 10.18). The feeling of the contact of the olive tip with the inner cortex of the bone ensures the proper positioning of the guide and helps to reduce the exposure to X-ray by reducing the need for frequent screening.

The guide rod is then centralised in the subchondral area of the distal tibia in both sagittal and frontal planes (Fig. 10.19a,b). Eccentric placement may lead to uneven reaming and possible malalignment. At this stage the length of the nail to be inserted should be determined. By placing a calibrated nail guide beside the reamer guide, ensuring that its tip is in the entry point in the tibial tuberosity, the correct length of the nail can then be determined by subtracting the protruded reamer guide length from the graduated nail guide (Fig. 10.20).

Reaming

Reaming starts with a 9-mm-diameter end-cutting flexible reamer. Use of a tissue protector decreases frictional injury to the surrounding soft tissue, par-

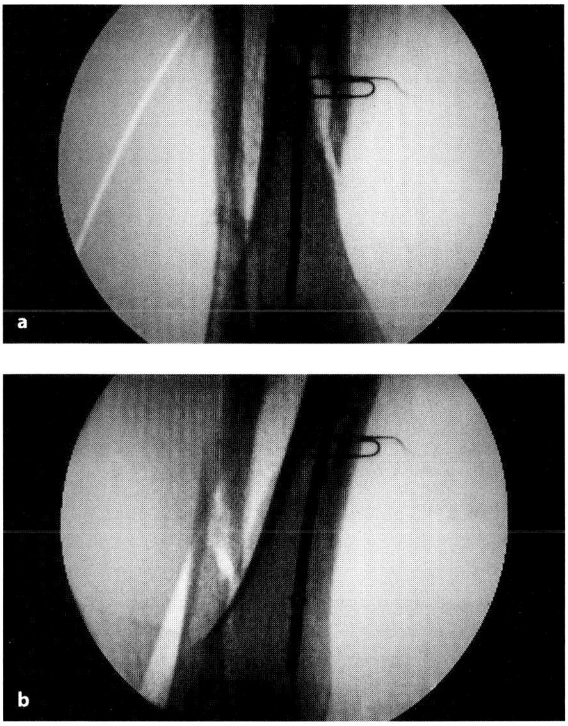

Fig. 10.19 a, b. The guide rod should be centralised in the distal tibia in both the frontal (**a**) and sagittal (**b**) planes

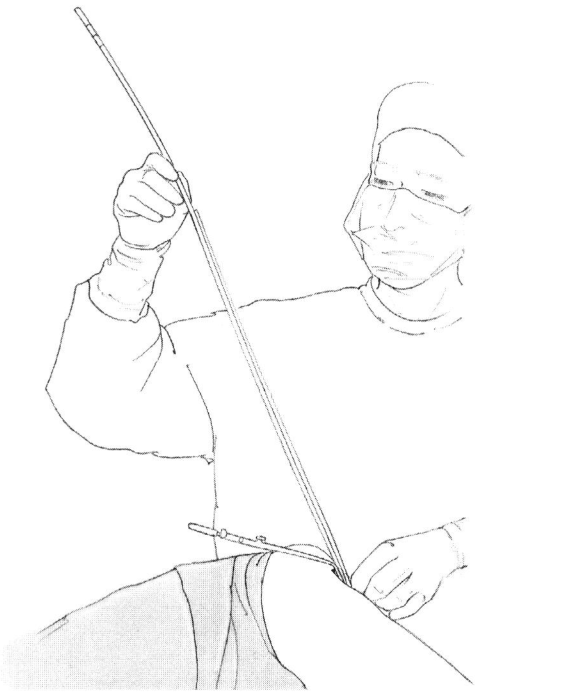

Fig. 10.20. The nail length is estimated by subtracting the protruded portion of the reamer guide from the length of the graduated nail guide

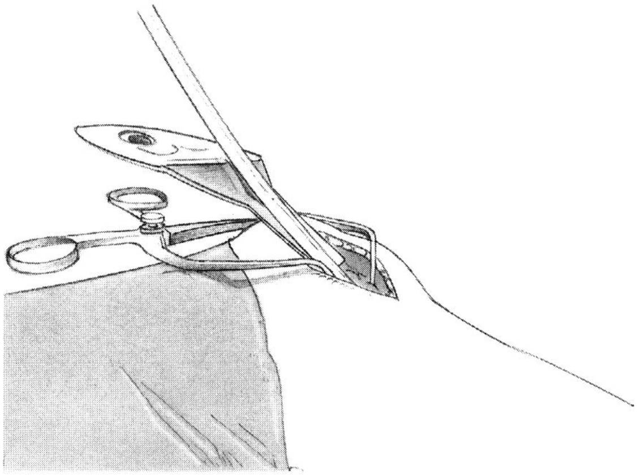

Fig. 10.21. The tissue protector protects the soft tissue and patellar tendon from frictional injury

ticularly of the patellar tendon (Fig. 10.21). Reaming should only be started when the reamer head is fully inserted into the medullary canal. The reamer should be passed following the curvature of the passage created in the proximal tibia (Fig. 10.22). Reaming in 0.5-mm increments is continued until 1.5–2.0 mm larger than the chosen nail diameter. Reaming should be done with minimal pushing and without excessive pressure. Repeating the reaming with the same reamer head should be done whenever there is resistance in the reaming process. The assistant should hold the guide rod with the guide rod holder throughout the process so as to avoid displacement of the guide rod, especially when the reamer is being extracted (Fig. 10.23). If the reamer guide is dislodged, it must be correctly replaced and its position checked radiologically prior to the next reaming procedure.

Nail Insertion

The curved olive-tipped reamer guide rod must be exchanged for a straight nail guide rod before insertion of the nail. This is done with a Teflon tube which is passed along the curved reamer guide to its end (Fig. 10.24). The reamer guide is then removed, leaving the Teflon tube in place. The straight nail guide rod can now be easily passed through the tube and the tube removed. The position of the nail guide is then checked with the C-arm.

The nail with the chosen diameter and length is mounted onto the driving device by tightening the nail-holding bolt with a socket wrench (Fig. 10.25). The nail is then introduced over the nail guide rod which protrudes posteriorly of the nail. The nail is pushed in manually as far as possible

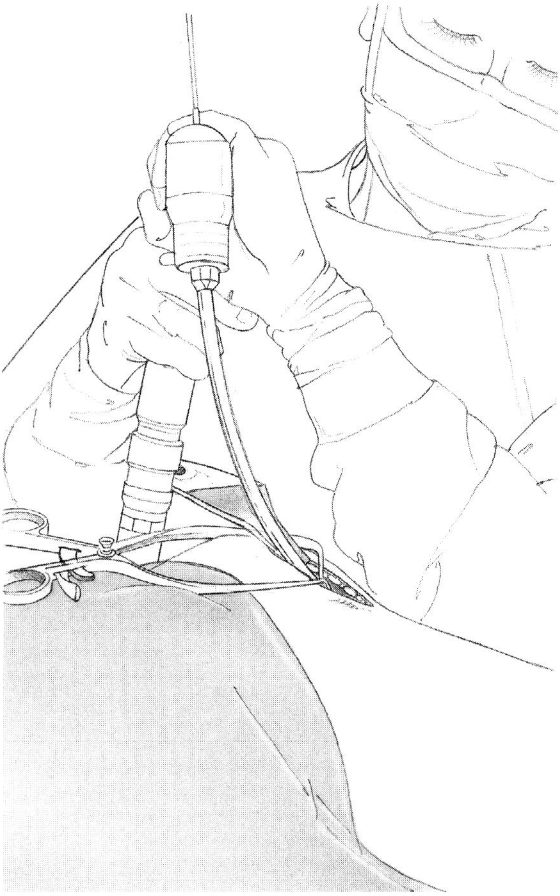

Fig. 10.22. The reamer should be passed along the curved passage created

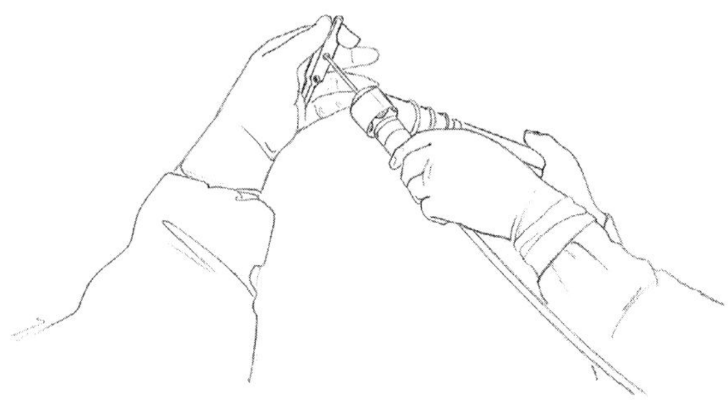

Fig. 10.23. The guide rod may be displaced, especially during removal of the reamer. The assistant must hold the rod in place by holding it with the rod holder

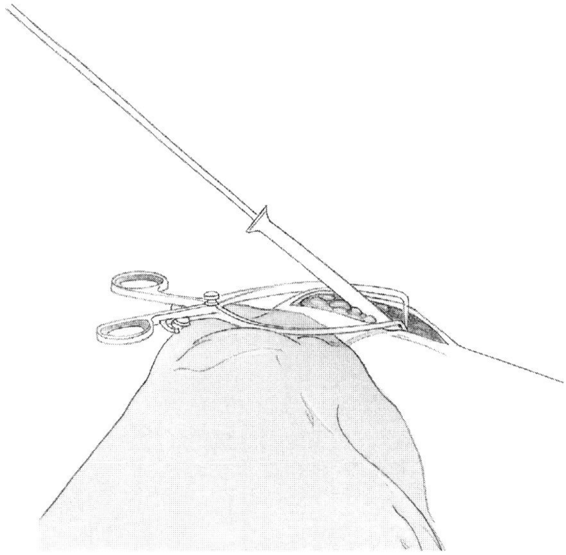

Fig. 10.24. A Teflon tube maintains the tract, allowing exchange of the reamer guide rod with the nail guide rod

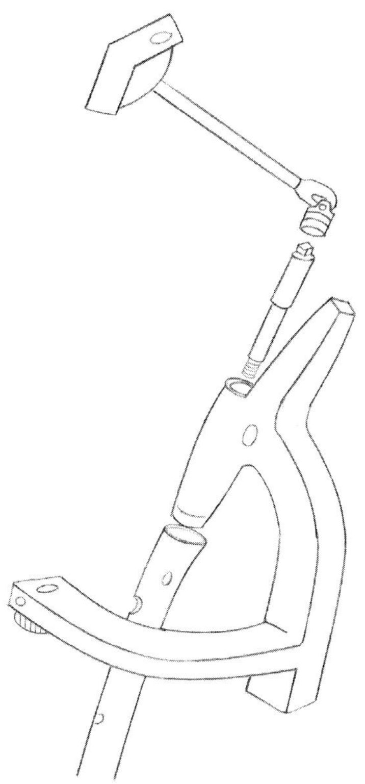

Fig. 10.25. The mounting of the nail on the driving/targeting device

before impacting gently with a mallet to its final position in the medullary canal (Fig. 10.26). The tip of the nail should be monitored constantly during insertion.

The nail guide can be removed after the nail has passed through the fracture site or removed during the last 5 cm of insertion. The proximal end of the nail should be inserted flush with the cortex at the entry site. A prominent nail end will cause impingement symptoms and irritation to the patellar tendon post-operatively.

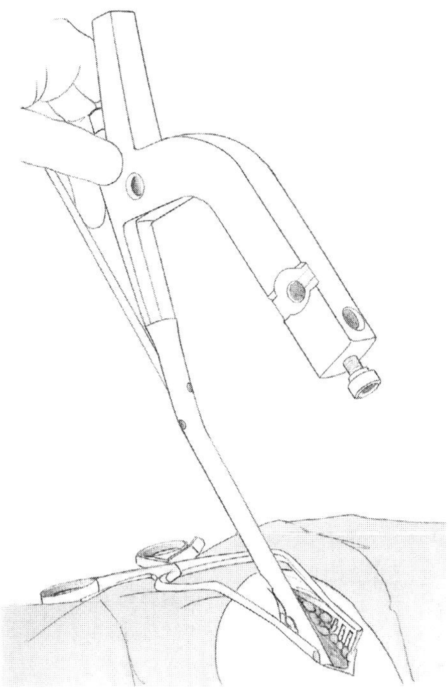

Fig. 10.26. The nail is inserted over the guide rod manually as far as possible

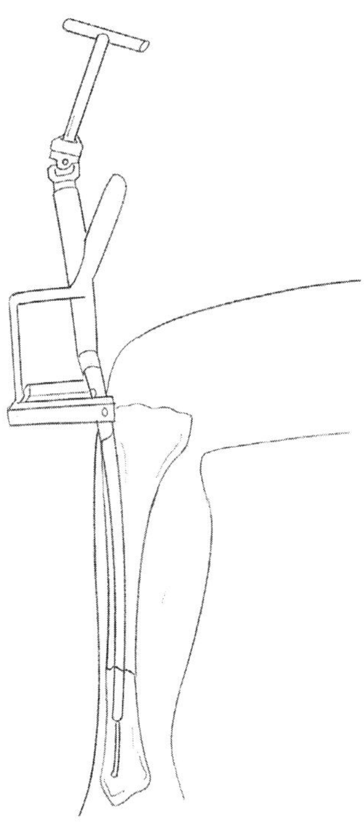

Fig. 10.27. The bolt should be tightened from time to time during hammering and before the targeting procedure to ensure accurate alignment

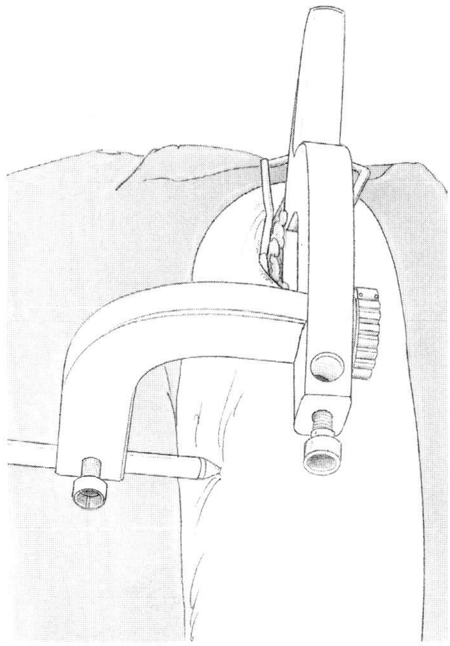

Fig. 10.28. Proximal locking is done through the targeting device

If there is over-distraction at the fracture site, the traction should be released before the final impaction.

Proximal Locking

Proximal locking is indicated in all unstable diaphyseal fractures and fractures in the proximal metaphysis/diaphysis which are rotationally unstable [3, 6, 8].

Always ensure that the nail guide has been removed before commencing the locking procedure.

The nail-holding bolt is tightened to ensure good targeting device alignment (Fig. 10.27). The tissue protector and obturator are put into the proximal sagittal hole and a small skin incision made to enable the sleeve(s) to come into contact with the cortex. The obturator is removed and the tissue protector is held in position by tightening the thumbscrew. A pointed awl pierces the anterior cortex with gentle hammering to ensure accurate drilling. A 3.7-mm drill sleeve (yellow colour code) is screwed into the tissue protector and both the near and the far cortices are drilled with a 3.7-mm drill bit (Fig. 10.28). The guide sleeve is removed and the length of the screw measured with a depth gauge. The required screw length is determined by using the depth gauge through the tissue sleeve. The near cortex is countersunk and the self-tapping 4.6-mm-diameter fully threaded screw of correct length is inserted through the tissue protector into both cortices. Secure purchase of the posterior cortex must be achieved as this gives the best mechanical stability in the proximal tibia.

The proximal transverse screw is inserted with the same technique from the medial surface of the tibia. Both screws should be inserted to give maximum mechanical stability.

The proximal targeting device can be removed. The wound is covered temporarily with saline gauze.

Distal Locking

Distal locking is indicated in all unstable diaphyseal fractures and distal metaphyseal/diaphyseal fractures which are rotationally unstable [3, 6, 8] (see Chap. 8, this volume).

The screws are inserted from the medial surface of the tibia. Care should be taken to avoid injuring the saphenous vein and nerve by retraction after skin incision.

Two 4.6-mm screws must be inserted to prevent rotational deformity and to achieve maximum stability.

Closure

The fixation is checked with the fluoroscopy before the wounds are closed. A proximal plug may be placed at the proximal end of the Grosse-Kempf nail to prevent bone ingrowth.

A drain may be placed in the proximal wound. The patellar tendon should be repaired with absorbable sutures and the skin closed with nylon.

The traction is released and the calcaneal pin removed. A light pressure bandaging is applied to the whole lower limb to control post-operative swelling.

Post-operative Management

The leg is elevated on a pillow or on a Braun's frame. Physical measures are taken to prevent occurrence of deep vein thrombosis, including anticoagulant in high-risk cases. Active movement of the ankles and the toes is encouraged immediately after the operation.

Radiographs are taken to ensure good reduction and stable fixation. In most cases, full weight bearing can be started immediately. Where there is poor bone contact, partial weight bearing is allowed until early callus formation, to decrease the stress on the nail, which could result in possible metal fatigue.

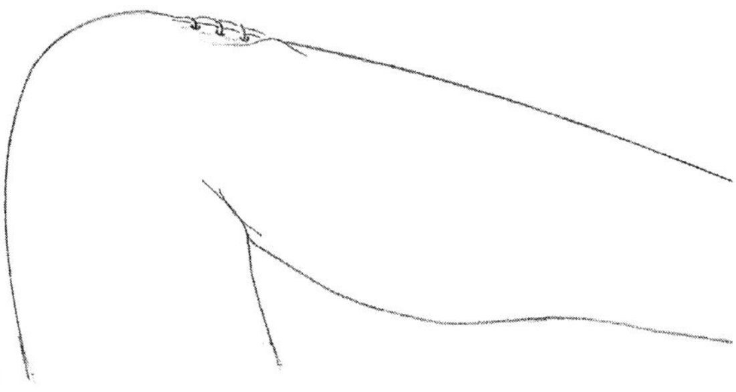

a

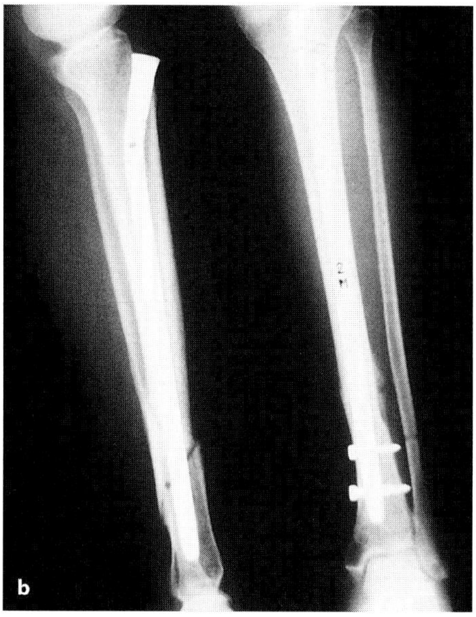

b

Fig. 10.29 a, b. Proximal protrusion of the nail will cause patellar tendon irritation. **a** Clinical illustration of the proximal tibia showing the subcutaneous protrusion of the nail and **b** X-ray film showing the protruded proximal end of the nail

Dynamisation

If delayed union is noted after 4–6 months, the nail may be dynamised by removing the two locking screws furthest away from the fracture site [6]. Removal of the proximal locking screws may lead to proximal protrusion of the nail and cause patellar tendon irritation (Fig. 10.29). It is recommended that whenever possible, the distal locking screws should be removed in the process of dynamisation.

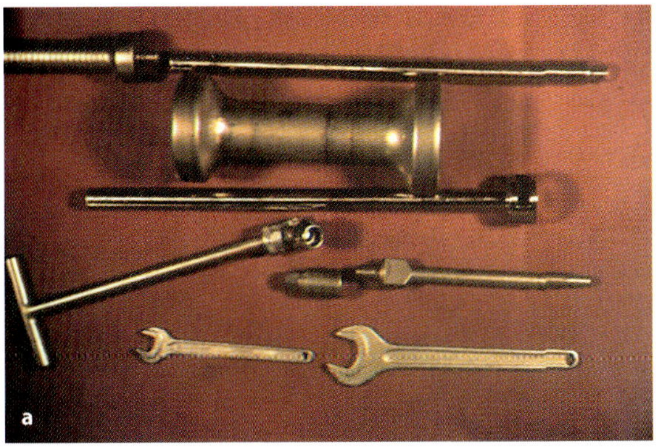

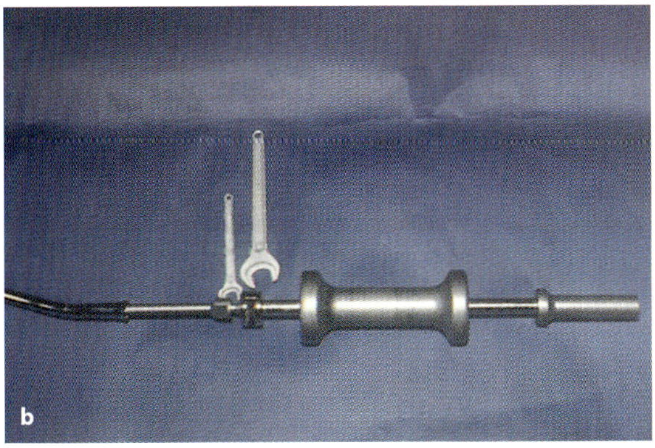

Fig. 10.30. Assembly of the extraction instruments. **a** The instruments for insertion of the extraction bolt and **b** the set-up of the extraction rod

Removal of the Implant

Removal of the implant is indicated when there is constant irritation to the surrounding soft tissue, patellar tendon impingement by the nail, or prominent screw heads. Removal should only be considered when there is clinical and radiological union with good corticalisation of the callus. The usual recommended timing is 2 years after the initial operation.

Both the proximal and distal locking screws are removed as the first step. The proximal nail end is approached as in insertion. Any bony overgrowth obstructing the proximal end of the nail may need to be removed to allow the introduction of the small extraction shaft. To assemble the extraction instruments, the adaptor is screwed onto the small extraction shaft which is then attached into the nail with a 10-mm socket wrench (Fig. 10.30). The adaptor is then removed and the long extraction shaft with a handle is attached to the small extraction shaft. The nail can then be extracted with the sliding hammer.

Errors and Potential Hazards

Positioning

The knee rest should always be put behind the distal femur. It must not be put behind the proximal tibia or in the popliteal fossa as this may cause anterior displacement of the proximal fragment as well as compressing the neurovascular bundle.

The degree of knee flexion should be adjusted to give good imaging with the fluoroscope. Special attention must be given to the imaging of the proximal and distal tibia so that both the anteroposterior and lateral views can be obtained. In many situations, a compromise has to be made between good imaging and easy manipulation of the instruments at the entry site by adjusting the degree of knee flexion and extension. The position should always be secured before proceeding to the operative procedure. Any adjustment of the position during operation may lead to loss of reduction and subsequent malalignment.

Compartment Syndrome

Pre-operative occurrence of compartment syndrome should be treated with fasciotomy before the nailing procedure.

Compartmental pressure may be increased with prolonged operation, excessive traction force for reduction, excessive reaming and concomitant severe soft tissue injury [10]. Compartmental pressure should always be estimated at the end of the nailing procedure. Fasciotomy should be made when there is a definite increase in the compartmental pressure. Prophylactic release is not indicated.

Locking

All locking should be done from the medial side of the tibia. Always put in two proximal locking screws to provide adequate fixation stability. The sagittal screw must have a good purchase in the posterior cortex. As the posterior cortex of the proximal tibia is slanting upwards posteriorly, excessive force in drilling may lead to bending the drill bit, resulting in breakage (Fig. 10.31). Excessive force also leads to loss of fine control and over-penetration of the drill bit into the posterior structures behind the tibia, risking injury to the neurovascular bundle. The use of a sharp drill bit

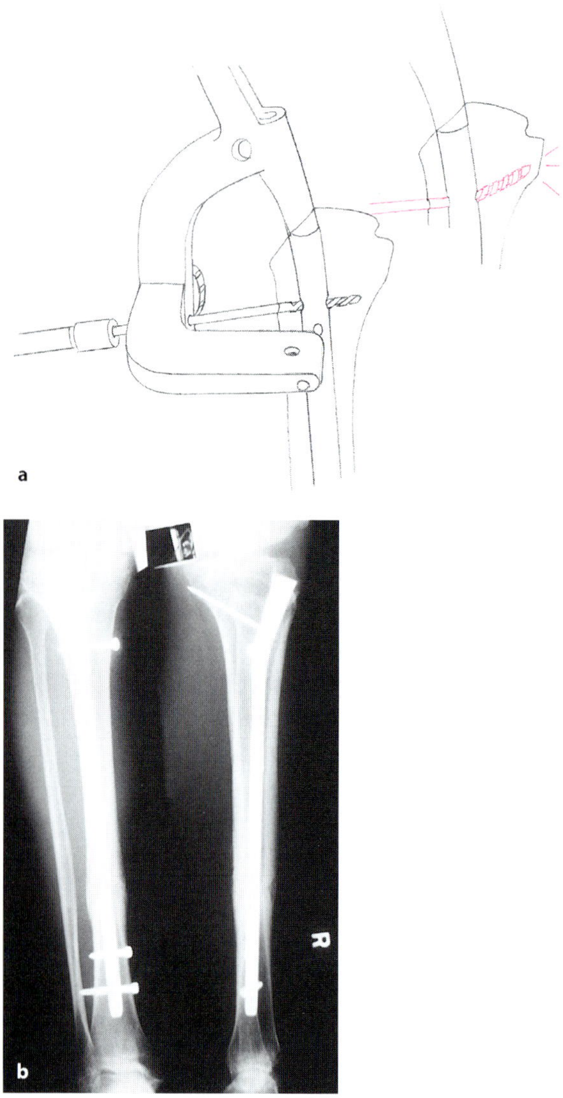

Fig. 10.31 a, b. Excessive force during drilling of the proximal sagittal screw hole in the hard, slanting posterior cortex may cause **a** slippage and **b** breakage of the drill bit

is important for the fine control of drilling in order to prevent complications.

Distal locking also requires two locking screws. The use of the Vecsei screws may be necessary in patients with osteoporotic bone [5] and in very distal fractures where locking has to be done in the distal metaphysis.

Proximal Tibia

The risk of proximal fragment anterior comminution is decreased by flexing the knee to more than 90° and placing the entry point very proximal and medial to the tibial tuberosity, in line with the medullary cavity.

Comminuted Fractures

X-ray of the contralateral tibia should be taken before the operation to estimate the normal tibial length. Reduction is achieved by axial traction, paying attention to correcting the rotational deformity. Bending the tip of the reamer guide helps pass it through the fracture site. During reaming, the reamer must be switched off while passing through the comminution segment. Reaming is resumed in the distal intact segment. Static locking is mandatory. Post-operative weight bearing needs to be graduated. Bone grafting is seldom required as many of the reamed products are dispersed through the fracture site and serve as an autogenous bone graft [8].

Segmental Fractures

During reaming, there is a risk that the intermediate segment may rotate with the reamer, causing periosteal stripping. This is prevented by holding the intermediate fragment percutaneously with a pair of reduction forceps (Fig. 10.32). Static locking should always be done to control rotational instability. Delayed union is common in either of the fracture sites and dynamisation is frequently required in such cases.

Intact Fibula

Tibial fracture associated with an intact fibula may be difficult to reduce. The important step is to reduce the rotatory deformity. The translational deformity can be reduced with the passage of the reamer guide.

Open Fractures

Most open fractures can be treated with the reamed locked nail. The use of unreamed nails may be indicated in highly contaminated open fractures. All fractures must be locked and non-weight-bearing walking must be strictly observed, as the risk of locked screw breakage is very high [5, 11] (see Chap. 5, other volume).

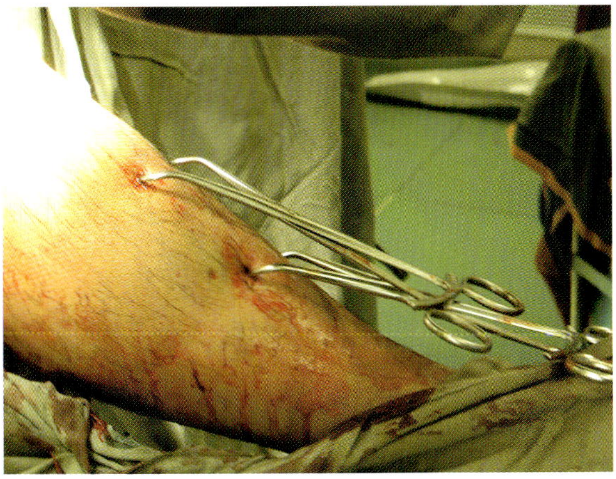

Fig. 10.32. Stabilising the segmental fracture during reaming with two pairs of reduction forceps

Non-union and Pseudoarthrosis

An intact or healed fibula should be osteotomised first. The fibrous tissue and callus can be penetrated by a pointed guide rod. Reaming and exchange nailing is indicated in hypertrophic non-union. Additional autogenous bone grafting may be required in atrophic non-union [13, 14].

Loose locking screws. Inadequate screw length and extension of fracture through the screw hole must first be excluded. In case of loosening due to osteoporosis, the Vecsei spreading screw can be used to create better anchorage on the nail and bone with the expansion bolt (see Chap. 9, this volume).

References

1. Bone JB, Johnson KD (1986) Treatment of tibial fractures by reaming and intramedullary nailing. J Bone Joint Surg Am 68:877–887
2. Browner BD, Cole JD (1987) Current status of locked intramedullary nailing – a review. J Orthop Trauma 1:183–195
3. Chao EYS, Aro HT (1994) Biomechanics of fracture repair and fracture fixation. current practice of fracture treatment, new concepts and common problems. Springer, Hong Kong, pp 9–58.
4. Chapman MW (1986) The role of intramedullary fixation in open fractures. Clin Orth 212:26–34
5. Duwelius PJ, Schmidt AH, Rubinstein RA et al. (1995) Nonreamed interlocking intramedullary tibial nailing: one community's experience. Clin Orthop 315:104–113
6. Grosse A, Taglang G (1993) Grosse and Kempf locking nail system – surgical technique. Howmedica, London
7. Küntscher G (1968) The classic: the intramedullary nailing of fracture. Clin Orth 60:5–12
8. Leung KS (1993) Intramedullary locked nail for fracture fixation. In: Surya B (ed) Recent advances in orthopaedic surgery (vol 1) Jaypee Brothers, New Dehli, pp 163–182
9. Maatz R et al. (1986) Intramedullary nailing and other intramedullary osteosynthesis. W.B. Saunders Company, Philadelphia
10. McQueen MM et al. (1996) Compartment monitoring in tibial fractures: the pressure threshold for decompression. J Bone Joint Surg Br 178:99–104
11. Riemer BL, DiChristina DG, Cooper A et al. (1995) Nonreamed nailing of tibial diaphyseal fractures in blunt polytrauma patients. J Orthop Trauma 9:66–75
12. Rockwood CA, Green DP (1996) Fractures in adults. (3rd edn.) Lippincott-Raven, Philadelphia
13. Rossen JW, Simonis RB (1992) Locked nailing for non-union of the tibia. J Bone Joint Surg Br 74:358–361
14. Sledge SL, Johnson KD, Henley MB et al. (1989) Intramedullary nailing with reaming to treat non-union of tibia. J Bone Joint Surg Am 71:1004–1019

CHAPTER 11

Proximal Femoral Fractures: Operative Technique for Peritrochanteric Fractures

G. TAGLANG

Introduction

The use of the Gamma nail is currently considered as standard for the treatment of pertrochanteric, intertrochanteric, and subtrochanteric fractures with an intramedullary device. It allows early weight bearing, whatever the type of fracture, in more than 80% of cases [1–3]. Of course, good results depend upon perfect operative technique. Everybody knows that intramedullary techniques are demanding and that the learning curve is often longer with this type of implant than with others [3]. For all these reasons, this chapter will attempt to answer a number of questions and provide the necessary technical details.

Positioning

Correct positioning is certainly the most important step towards achieving a perfect reduction of the fracture. In our department, the procedure is performed under spinal anaesthesia in a high percentage of cases (84%) [1], and always on a fracture table in a supine position. Theoretically, the lateral decubitus can give better access to the greater trochanter area, but the rotational deformities are less well controlled. In addition, under spinal anaesthesia, the lateral decubitus is not well tolerated by patients, especially those with pulmonary problems. It is therefore our opinion that the supine position is ideal for such patients (Fig. 11.1).

Fracture Reduction

Using a fracture table is also required to achieve an anatomical reduction of the fracture. The traction on the fractured limb is applied by the shoe; the limb must be in a perfectly straight position with no abduction or adduction. Excessive adduction may lead to a varus deformity, even if the access to the greater trochanter is facilitated. Excessive abduction will, on the other hand, result in a valgus in the fracture line and good access to the tip of the trochanter major will be difficult.

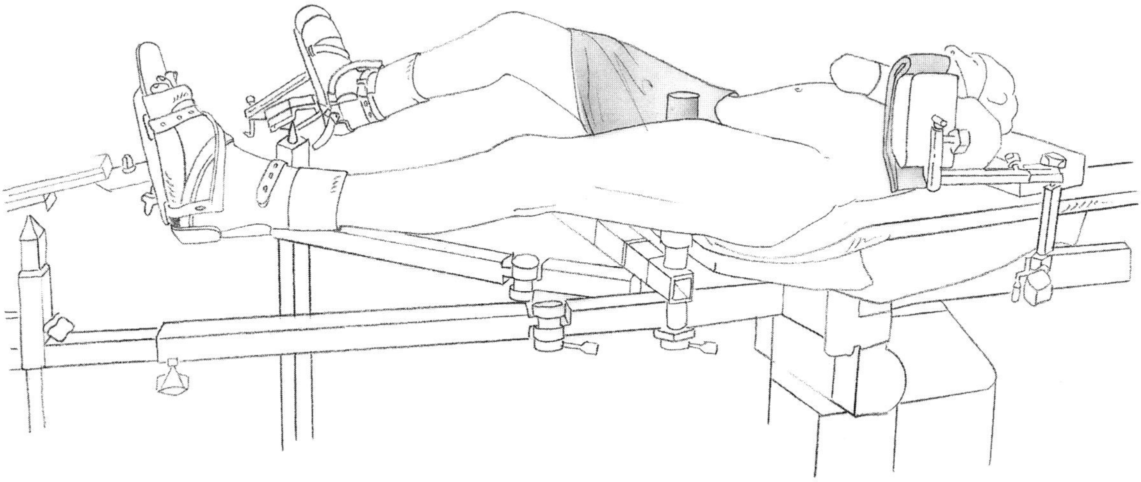

Fig. 11.1. Position of the patient on the fracture table in supine position for a Gamma nailing. Observe the thoracic support adapted on the table

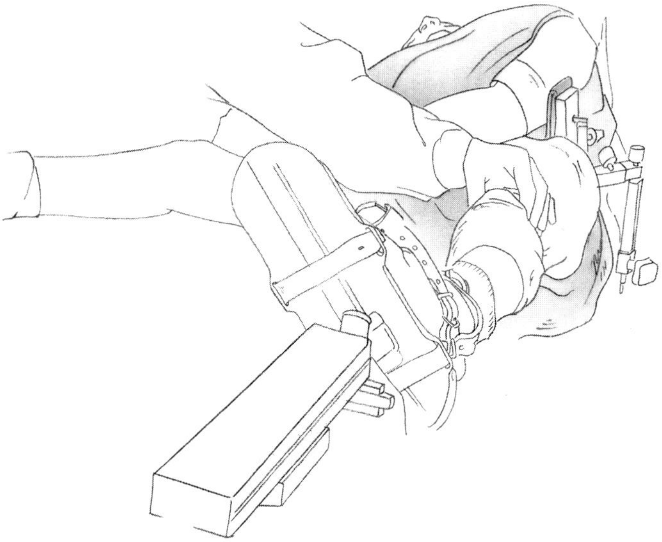

Fig. 11.2. The lower limb is in internal rotation but the patella is horizontal

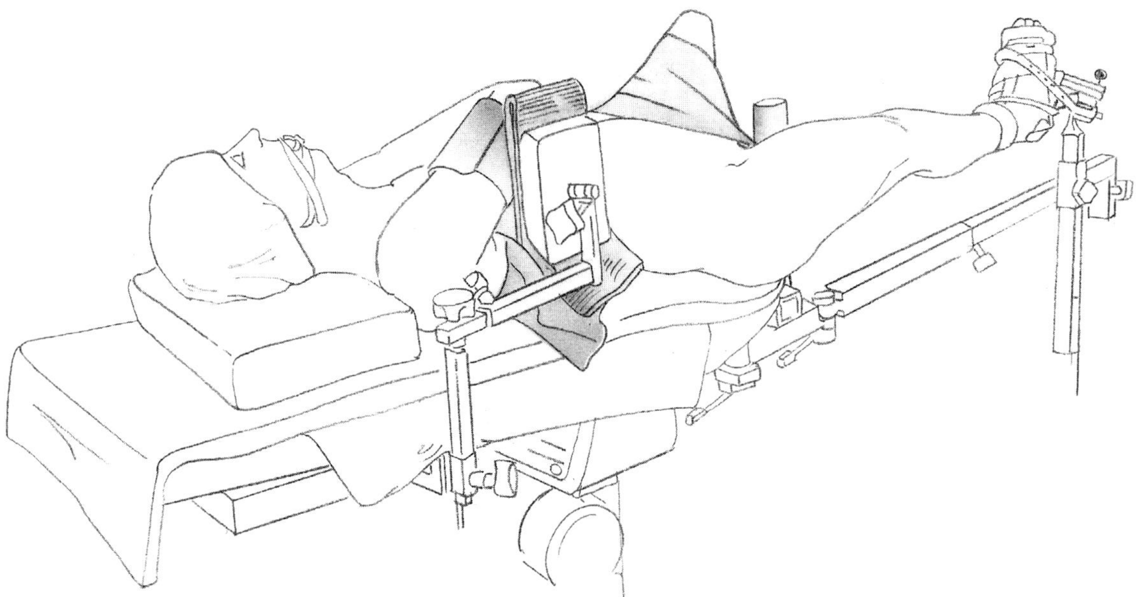

Fig. 11.3. The thoracic support in place, the trunk is bent to the opposite side

Most fractures are displaced with an excessive external rotation of the distal fragment, the reduction must therefore be made in internal rotation of the distal fragment. Positioning the patella in a perfectly horizontal plane, parallel to the floor, gives the best clinical control (Fig. 11.2). The greatest complications observed were those that had no correction of rotation, but with a certain percentage of external rotation of the distal part.

Putting the lower limb in a straight position and reducing the fracture by pulling on the foot results in bringing the trunk in alignment with the hip joint. This can cause problems during the reaming procedure. It therefore seems important to bend the trunk to the opposite side: it will then be maintained by a thoracic support fixed on the fracture table (Fig. 11.3).

Even after scrupulously following these rules, repositioning the fracture may at times be difficult. In our experience, two situations occur the most frequently:

1. A subtrochanteric fracture with an oblique fracture line on the lateral view. This fracture keeps the anterior part of the proximal femur

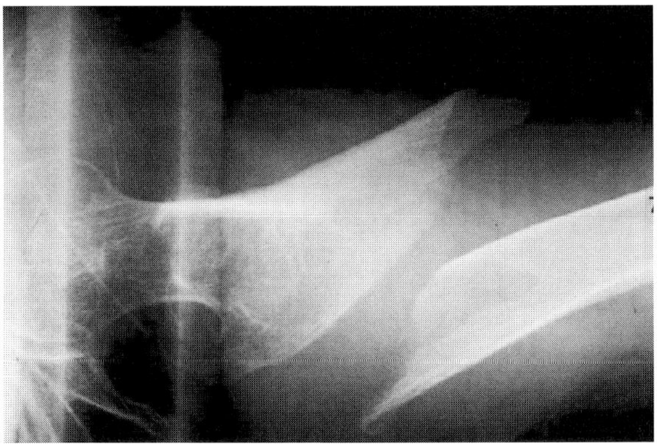

Fig. 11.4. Typical deformity of an oblique sub-trochanteric fracture with bending of the proximal part due to the psoas muscle

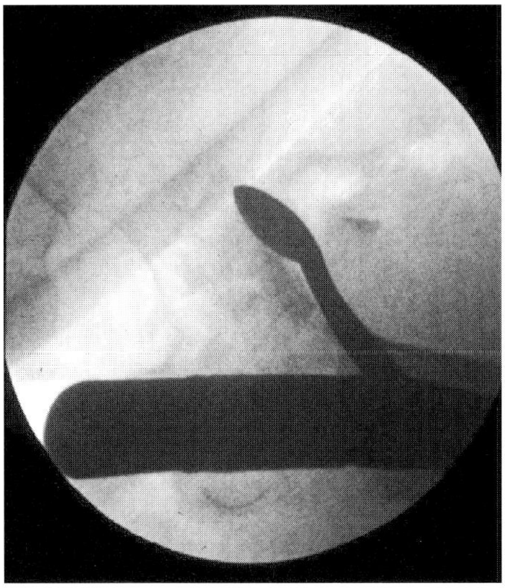

Fig. 11.5. Use of a spatula to reduce the proximal fragment

intact. This proximal fragment is in flexion due to the action of the psoas muscle which is still attached to the lesser trochanter (Fig. 11.4). Küntscher's technique to reduce this fragment with a closed procedure, using a small diameter nail, is not possible in this situation. Indeed, the posterior part of the proximal fragment is very short and often refractured; therefore the small nail cannot reduce the fragment in extension because it lacks support. In this type of fracture, the reduction can be done with minimal opening of the fracture site and the application of a clamp. Better still, it can be done using a Wagner spatula through the same incision to reduce the anterior bending of the proximal fragment. This spatula is held by the assistant during the beginning of the procedure, until the lag screw is positioned (Fig. 11.5).

2. The lack of reduction in transverse subtrochanteric fractures in obese patients. The weight of the thigh causes posterior displacement of the distal part of the femur. The easiest and most elegant solution to this problem is to put a knee support under the posterior aspect of the thigh to lift the distal part. This support must not be in conflict with the image intensifier.

Positioning of the Image Intensifier

Using two image intensifiers, it is important to abduct the unaffected leg to position the first C-frame between the two limbs for lateral control. This C-frame is positioned over the thigh so that during the reaming procedure the image intensifier and the guide wire are kept clear of each other. The second image intensifier comes from the opposite side and controls the reduction in the anterior-posterior plane. Positioning with two image intensifiers makes it easy to use a single sterile drape (Fig. 11.6).

With only one image intensifier, we recommend the same positioning as for a conventional G&K nail. The opposite limb must be flexed 90° in the hip joint and 90° in the knee joint, with a maximum abduction in the hip joint. The lower limb is positioned on a Koeppel support. This positioning allows the optimal use of the image intensifier either in the anterior-posterior or in the lateral view.

Draping

The patient is prepared and draped as for a standard fixation of a hip fracture. We use a single sterile drape, covering the thigh and both lower limbs with the image intensifier(s) (Fig. 11.7).

Skin Incision

The tip of the greater trochanter is located by touch; in obese patients the use of the image intensifier may be necessary (Fig. 11.8). The incision begins at the level of the tip of the trochanter major and extends proximally to about 5–8 cm, depending on the size of the patient. The incision is deepened through the fascia lata, splitting the abductor muscle for approximately 3 cm immediately above the tip of the greater trochanter, thus exposing its tip.

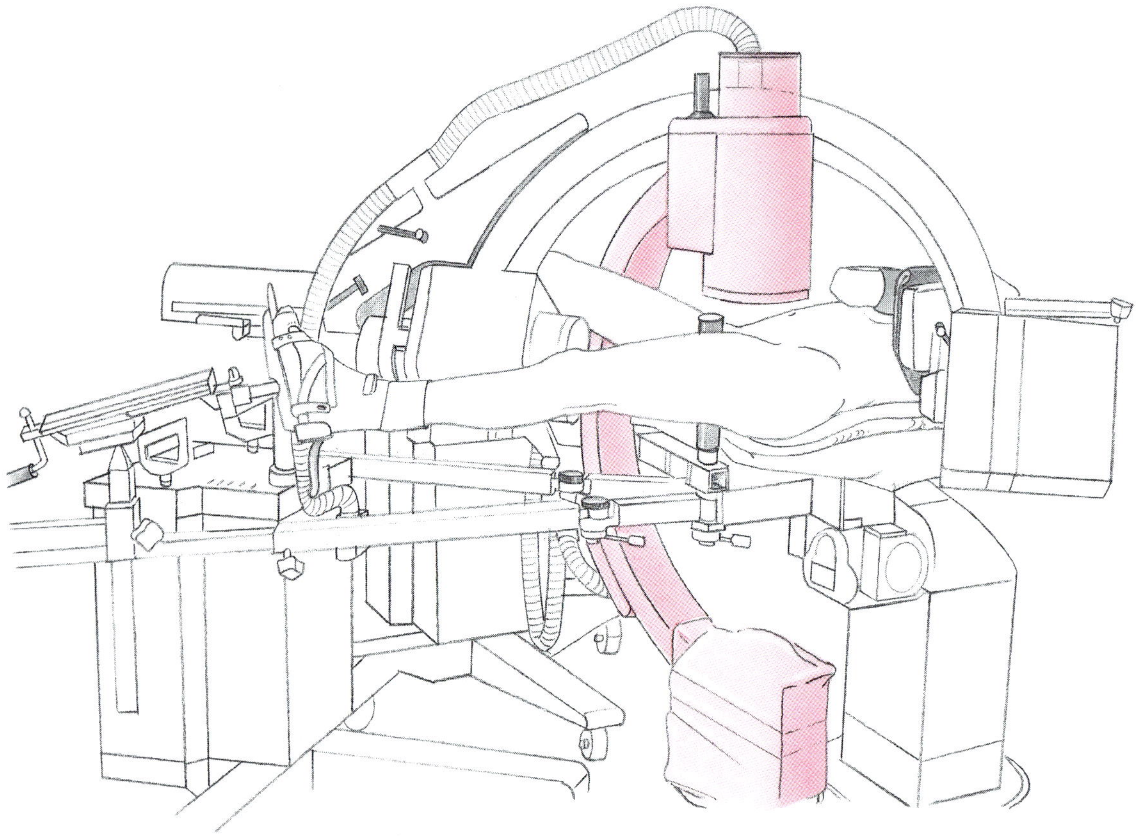

Fig. 11.6. Positioning with two image intensifiers. Observe that the C-frame for the lateral view is positioned over the thigh

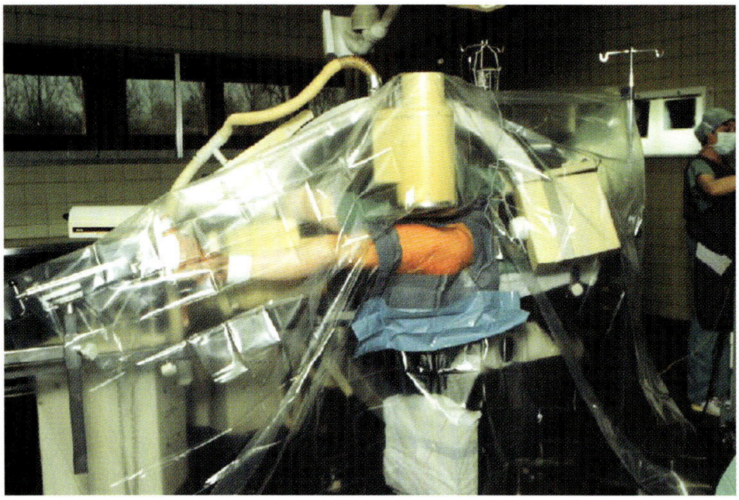

Fig. 11.7. Positioning of the patient with the sterile draping

Bone Entry Point

The tip of the greater trochanter is identified with the finger and the pointed awl is positioned 2 cm above the finger: the junction of the anterior third and posterior two-thirds of the tip of the greater trochanter. At this stage, it is important to check the position of the pointed awl on the anterior-posterior view (Fig. 11.9) with the image intensifier. If there are any doubts, the lateral view should also be checked.

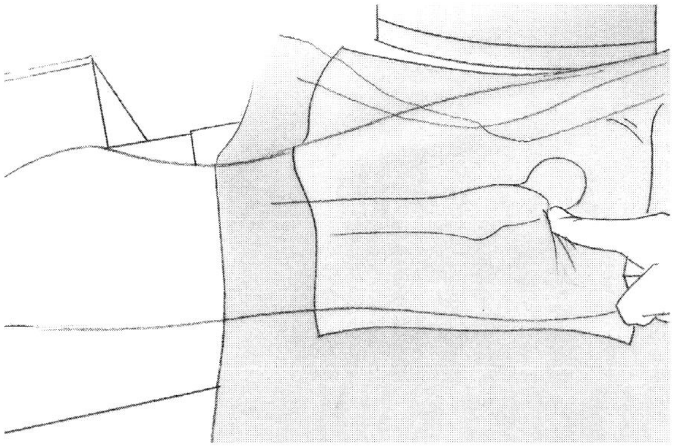

Fig. 11.8. Identifying the greater trochanter before the skin incision

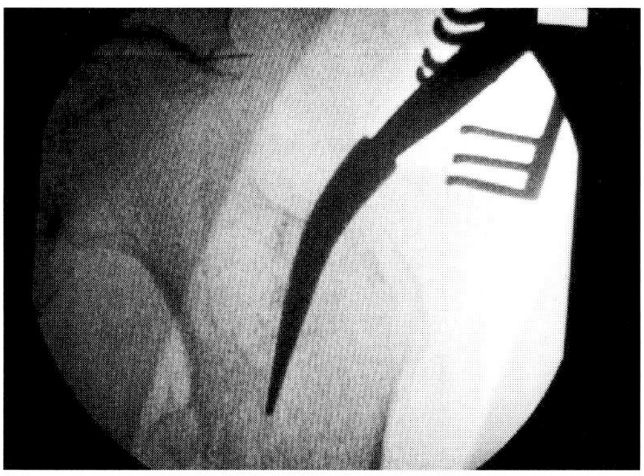

Fig. 11.9. Verification of positioning the pointed awl on the anterior-posterior view

The optimal point of entry is the tip of the greater trochanter and never the piriform fossa. Problems occur when conventional nails are inserted into the fossa (avascular necrosis of the femoral head, refracture after nail removal, septic complications) and the same can occur with the standard Gamma nail. Also, due to the valgus design (10° mediolateral curvature), the wrong entry point can increase the contact between the distal tip of the nail and the lateral cortex. The entry point must not be too lateral because this can make it difficult to optimally place the lag screw in the lower part of the femoral neck and head. Using a new model of the Gamma nail, the Trochanteric Gamma Nail (TGN), the distal tip of the nail is less frequently in contact with the lateral cortex because this new model is shorter (18 cm), thinner (11 cm) and the mediolateral curvature is only 4°. In addition, this nail has only one distal hole to ensure the distal locking to the bone.

Placing the Reaming Guide Wire

To facilitate the insertion of the guide wire, it is bent so there is no conflict with the soft tissues at the proximal part of the thigh. The guide wire is inserted, using the Jacob's chuck. The bowed shape of the femur and a posterior comminuted fracture in most cases requires internal rotation of the guide wire. This will avoid the the guide wire coming out posteriorly (Fig. 11.10). The guide is then pushed down to the condyle area so that reaming can begin.

Reaming Technique

The patient's bone quality greatly influences the reaming technique. Flexible reamers with sharp heads and deep flutes are used. In elderly people, four reamers are routinely used: 10, 12, 14 and 17 mm for the proximal part of the femur. In younger patients, we use the power and reamers in 0.5 mm increments, from 10 mm to 14 mm for a 12 mm standard Gamma nail. Care must be taken with flexible reamers to ensure that the guide wire is not displaced laterally during reaming. This could lead to resection of more bone on the lateral side of the wire, which in turn would lead to an offset position for the nail and the risk of fracturing the shaft. In subtrochanteric fractures in young people, it is absolutely necessary to over-ream to the greater trochanter area up to 17 mm. With the Trochanteric Nail (TGN), we also ream the shaft up 14 mm, even if the diameter of this nail is only 11 mm. This gives greater security during the insertion of the nail.

Insertion of the Nail

The selected nail (most often 11 mm in diameter for the Standard or the Trochanteric Nail) is now assembled onto the carbon fibre targeting device. The locating peg slots must correspond to the notches. The nail is held by the nail-holding screw, and tightened using the socket wrench and the driver extension.

Nail/Lag Screw Positioning

Nail insertion is monitored with the image intensifier C-arm. The projected axis of the lag screw can be measured with a ruler on the monitor to ensure that the lag screw will be positioned ideally. Visual estimation has proved to be unreliable.

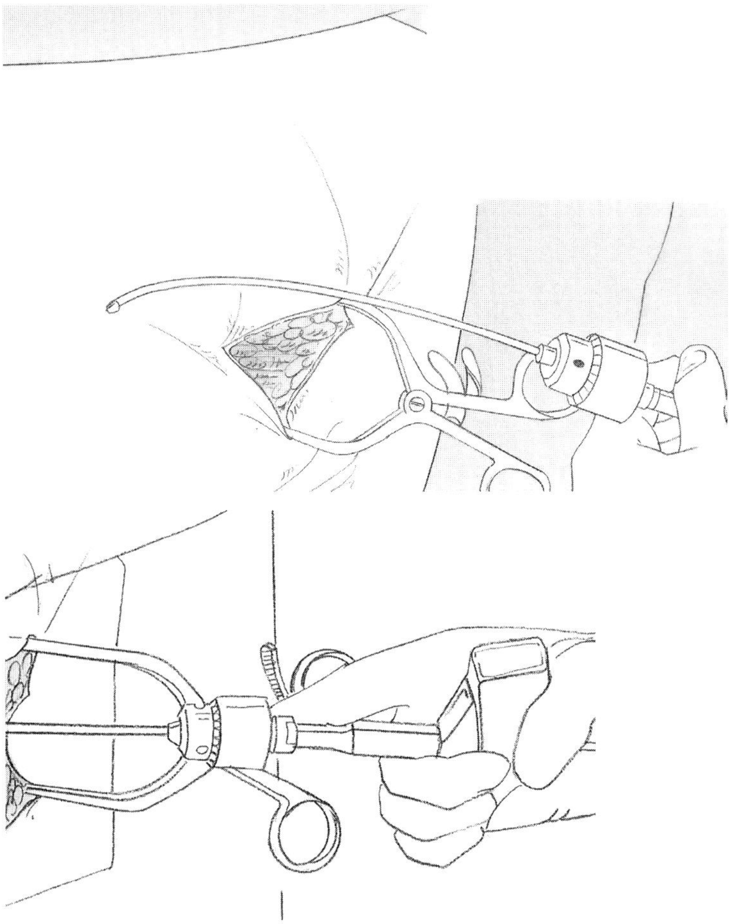

Fig. 11.10. Introduction of the guide wire

To ensure correct positioning of the lag screw, close attention must be given to the anteversion angle and to the depth of nail insertion into the femoral canal. The Gamma nail must be inserted with external rotation (10°–15°) to be sure that the K-wire will hit the femoral neck.

The Gamma locking nail is inserted by hand (Fig. 11.11), and *never with a mallet*, until the lag screw holes (visible as crescent shapes on the monitor) are lined up with the inferior half of the femoral neck. The desired result of this is to ultimately position the nail. When the Gamma locking nail is inserted to its final depth, the plane of the targeting device will be parallel to percutaneous guide wire, which can be put through the two small holes of the target device. (A 2-mm Kirschner wire can be inserted percutaneously anterior to the shaft and parallel to the axis of the femoral neck and head.) This ensures the correct degree of rotation to align the lag screw holes with the anteversion angle of the femoral neck. It is sometimes difficult to fully insert the nail into the femur; one reason could be that the medullary canal is too narrow. As the Gamma locking nail is a very strong, rigid implant, it must not be forced into the femur, e.g. by hammering, as there is a danger of fracturing the femur [3, 4]. If the nail will not go into the femoral cavity far enough to allow proper positioning of the lag screw, the nail should be removed and the canal reamed 0.5 or 1 mm more. Do not forget the possibility of using a 11-mm nail (we have used only 11-mm nails in our unit for the last 3 years, particularly the TGN, which only exists in the 11-mm size).

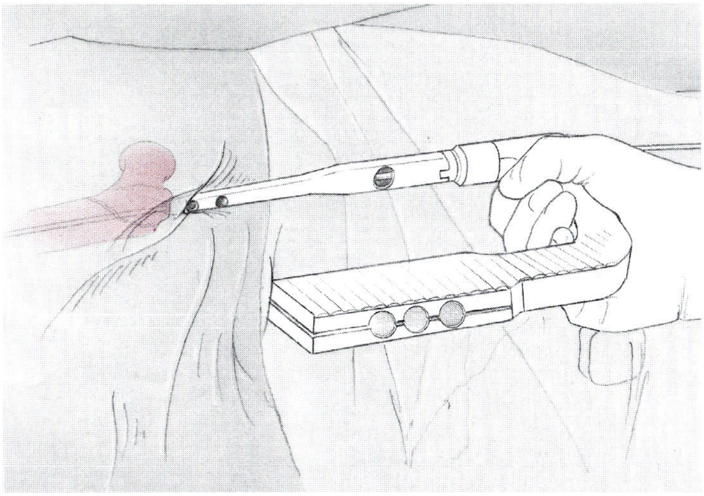

Fig. 11.11. The Gamma nail must be introduced by hand

Lag Screw Targeting

Remove the reaming guide wire using the Jacob's chuck, ensuring that the jig is supported to prevent external rotation of the Gamma nail. With the nail inserted to the proper depth, it is now necessary to slide the targeting sleeve, corresponding to the nail angle of the selected Gamma locking nail, onto the end of the carbon fibre targeting device (Fig. 11.12). Note that for the TGN the colour of the targeting sleeve is different (green); this is important so that the sleeve before the Standard Nail is not exchanged with the Trochanteric Nail. Before proceeding, be sure that the nail-holding screw is fully tightened. The targeting device may require support by an assistant, to prevent its weight from externally rotating the nail, until the next stage is completed. The soft tissue protector and the guide sleeve for the lag screw are assembled, and passed through the targeting sleeve to the level of the skin (Fig. 11.13). This indicates the position for the small incision to be made, which is made down to the bone.

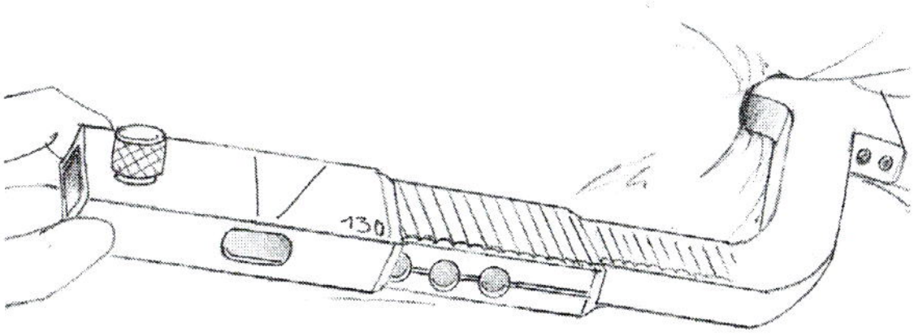

Fig. 11.12. Putting the targeting sleeve in place

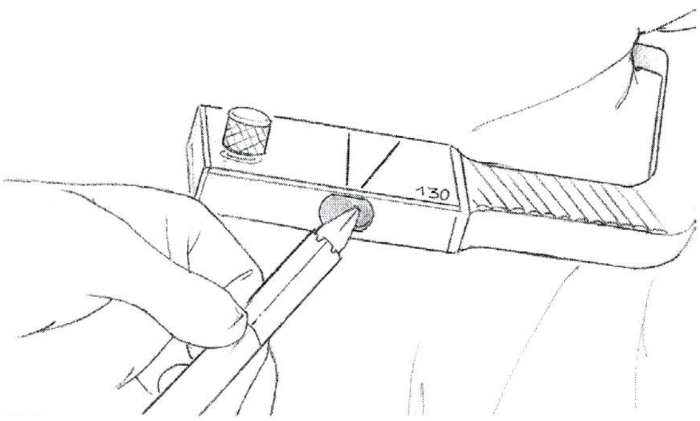

Fig. 11.13. The soft tissue protector and the guide sleeve for the lag screw are assembled and passed through the targeting sleeve to the level of the skin

The guide sleeve and tissue protector assembly is now passed through the incision to press firmly against the lateral cortex. The percutaneous anteversion guide can now be inserted if this has not already been done.

The soft tissue protector is removed and the lag screw guide is brought in contact with the lateral cortex. The thumb wheel on the targeting sleeve must be tightened to lock the guide sleeve in place and further stabilise the jig assembly (Fig. 11.14).

With the guide sleeve firmly in contact with the cortex, the awl should be inserted and turned, in order to pierce the lateral cortex (it is strictly forbidden to mallet on the handle of the pointed awl) (Fig. 11.15). Check for proper positioning on both anterior-posterior and lateral intensifier views. Before proceeding, check that the guide wire for the flexible reamer used earlier has been removed.

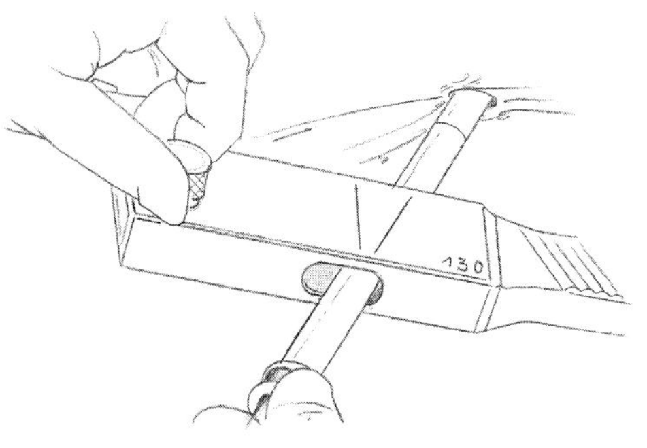

Fig. 11.14. The thumb wheel on the targeting sleeve must be tightened to lock the guide sleeve in place and further stabilise the jig assembly

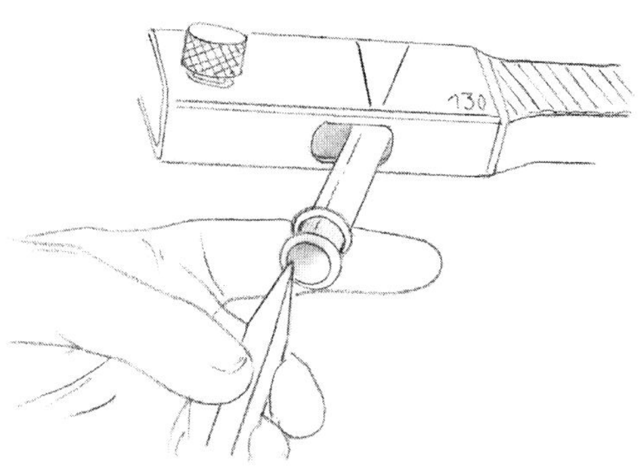

Fig. 11.15. The awl should be inserted and turned in order to pierce the lateral cortex

The soft tissue protector is now re-inserted to act as a guide sleeve for the lag screw guide wire, which is inserted using the Jacob's chuck.

The guide wire should be screwed into the subchondral bone, checking for position on both the anterior-posterior and lateral intensifier views (if the thread of the guide wire is in the subchondral bone, the lag screw will stop 1 cm before).

The tip of the guide wire must be placed in the inferior half of the femoral head in the frontal plane, and on the middle in the lateral plane; the objective is to place the lag screw below the centre of the femoral head on the anterior-posterior view and central on the lateral view, otherwise the risk of it cutting out of the head is increased [4].

If the guide wire is wrongly positioned, the first step is to withdraw the guide wire itself and then to withdraw the nail. Rotate the nail in the appropriate direction and re-insert as before. The guide wire is then redrilled and control screening is carried out as before.

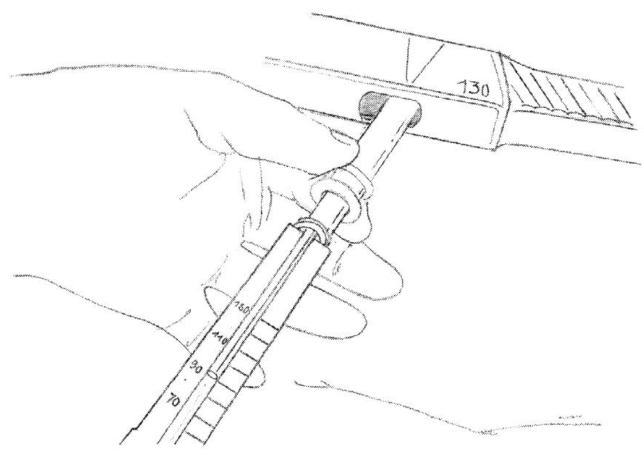

Fig. 11.16. The lag screw length required is measured, using the depth gauge

Lag Screw Reaming

When the guide wire is in a perfect position, the required lag screw length is measured, using the depth gauge (Fig. 11.16). Before starting to measure, ensure that the guide sleeve is pressed firmly against the lateral cortex of the femur; if you do not do so, it will be too short. Take the depth gauge and place it directly under the guide wire.

The measurement on the gauge is transferred to the adjustable stop on the lag screw step drill. It should be noted that the adjustable stop is positioned with the chosen length next to the stop on the side towards the drill tip. The collar is used to lock the stop in position (Fig. 11.17).

The soft tissue protector is removed and the lag screw step drill is passed over the guide wire, through the guide sleeve. The path for the lag screw is thus reamed, using the Jacob's chuck. If exceptional resistance is encountered, a power drill may be used with great care. Drilling should continue until the stop impacts against the guide sleeve (Fig. 11.18), ensuring that the targeting device is supported to prevent movement.

If insertion of the guide wire is repeated in order to get a satisfactory position, the wire may have become bent, due to its passing through a previous track. This makes it difficult to pass the step drill over the bent wire. If the guide wire is only slightly bent, then the step drill can be passed over it, using a to-and-fro movement. If the guide wire is markedly bent then it should be removed and a new guide wire inserted; alternatively, the step drill can be passed smoothly up to the subchondral bone without wire.

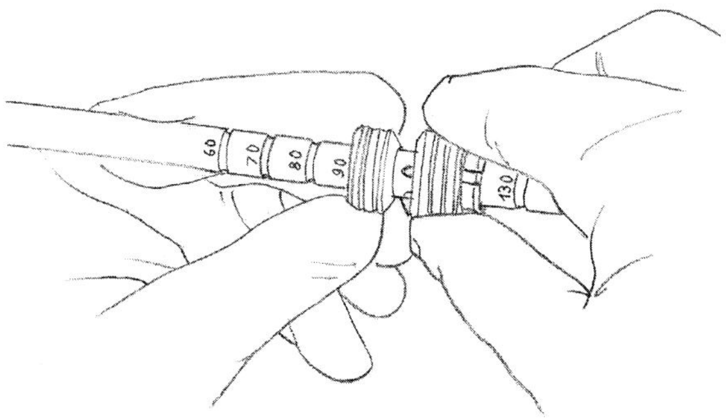

Fig. 11.17. The measurement on the gauge is now transferred to the adjustable stop on the lag screw step drill

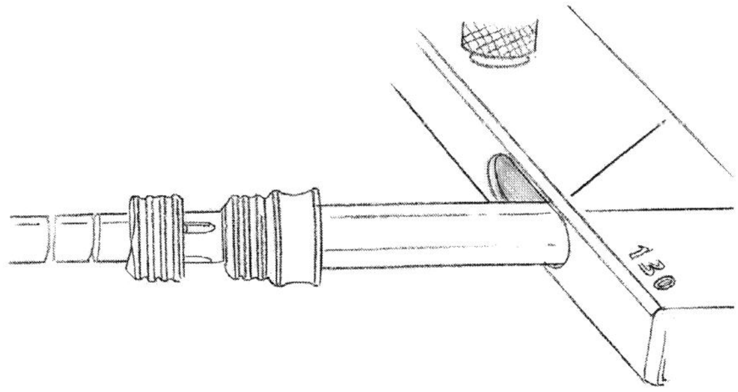

Fig. 11.18. Drilling should continue until the stop impacts against the guide sleeve

Lag Screw Selection and Insertion

The proper length lag screw is chosen by selecting a size at least 5 mm longer than the measurement previously made on the lag screw gauge for reaming. It is important that the lag screw protrudes at least 5 mm from the lateral femoral cortex to retain rotational stability and to permit sliding (on the current system the lag screw exists in 5 mm steps from 85 to 110 mm, the most frequently used lag screws are 95, 100 and 105 mm in length for a 130° nail). The lag screw of the right size is now assembled with the lag screwdriver. The end thumbhole must be pulled back, and the screw and driver connected. The lag screw is now passed over the guide wire, through the guide sleeve, and threaded up to the subchondral part of the head. When the thread on the screwdriver comes in contact with the stop on the guide sleeve, then the screw is distally in the right position in the subchondral bone.

After tightening the screw, ensure that the handle of the lag screwdriver is either parallel or perpendicular to the targeting device (Fig. 11.19), so that the set screw will engage in one of the four lag screw grooves.

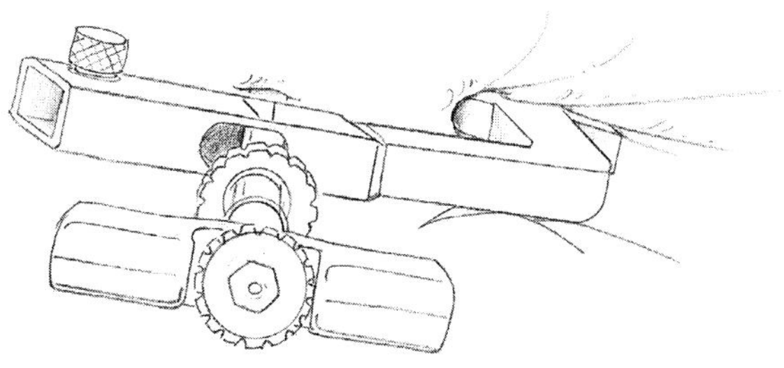

Fig. 11.19. After tightening the screw to ensure that the handle of the lag screwdriver is either parallel or perpendicular to the targeting device

Set Screw Insertion

The set screw is inserted through the opening in the nail-holding screw at the proximal end of the target device (Fig. 11.20). It is then tightened fully, using the set screwdriver and socket wrench. This will be a little stiff because the nail has a nylon insert in the threads to prevent spontaneous loosening.

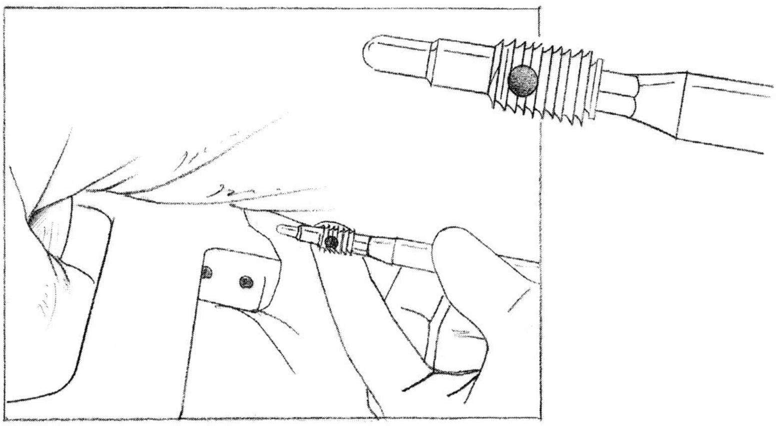

Fig. 11.20. The set screw is inserted through the opening in the nail-holding screw at the proximal end of the target device

The screw should then be unscrewed one quarter of a turn to ensure free sliding of the lag screw. Ensure that the set screw is still engaged in the groove by checking that the lag screw cannot now be rotated with the lag screwdriver. If distal locking is not indicated, disconnect the lag screwdriver using the end thumbhole, remove the lag screwdriver, guide sleeve, guide wire, targeting device, and sleeve, then complete the operation as described. If distal locking is indicated, then leave the targeting device in position and continue.

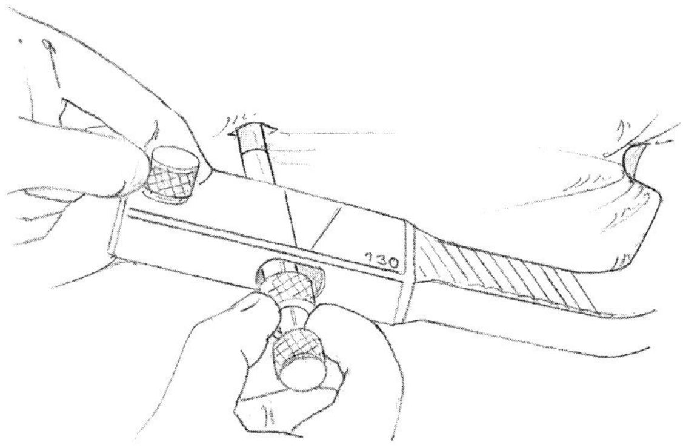

Fig. 11.21. The soft tissue protector is now removed and the guide sleeve is pushed into contact with the cortex

Distal Locking Screw(s)

The distal soft tissue protector has to be inserted into the distal guide sleeve. Slacken the thumbwheel on the targeting sleeve, then pass the guide sleeve and protector through the proximal hole in the targeting device. This indicates where the first small incision is to be made. The incision is developed down to the lateral cortex, and the tissue protector sleeve assembly is passed through. The soft tissue protector is now removed and the guide sleeve is pushed into contact with the cortex (Fig. 11.21).

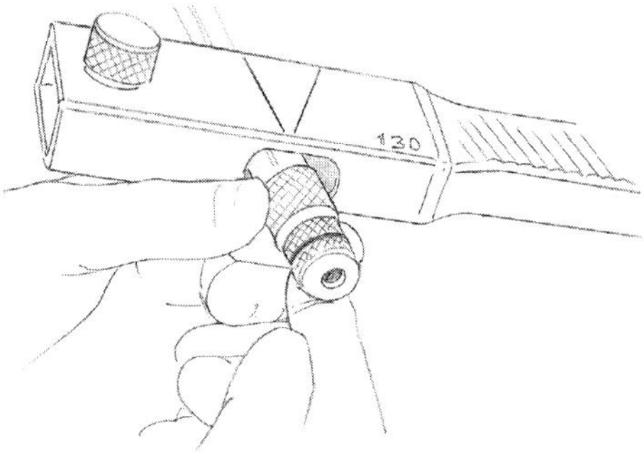

Fig. 11.22. The 5.5-mm guide sleeve is inserted (colour code: blue)

The guide sleeve should be locked into position using the thumbwheel provided. We think that the pointed awl is no longer necessary since we use the new 5.5-mm drills, and we are convinced that some of the complications described were a consequence of fissures made during this step.

The 5.5-mm guide sleeve is inserted (colour code: blue) (Fig. 11.22). The 5.5-mm distal drill for fully threaded screws is used, making sure that the distal guide sleeve is held firmly engaged in the cortex at all times during the drilling.

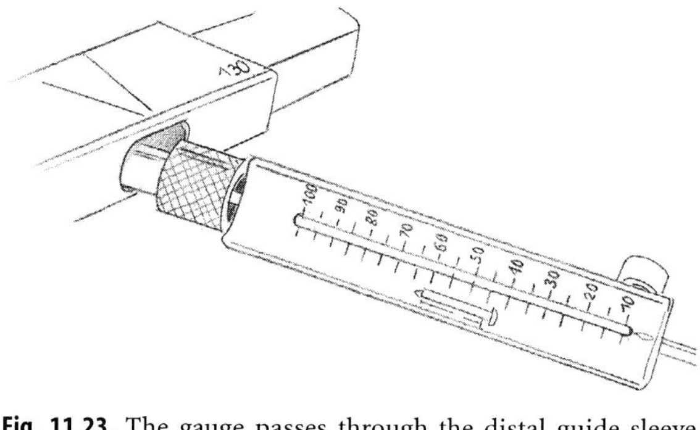

Fig. 11.23. The gauge passes through the distal guide sleeve with its tip passing into the medial cortex

After drilling, measurement of the distal screw length is made by using the distal screw depth gauge, but first remove the distal drill guide. The distal screw depth gauge gives the indication of the working length of the screw, i.e. without the head and the tip. The gauge passes through the distal guide sleeve with its tip passing into the medial cortex (Fig. 11.23).

A measure of the distal screw length is therefore taken from a direct reading on the depth gauge. The most commonly used screw lengths are 25 and 30 mm. The proper size of distal self-tapping screw (6.28 mm in diameter) is introduced through the distal guide sleeve and tightened, using the distal screwdriver (Fig. 11.24).

After biomechanical and clinical experiments, we currently use only one screw to lock the Gamma nail distally. In cases of very low subtrochanteric fractures, using the long Gamma nail is now indicated. For the TGN, the locking is done distally through the single hole dedicated to the locking procedure.

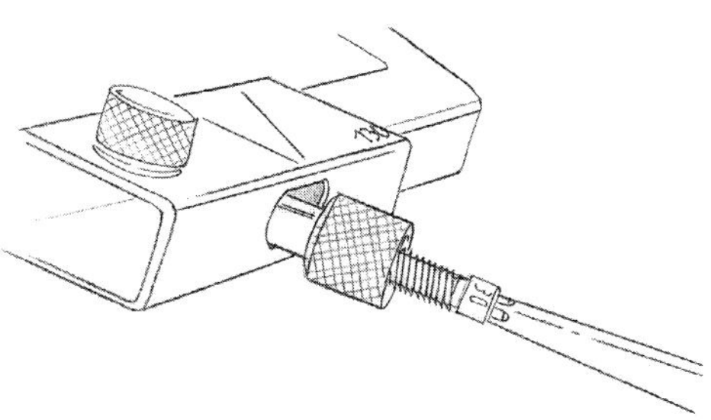

Fig. 11.24. The proper size of the distal self-tapping screw (6.28 mm in diameter) is introduced through the distal guide sleeve and tightened, using the distal screwdriver

Final Checking

Remove the guide sleeves and targeting device. Check the final position of the implant using the image intensifier in the anterior-posterior and lateral planes. Close the wounds proximally with one drain, without forgetting the small stab wounds.

Extraction of the Nail

In young patients or in cases of local impingement, nail or lag screw protrusion is an indication for Gamma nail extraction. The patient can either be in a supine position on a fracture table, if the image intensifier is needed to localise the nail, or on a conventional table in lateral decubitus. The following steps must be observed for the extraction procedure:

First the distal screw or screws must be removed. A small incision through the old scar must be made on the lateral cortex of the femur, to expose the outer end of the lag screw. The lag screw guide wire is then passed up to the lag screw, to act as a guide for the screwdriver. Without using the lag screw guide wire, it is sometimes difficult to perfectly place the screwdriver in an optimal position on the lag screw. The lag screwdriver is then passed over the guide wire and engaged with the distal end of the lag screw.

An incision is made over the proximal tip of the nail and the set screwdriver is engaged with the set screw and the screw is rotated anticlockwise with the socket wrench far enough to disengage the screw from the lag screw groove. The set screw is then completely extracted. The lag screw is extracted by rotating the lag screwdriver in an anticlockwise direction. The lag screw guide wire must also be removed. The nail extraction rod is then threaded into the proximal end of the nail. A sliding mallet is attached and the nail extracted. Finally the wounds are closed.

Technique of the Long Gamma Nail

After experience and good results with the standard Gamma nail, we decided to extend the indications of this nail to the combination of diaphyseal femoral fractures and neck fractures [5, 6]. This is the origin of the longer implant. Like the standard nail, this nail is an unslotted, cannulated nail with a clover leaf profile (in the first generation, the actual Long Gamma Nail had a round profile, as the clover leaf profile seems not to be important in an unslotted nail). The proximal diameter is 17 mm because the distal diameter is only 11 mm. The neck angles are 125°, 130° and 135°. The nails incorporate proximal anteversion of 10°, which has led to the design of right and left forms. The lengths available are between 340 mm and 440 mm. As for the TGN the mediolateral angle of the nail is 4°. The best indications for this device are:

1. Long subtrochanteric fractures
2. Pertrochanteric fractures associated with shaft fractures
3. Pathologic fractures extended to the diaphyseal area, including imminent fractures
4. Revision procedures

For most procedures, the long Gamma nail technique is similar to that of the standard (or TGN) technique. The differences are especially important for the positioning and the distal locking procedures. For positioning, we usually apply transcondylar traction using a Steinmann pin and a stirrup. This system allows good stability of the thigh, especially for the distal locking procedures. The Steinmann pin is positioned just before and removed just after the operation in the operating theatre. As in the standard technique, the trunk is bent to the opposite side and the patella must be horizontal.

Reaming is performed as usual, but it is particularly important to ream to the trochanter area up to 17 mm. This step is important for cases of subtrochanteric fractures in young patients with an intact greater trochanter. Nailing and proximal locking techniques are no different from the standard technique. For distal locking, the target mounted on the C-frame or the free-hand techniques are indicated, as for the femoral G&K nail. (Please refer to Chap. 8, this volume, on distal locking techniques for more details.)

References

1. Kempf I, Grosse A, Taglang G, Favreul E (1993) Gamma nail in the treatment of closed trochanteric fractures. Results and indications a propos of 121 cases. Rev Chir Orthop Reparatrice Appar Mot 79:29–40
2. Eberle C, Guyer P, Keller H, Metzger U (1993) The Gamma nail: an ideal implant for treatment of unstable fractures in elderly patients. Helv Chir Acta Mar 59:527–531
3. Leung KS, So WS, Shen WY, Hui PW (1992) Gamma nails and dynamic hip screws for peritrochanteric fractures. A randomised prospective study in elderly patients. J Bone Joint Surg Br 74:345–351
4. Mahaisavariya B, Laupattarakasem W (1992) Cracking of the femoral shaft by the gamma nail. Injury 23:493–495
5. Leung KS, So WS, Lam TP, Leung PC (1993) Treatment of ipsilateral femoral shaft fractures and hip fractures. Injury 24:41–45
6. Stapert JW, Geesing CI, Jacobs PB, De Wit RJ, Vierhout PA (1993) First experience and complications with the long Gamma nail. J Trauma 34:394–400

CHAPTER 12

Humeral Fractures

H. Seidel

Introduction

Stabilisation of humeral fractures with rods placed in the medullary canal was introduced by Küntscher [2], Rush and Rush [6], and Hackethal [1]. The entry to the medullar canal was made either from the distal or the proximal end of the humerus.

Küntscher proposed the slotted elastic nail with the classical self-fitting technique. He used both the proximal and the distal entry to the medullar canal. Rush proposed two elastic rods with three-point fixation. He preferred the proximal entrance. Hackethal used a bundle of elastic rods and preferred the proximal approach. But the operative treatment of humeral fractures has been dominated by the plating technique of the AO group of Müller, Allgöwer, Schneider and Willenegger [3].

Our analysis of Küntscher's technique with our patients has shown that more complications are experienced with the distal entry point than with the proximal entry point. The greatest disadvantages of the Küntscher technique have been the proximal instability with distraction or telescoping, rotation instability and pseudarthrosis, misalignment and protrusion of the nail on the top of the shoulder joint. Problems of the rotary cuff in combination with limited motion and pain at the shoulder were not unusual with the Küntscher nail.

The advantage of this technique was the closed procedure and the biological callus consolidation of the fracture. The disadvantage of the Küntscher nail is the impossibility of fixation of both the small distal humeral bone and the large proximal humeral bone with one self-fitting elastic nail (Fig. 12.1).

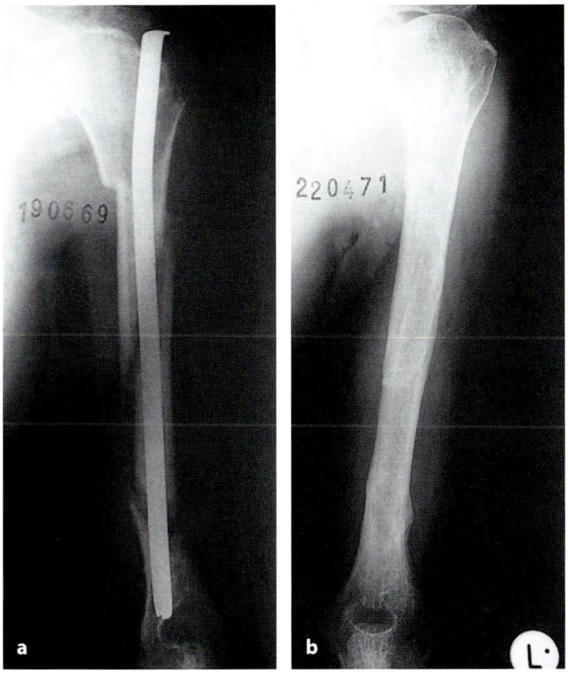

Fig. 12.1 a, b. Comminuted fracture of the humeral diaphysis treated by a classic Küntscher nail

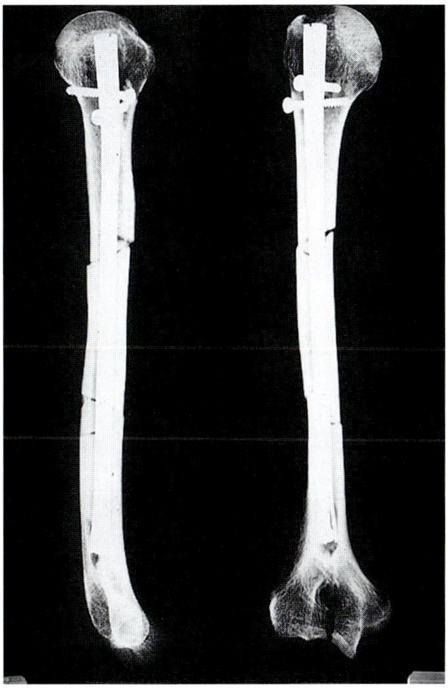

Fig. 12.2. Proximal third humeral fracture fixed by the Seidel humeral locking nail (HLN)

The humeral locking nail was first proposed by Seidel [7]. The entrance is at the proximal end of the humerus and penetrates the rotator cuff. With this nail, the proximal fragments can be stabilized with locking screws guided through the nail (Fig. 12.2). The rotator cuff is protected because the nail is safely fixed with the locking screws below the level of the rotator cuff. Very proximal humeral shaft fractures and humeral head fractures are safely stabilized with the nail, in combination with the washer technique.

This nail is suitable in different sizes for humeral shaft fractures and humeral head fractures. Since 1992, the second generation of the nail and instrumentation has been in development and clinical test. It has been widely available since 1995. The second generation of instrumentation is safer in every step of the operation and the rotational stability of the nail is 50% higher than with the first model and technique (Fig. 12.3 a, b).

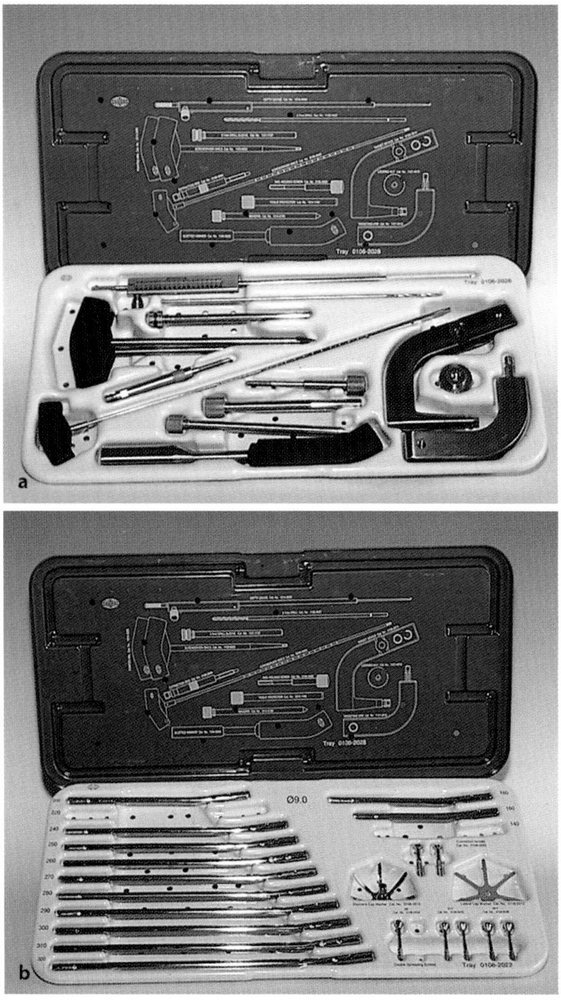

Fig. 12.3. a Humeral locking nail: instruments. **b** Humeral locking nail: implants

Nail Design

The second generation of nails have three different nail diameters: 7, 8, and 9 mm and they are available in lengths between 14 cm and 32 cm.

The wall of the nail is solid; it has no slot and it is cannulated. The nail is stiff and resistant to torsion and bending deformation. The shape of the nail is retrocurved in the proximal portion with a 7.5° angle. This curvature corresponds to the anatomical retroversion of the humeral head and prohibits nail protrusion on the front side of the humeral head. It is resistant and stabilises even long comminuted fractures without loss of alignment.

The nail is guided into position like the classical Küntscher nail using a guide wire. The nail has three proximal locking screws (HS1, HS2, HS3). The first screw hole in the proximal part of the nail (for the screw HS1) has a thread in the nail hole and goes from the lateral to medial direction.

The second screw hole (for screw HS2) is unthreaded and has the frontal-dorsal direction. The third screw hole is also unthreaded (HS3) and has again the lateral-medial direction (Fig. 12.4). As the screw holes for HS2 and HS3 have no thread in the nail, they can be utilised like compression screws. The screw hole for HS1 can only be used as a fixation screw. For humeral shaft fractures the screws HS1 and HS3 are mostly used. The HS2 screw is used if compression to the dorsal fragment is required The distal locking of the nail is performed with a special technique of expansion of the tip of the nail.

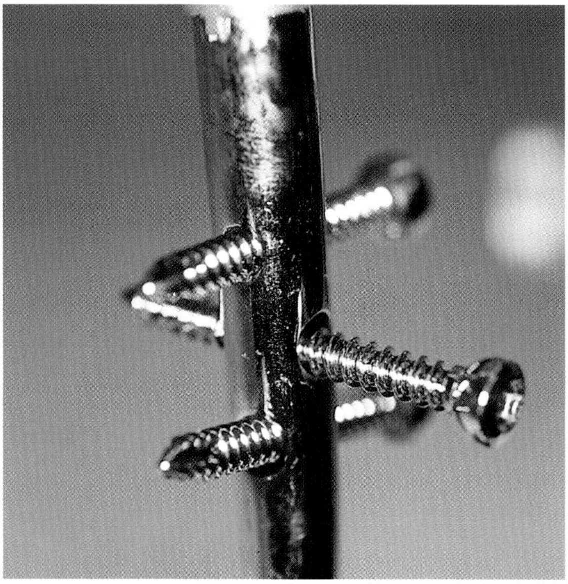

Fig. 12.4. Humeral locking nail: proximal locking. Three locking screws: HS1, HS2, HS3

Distal Locking

The distal end of the nail has three slots and is expandable. Distal locking is achieved with an internal screw-spreading mechanism, using a double spreading screw (DS) which is available in five sizes in order to achieve the optimum spreading. The stability of the distal locking mechanism has been tested in the laboratory and the rotational stability is 50% higher than with the old distal mono-locking screw (MS) used in the first series of implants.

The tests have also shown the best final position of the distal locking screw. This position is achieved if the spreading screw is just dipped in the nail. If the spreading screw is too deep in the nail, the fixation is less stable. With the range of diameter of the spreading screw from 7 to 11 mm, the optimum position can be achieved for every humeral medullary canal.

Instrumentation: Nails and Screws

Only a few instruments are necessary for nail insertion. All of them are stored on the instrumentation tray.

1. **The target device**
   (complete, transverse, frontal)
   The target device is mounted on the top of the nail. Two slots in the nail correspond to two lugs on the target device, thus ensuring the correct alignment of the nail and target device. The bow of the nail must be orientated towards the dorsal side of the humerus.
2. **The nail holding screw**
   The nail holding screw fixes the target device to the nail. The screw is tightened by hand and has to fix the target device securely onto the nail. If this is not done correctly, difficulties with proximal locking of the nail will be encountered.
3. **The long screwdriver** (spreading screw)
   The long screwdriver is introduced through the cannulated nail holding screw and passed down through the nail into the spreading screw. The spreading screw is then rotated anticlockwise in order to spread the distal portion of the nail.
4. **The nail guide pin** (2 mm)
   The 2-mm-diameter nail guide pin is used to introduce the nail while maintaining reduction of the fracture after the reaming has been carried out with a standard reaming guide wire (3 or 3.4 mm).
5. **The tissue protection sleeve**
   The tissue protection sleeve is used to target the proximal screw holes. It is guided through the holes of the target device and is passed through the soft tissue down to the cortex.
6. **The holding screws for the protection sleeve**
   The thumb screw is used to fix the tissue protection sleeve in position when it is up against the cortex.
7. **The awl**
   The awl is introduced through the protection sleeve and prepares the cortex prior to drilling for the locking screw.
8. **The drill guide sleeve**
   The drill guide is colour coded yellow. It is secured on the tissue protection sleeve by a screw thread in the protector. This sleeve ensures the accurate drilling of the holes for the cross locking screws.
9. **The drill bit** (3.7 mm)
   The drill bit (3.7 mm) is also colour coded yellow.
10. **The screw gauge**
    The screw gauge determines the length of locking screw required. It measures the working length of the screw, i.e. the length from cortex to cortex. Both the screw head and screw tip are excluded from this measurement.
11. **The extraction adapter**
    The extraction adapter is connected to the proximal part of the nail for removal of the implant. It screws into the internal threaded portion of the nail. The nail cannot be extracted without unlocking proximally and distally first. For the distal unlocking, the long screwdriver is reintroduced through the cannulated nail into the spreading screw and rotated clockwise to unlock the spreading screw. The target device is not necessary for nail extraction.
12. **The standard capwasher**
    The standard capwasher is used in very rare cases of humeral head fractures.
13. **The connection screw**
    The connecting screw fixes the standard capwasher on the top of the nail.
14. **The lateral capwasher**
    The lateral capwasher is intended to stabilise humeral head fractures and very proximal shaft fractures. It attaches to the lateral aspect of the humerus, its five flanges can be curved to hold the fracture fragments in place without impinging on the rotator cuff.
15. **The nail collection**
    The nails have diameters of 7, 8, and 9 mm and range in length from 140 to 320 mm. The

nail has three holes proximally for the locking screws. The first (HS1) is transversal from the lateral to the medial side. The second (HS2) is crossed to the first running in the frontal-dorsal direction and the third (HS3) is parallel to the first. The first hole has a thread which allows the first screw to be used as a fixation screw. With this screw the lateral capwasher is attached to the nail. The second and the third holes are unthreaded and so screws placed in them act as compression screws. The second screw is also useful in obtaining better fixation in special fracture types of the humeral head.

16. **The spreading screws**
The spreading screws lock the nail distally by expansion of the tip of the nail. The nail has three slots distally and the spreading screw is inserted by use of the long screwdriver. Spreading screws with a range of 7–11 mm in diameter are available. The new generation of spreading screws is a double spreading screw with a higher fixation stability.

Indications for the Humeral Locking Nail

All humeral shaft fractures from S1 to S5 can be treated with the nail (Fig. 12.5). For good fixation, the distal fragment must be at least 5 cm in length. The indication is given for A1–A3, B1–B3 and C1–C3 fractures (AO Classification).

The absolute indications for operation are open fractures, polytraumatised or multiple injury patients, fractures with traumatic nerve lesion, obese patients, alcoholics, patients who are dependent on drugs and aged patients who are unable to comply with functional treatment.

Operative Technique

The operative technique is closed. After preparation of the entrance into the humerus, the instrumentation follows a step by step sequence: reduction, reaming, nailing, distal locking, and proximal locking.

Positioning and Draping

The position of the patient is half sitting on the operation table in the so-called beach chair position. The upper part of the body is positioned on the fracture side and the shoulder and forearm are away from the table. The upper arm is not supported and is free for fluoroscopic X-ray control. The upper arm is reclined at 30°–60° and the forearm is in 60° flexion. With this positioning the head of the humerus is in a good position for the approach to prepare the entrance and for the rotator cuff to introduce the nail (Fig. 12.5 b).

Only the humerus and the shoulder are undraped. The assistant holds the forearm for reduction of the fracture. The surgeon stands directly in front of the shoulder. The instrumentalist is on the right side of the surgeon, the assistant on the forearm side. The C-frame comes from the surgeon's side and stands between the surgeon and the assistant (Fig. 12.6).

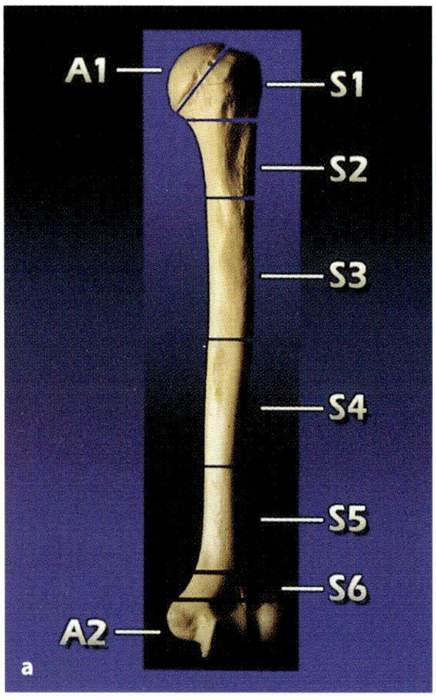

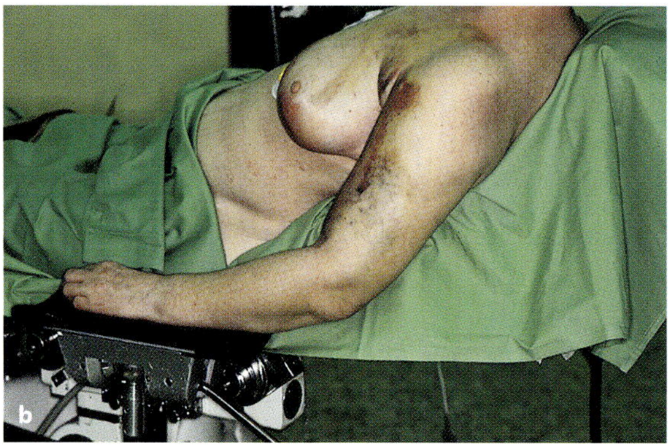

Fig. 12.5. a Fractures from S1 to S6 can be treated with the humeral locking nail. **b** Positioning of the patient

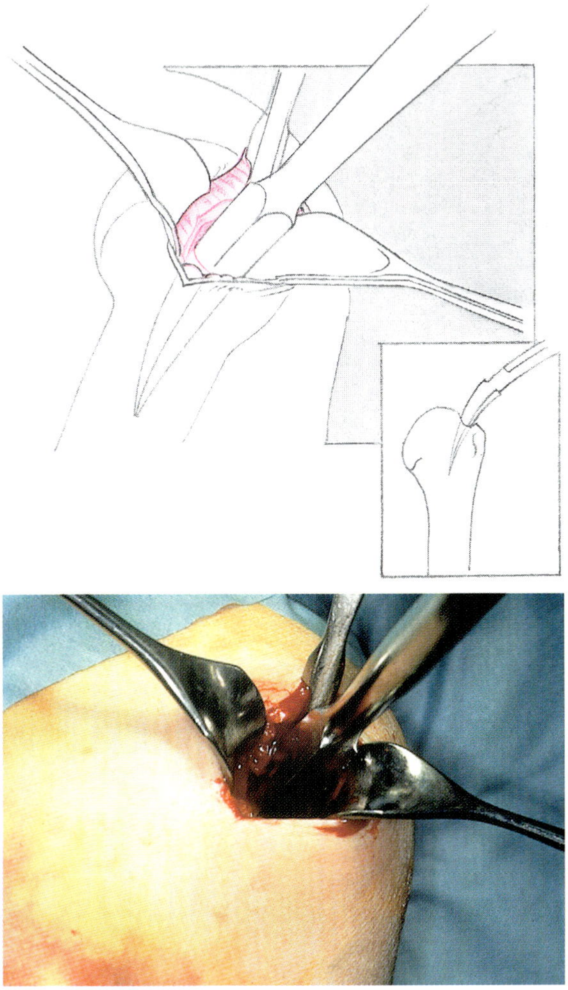

Fig. 12.10. Introduction point and entrance with the pointed awl

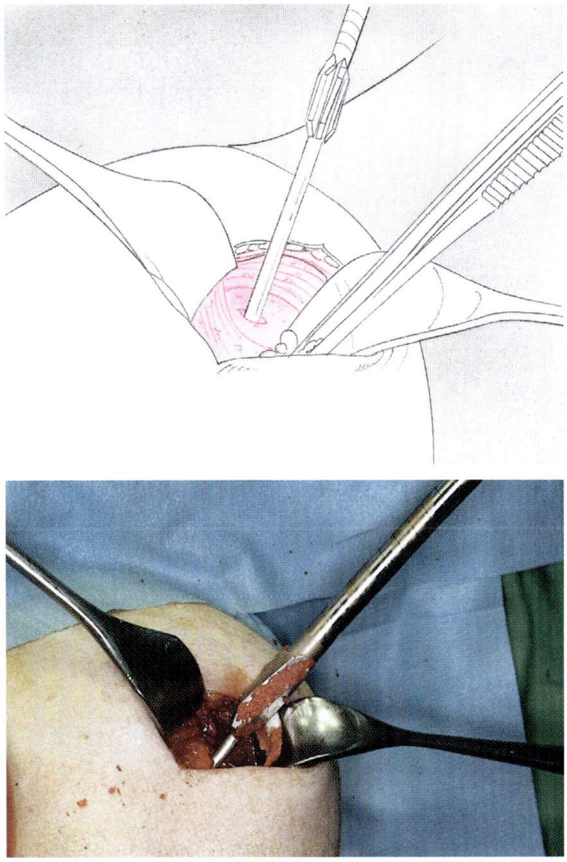

Fig. 12.11. Introduction of guide wire and reamer

At the end of the reaming procedure, the entrance portal is cleaned and washed to prevent calcification in the soft tissue due to the reaming products.

Nail Preparation with Target Device

The nurse prepares the chosen nail for introduction. The targeting device is screwed onto the nail with the fixation screw. The concave curvature of the nail must face the posterior side. The alignment of the target device is checked before insertion (Fig. 12.13). The spreading screw is screwed into the nail with clockwise turns. The correct position of the spreading screw is just on the tip of the nail, without causing expansion (Fig. 12.14).

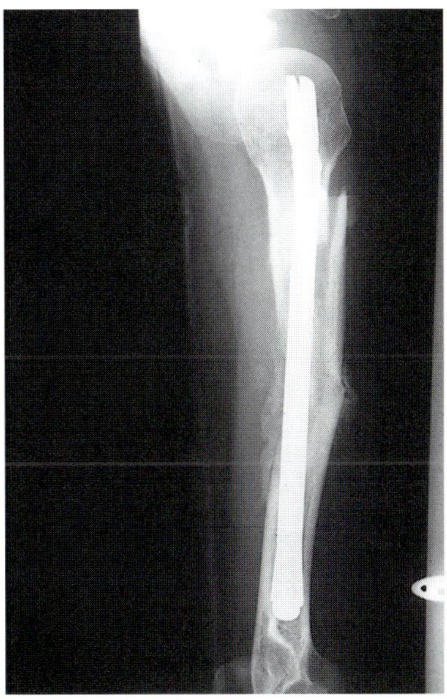

Fig. 12.12. The longest nail should be selected

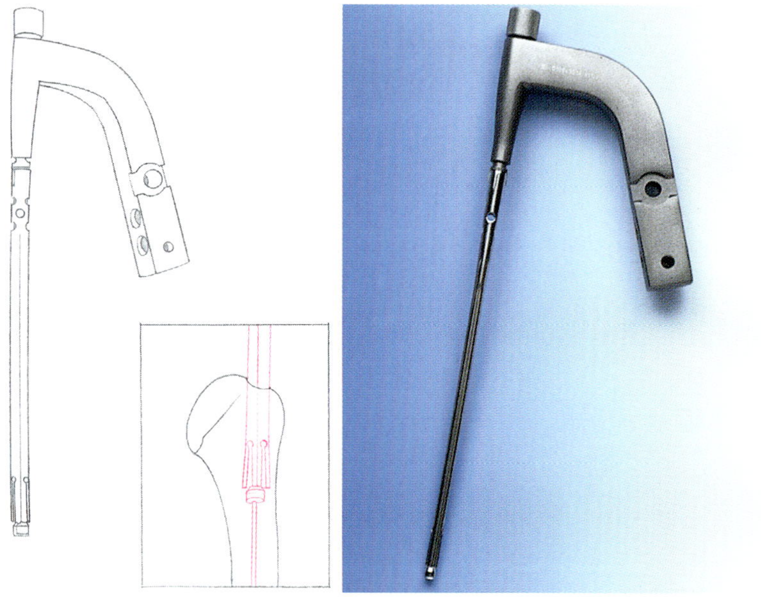

Fig. 12.13. The targeting device and the spreading screw that were screwed onto the nail

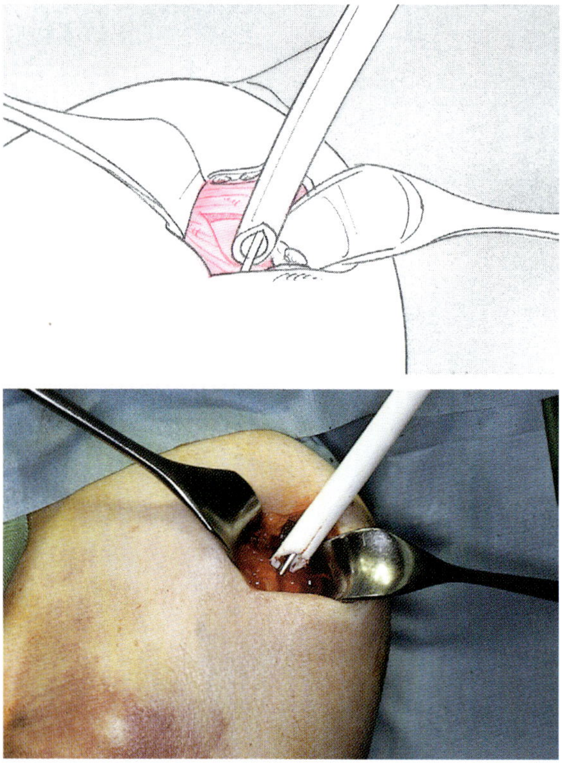

Fig. 12.14. The position of the spreading screw just at the tip of the nail

Nail Introduction and Nail Position

The reaming wire is exchanged, using a polyethylene tube for the 2-mm-diameter nailing guide (Fig. 12.15 a). The nail is introduced by hand, ensuring the bend of the nail is dorsal, with a small amount of rotation. Hammering has a high risk of splitting the bone and is forbidden. The proximal edge of the nail must be inserted just inside the cortex. This position is identifiable on the target device, which has a notch to indicate the correct level of insertion. The notch should be level with the cortex when insertion is complete. Thus, the instrumentation guarantees that the nail is inside the cortex and cannot irritate the soft tissues (Fig. 12.15 b, c).

Distal Locking

The long hex screwdriver is passed down through the nail holding the screw and the cannulation in the nail into the spreading screw. The surgeon is able to feel the contact of the screwdriver with the spreading screw as a click. By rotating the screwdriver to the left (anticlockwise), the spreading screw is drawn back into the nail. The final position of the screw is checked with the image intensifier. The best position is with the screw-end level with the nail-end. The surgeon can feel the locking stability of the screw as the resistance to expansion increases when the nail tip engages the cortex. In our experience, this expansion has never caused bone splitting (Fig. 12.16).

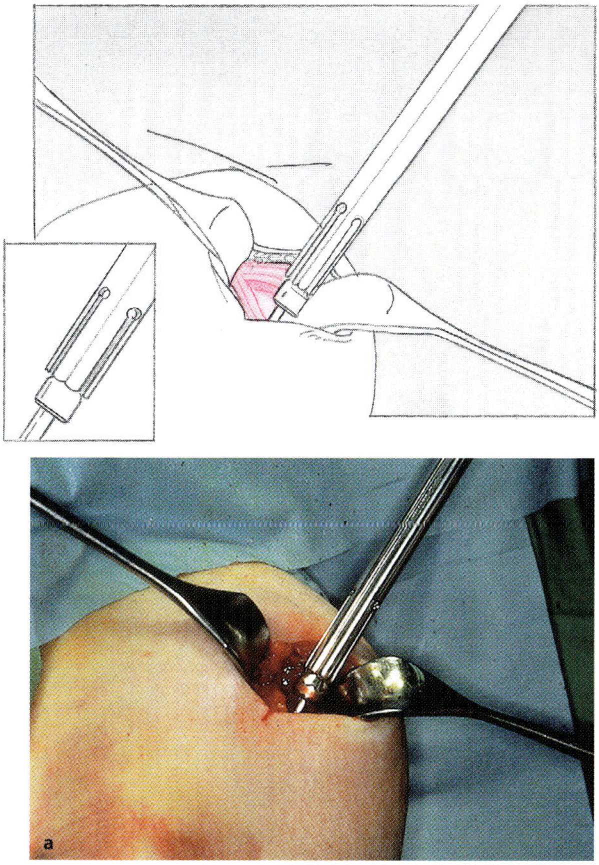

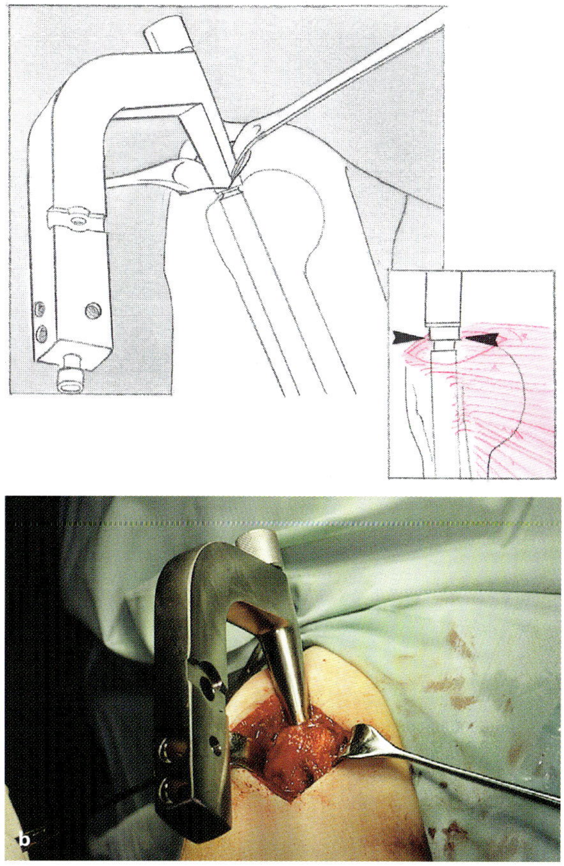

Fig. 12.15. a The reaming guide is changed with a polyethylene tube. **b, c** The proximal edge of the nail must be inserted just inside the cortex

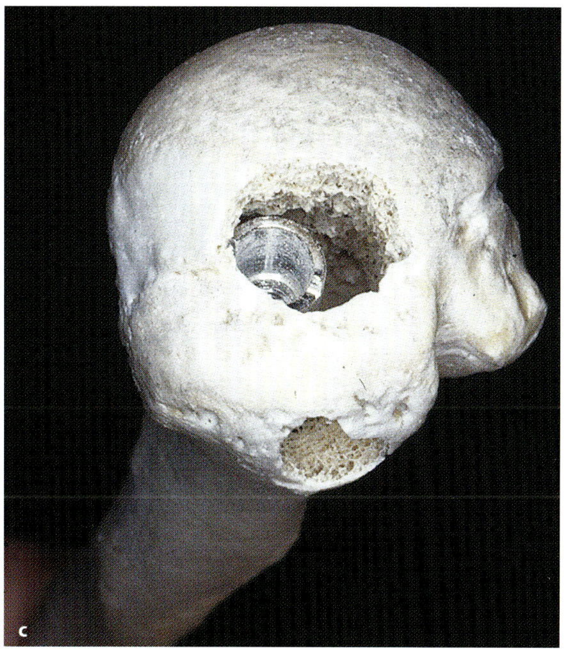

Proximal Locking

After distal locking, the proximal screws are positioned to complete the locking of the nail. Two screws are recommended for the best stability. Only with two screws is the rotational stability of the proximal fragment ensured (Fig. 12.17). With a single screw, rotation of the head fragment around the screw is possible. Care must be taken in positioning the AP screw, as it can come into conflict with the long biceps tendon. Therefore, carefully preparing the setting is recommended.

The proximal locking procedure starts with the insertion of the sleeve system into the transverse targeting device. First, a small skin incision is made and the muscle is divided. The tissue protector sleeve is positioned in the lower hole (HS3) of the lateral targeting device. The sleeve is pushed into contact with the lateral cortex.

The sleeve is then fixed into position, using the thumb screw in order to ensure that the correct alignment is maintained. To ensure accurate drilling, the pointed awl is introduced, tapped, and turned to pierce the lateral cortex. The drilling guide sleeve (colour coded yellow) is introduced

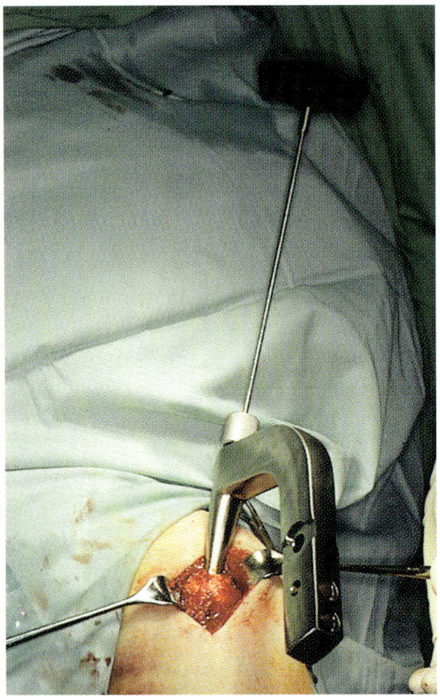

Fig. 12.16. Distal locking with the long screwdriver

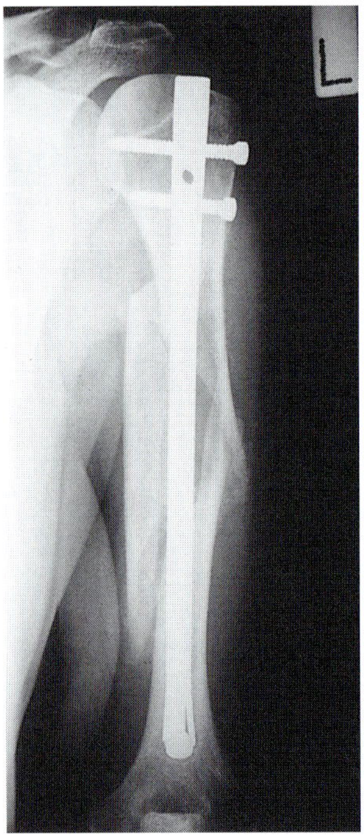

Fig. 12.17. Two screws ensured the proximal rotational stability

and both cortices are drilled using the yellow 3.7-mm-diameter drill bit (Fig. 12.18).

The screw length is measured with the depth gauge and the self-cutting screws (4.6 mm) are introduced. These screws do not require a tap (Fig. 12.19). In cases of shaft fractures, the second screw (first screw hole on the nail HS1) is also in-

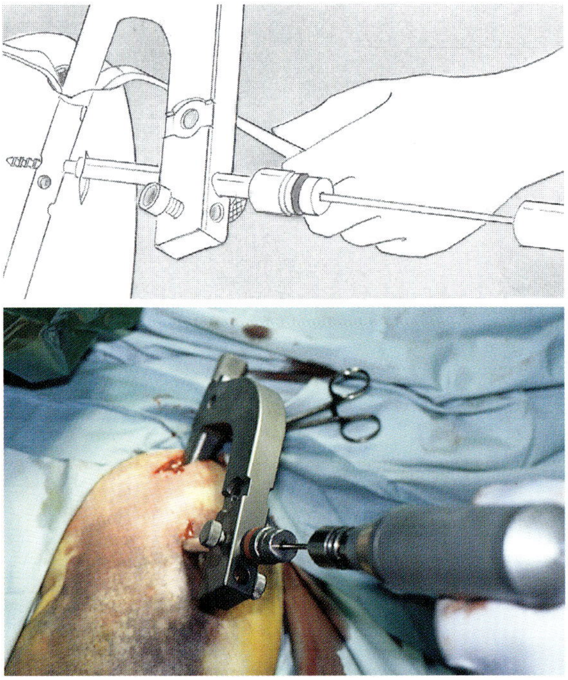

Fig. 12.18. Proximal drilling through the drilling guide sleeve

serted, using the same procedure. The final image intensifier control confirms the correct position of the nail and the fracture reduction.

If the required frontal target arm is attached to the targeting device, the procedure is repeated for the AP screw. The long biceps tendon must be prepared so that the locking screw does not penetrate the tendon.

Proximal Fractures

For proximal fractures with two, three, or more head fragments, open reduction is recommended [4]. The typical subcapital fracture without fragmentation on the minor or major tubercle can be treated with the closed technique. If the bone quality is good enough to allow screw fixation in the humeral head, the locking technique with one screw, two or even three screws is performed. The fracture type determines the number of screws required.

The first nail hole has a thread which allows the screw in this hole to provide more stability to the system than the other screws which can slip in their holes. The top of the nail must be embedded in the head, to prevent impingement and pain (Fig. 12.20 a, b). For this osteosynthesis, short nails (14–20 cm) are used. The top of the nail prevents dislocation of the head fragment in the form of rotation or valgus and varus disloca-

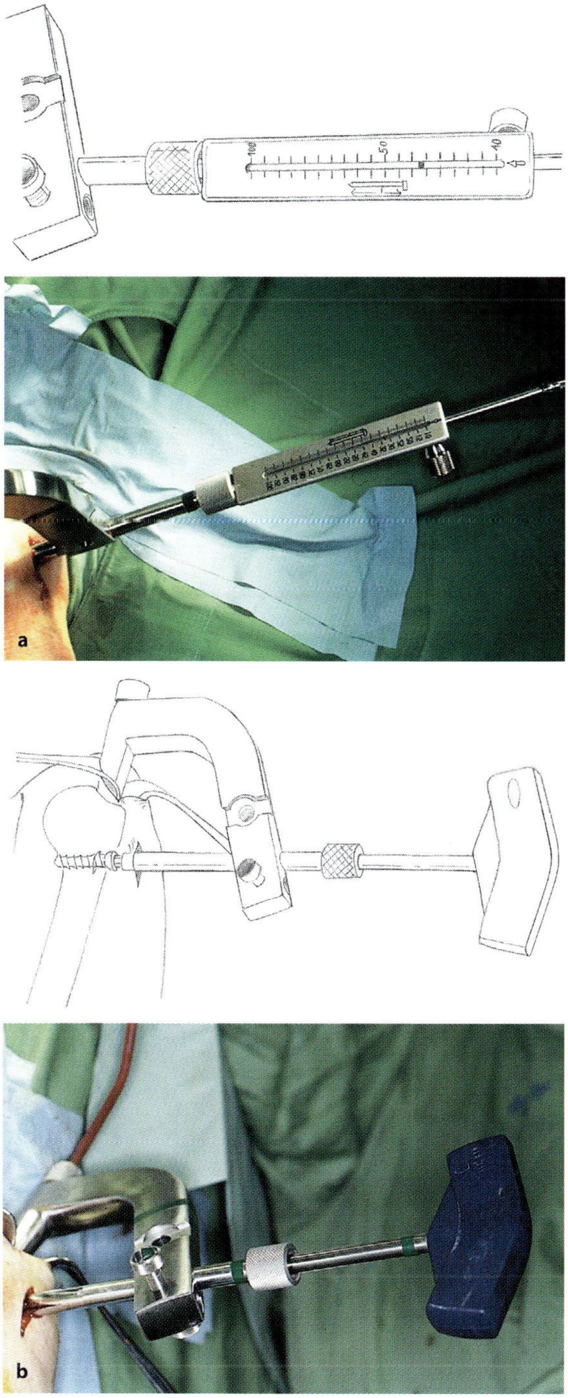

Fig. 12.19. a Measuring the screw length with the depth gauge. **b** Self-cutting screw is introduced

tion. The screw guides the head fragment during flexion and rotation. In addition, the screw fixes any fragments of the greater tuberosity. If an excessive fragmented fracture with accompanying retraction of the rotator cuff with dislocation is presented, open reduction is imperative.

Humeral Head Fractures

The skin incision is 10–15 cm long and runs in the same direction as for humeral shaft fractures (Fig. 12.21). The deltoid muscle is split longitudinally on its medial side. Preparation and loosening of the muscle on the clavicle is not performed; it is retracted to the lateral side. The subacromial bursa is resected and the fracture is reached.

The first step is to place the humeral head in articulation, then the different bone fragments and the rotator cuff are identified. The long biceps tendon is used to orientate the reconstruction and indicate the relative positions of the greater and minor tuberosities. The nail is put in the medullary canal through the fracture. Reaming is not used in the proximal section because the medullary canal is large. The top end of the nail is inserted below the level of the humeral head. Distal locking is performed. The rotator cuff and bone fragments are placed in position. The *lateral washer* fixes both the cuff and the bone fragments, making a functional and stable unit. The lateral washer is fixed in position with the first screw of the nail, using the transverse targeting device.

The rotator cuff is located under the lateral washer. The lateral washer with five flanges has the same function as a hand holding an egg. It guides, without additional trauma, the humeral head and prevents the dislocation of the head (Fig. 12.22).

This very individual operation corresponds to the large variation in humeral head fractures. For adequate fixation, the flanges are bent individually for each patient. The tips of the flanges are bent and pressed in the bone. If all five arms of the lateral washer are not required, one or two can be removed before final insertion. In addition to the washer fixation, sutures are used to attach the rotator cuff to the washer. Using this technique, a resection of the humeral head is avoided.

The Neer acromioplasty facilitates the healing of the rotator cuff. For this reconstruction, short nails (14–20 cm) are used. At the end of the operation, it is important that the rotator cuff is thoroughly cleaned to ensure that all bone-debris is washed out. The articulation is drained with a Redon drain.

Summary of Operative Technique

Diaphyseal Humeral Fractures: Closed Reduction

1. Short frontal skin incision
2. Preparation of deltoid muscle

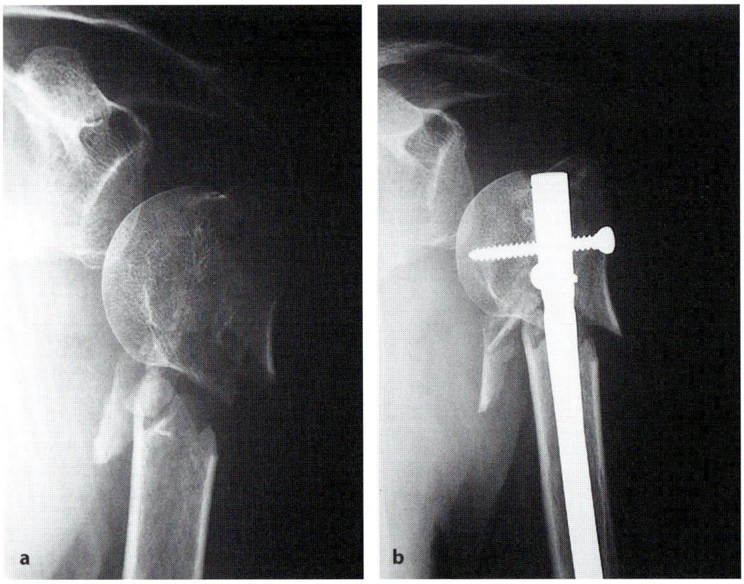

Fig. 12.20 a, b. Subcapital fracture treated by the closed technique with the humeral locking nail

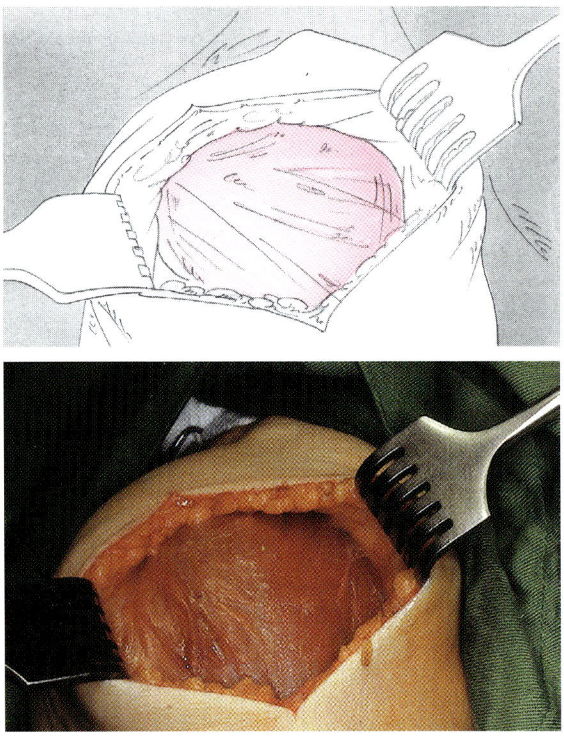

Fig. 12.21. Incision for humeral head fractures

3. Resection subacromial bursa
4. Incision of rotator cuff
5. Entrance point in the sulcus in the humeral head
6. Fracture reduction
7. Reaming in 0.5-mm steps
8. Over-reaming by 2 mm
9. Change reaming wire to nail guide wire
10. Nail concavity dorsal
11. Spreading screw into the nail end
12. Nail insertion by hand
13. Distal locking left turn
14. Proximal locking two screws
15. Cuff cleaning
16. Joint drainage – Redon drain

Proximal Humeral Fractures: Open Reduction

1. Longer frontal skin incision
2. Muscle preparation
3. Resection of subacromial bursa
4. Reduction of humeral head
5. Short nail insertion through fracture
6. Distal locking
7. Reduction of fragments and rotator cuff
8. Pre-bending of lateral washer
9. Positioning of lateral washer
10. Screw fixation in lateral washer
11. Cuff suture onto lateral washer
12. Joint drainage

Postoperative Management

The postoperative treatment is divided into four periods: the acute wound period, the fresh wound period, the soft callus period, and the fixation callus period.

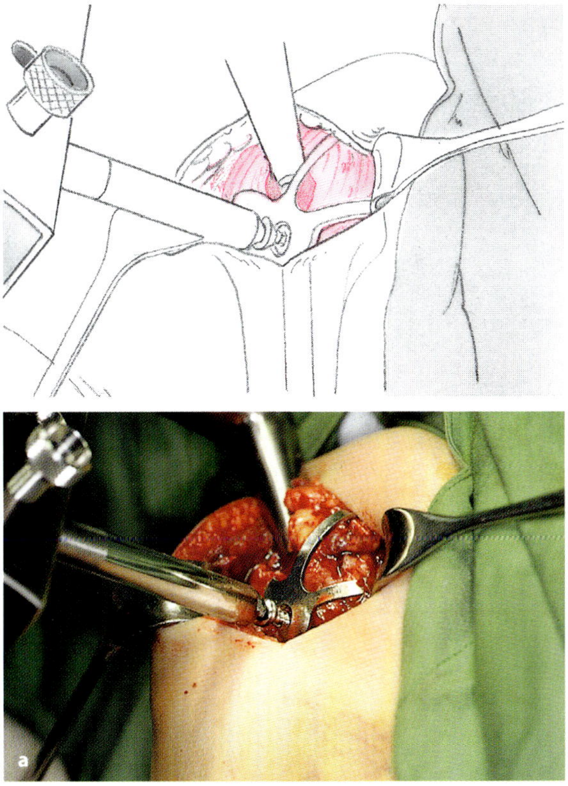

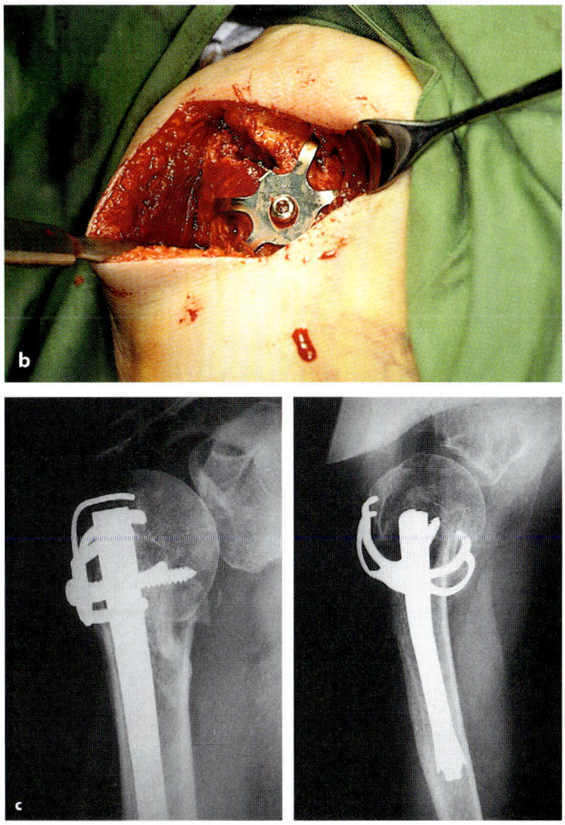

Fig. 12.22 a–c. Humeral head fracture fixed by lateral washer

Acute Wound Period (0–8 Days)

The damage to the soft tissue limits the immediate postoperative management. Both the haematoma and the soft tissue swelling restrict free motion, as does the pain of the wound. In order to reduce the swelling, cooling techniques are used; medication is generally not required. In the first few postoperative days, analgesics may become necessary when physiotherapy and movement of the injured limb begin. No external plaster or splint is used. The upper limb is supported with a collar sling. Immediately after the operation, active exercises and isometric muscle contraction without passive resistance are started. Isometric muscle contractions (500 times per day) are required.

After 3–4 days the patient begins to elevate himself on the climbing ladder. After 2 weeks an elevation of 90° is achieved. In this period external rotation at the elbow is not allowed; however, flexion is unrestricted.

Fresh Wound Period (1–2 Weeks)

Ten to twelve days after the operation the stitches are removed. The patient begins hydrotherapy and is encouraged to swim. The isometric muscle training is continued at the rate of 500 times per day, active elevation, abduction and rotation of the shoulder joint is encouraged. External rotation of the elbow is allowed without resistance to the rotation.

Soft Callus Period (2–6 Weeks)

When the first soft callus is evident on X-ray, more active motion can begin. The patient is able to perform all normal everyday activities and can drive a car. Active sport and heavy weight bearing is not allowed. The isometric muscle exercises are increased by the use of weights from the fourth postoperative week.

Fixation Callus Period (>3 Months)

When there is X-ray evidence of stable overbridging callus, full weight bearing is possible. This consolidation normally takes 8–12 weeks. The implant is removed after 6–12 months postoperatively in young patients (less than 70 years) with shaft fractures. Where the proximal capwasher has been used, it must be removed in every case, 6–12 weeks after the operation. If the lateral washer has been used it can be removed at the same time as the nail.

Errors and Potential Hazards of Operative Technique

Entrance

The approach must be frontal. The lateral approach has the risk of fracture of the medial cortex and causes displacement of the fracture. The entry point has to be just behind the top of the major tubercle. If the entry point is too ventral, damage to the frontal head and the rotator cuff will occur. It is also a problem in proximal fractures, because the bone stability is too weak. Also the vascularity can be damaged frontally but not dorsally in the rotator cuff. The longitudinal incision of the rotary cuff has to be long enough (1.5–2 cm). If the incision is too small the rotary cuff will be damaged by the reamer.

Reaming

The reaming has to be done carefully. Sharp reamer heads are necessary. Reaming has to be performed in 0.5-mm steps. The reaming products on the rotator cuff produce calcification. Absolutely no bone debris must be left in the rotator cuff. Never ream in a comminuted fracture area. Never nail if the radial nerve could be involved in the fracture. This must be prepared by open reduction prior to nailing.

Nails

The longest nail for unstable fractures is the best nail. The bow of the nail is placed to the dorsal side. The nail insertion must be done carefully, pushing by hand. It is very important to avoid hammering. The nail has to be 2 mm smaller than the reamed canal. Respecting this condition, the nail diameter must be calculated between 7 and 9 mm.

Locking

The highest stability of distal locking is achieved if the locking screw is just in the nail. The canal has to be 2 mm larger than the nail. First distal locking, followed by proximal locking. In order to lock the distal screw, rotate the long screwdriver anticlockwise. When unlocking turn the screwdriver clockwise. Proximal AP locking can be dangerous for the long biceps tendon. The tissue protector must be in direct contact with the bone. If the situation is not clear, the tendon must be made visible by making a longer incision. The first proximal and the third locking screws must always have a strictly transverse direction. If they are allowed to go in the diagonal direction there is a risk of hitting the branch of the axillary nerve. The lateral washer must be bent onto the bone and it must fixed to the rotator cuff. Sutures from the rotary cuff onto the lateral washer secure the rotary cuff. The rotator cuff is under the lateral washer.

Pseudarthrosis

Large displacement over the nail could cause pseudarthrosis. In long spiral fractures with large fracture cracks, muscle can be interposed and can hinder the consolidation. If the fracture gap in transverse fractures is too large, there is a high risk of pseudarthrosis. This can be avoided by compression of the fracture before proximal locking.

References

1. Hackethal KH (1961) Die Bündelnagelung. Springer, New York Berlin Heidelberg Tokyo
2. Küntscher G, Maatz R (1945) Technik der Marknagelung. Georg Thieme, Leipzig
3. Müller ME, Allgöwer M, Schneider R, Willenegger H (1991) Manual of internal fixation. Springer, New York Berlin Heidelberg Tokyo
4. Neer CS (1970) Displaced humeral fractures. Part I: Classification and evaluation. J Bone Joint Surg Am 52:1077–1089
5. Poelchen, R (1930) Die Behandlung der Frakturen der oberen Extremität ohne Fixation, nur mit aktiver Extensionsbehandlung. Monschr Unfallheilkd 37:193–219
6. Rush LV, Rush HC (1950) Intramedullary fixation of fractures of the humerus by longitudinal pin. Surgery 27:268–273
7. Seidel H (1989) Humeral locking nail: a preliminary report Orthopedics 12:219–226

CHAPTER 13

Ulnar Fractures

C. LEFÈVRE and D. LE NEN

Introduction

The goal of treatment of fractures of both forearm bones is, besides consolidation, to preserve the function of prono-supination of the upper limb; this implies that the lengths and curvatures of both bones have to be considered [1, 11]. Indeed, if this anatomical requirement is respected initially, the function of prono-supination can be preserved after the consolidation of the fracture site. Because of this anatomical requirement, the diaphyseal fractures of the forearm, isolated or associated, usually require surgical treatment. The method used most often is still osteosynthesis with screws and plates. We, however, find it unsatisfactory that during the implanting of such a plate it is necessary to expose the fracture site, which triggers bone destruction, added trauma to the soft tissues and a risk of secondary synosteosis. Moreover, the implant can cause discomfort to the patient (especially at the level of the ulna, which is the superficial bone) under a scar of more than 10 cm in length. Finally, the removal of the implant requires the same initial approach and is sometimes followed by a recurring fracture because of the "stress protection" of the cortical areas bridged by the plate. Hence, closed intramedullary osteosynthesis seems to be an interesting alternative. This chapter will deal with the problems posed by ulnar nailing.

Historical Background

One of the first descriptions of intramedullary osteosynthesis of the forearm dates back to a publication of Shone [6], who proposed aligning the diaphyseal fragments with thin metallic wires requiring a minimal approach. The non-invasive character of this new method had great success. Since then, it has been adopted by Lambotte and Danis.

In 1920, Kirschner took up this idea but noticed that there was no great difference with immobilization in plaster which led to 12% pseudarthrosis: pinning led to 17%! He did notice, however, the excellent control of the fragment alignment thanks to his method.

At the end of the 1930s, Rush [5] proposed a larger triangular section wire (3 mm) with which excellent control of the fragment rotation could be achieved. Unfortunately, the clinical results were quite disappointing, as the rate of pseudarthrosis reached approximately 16%.

The insufficient calibre of these implants led to an absence of bone-implant contact. This caused lateral displacements of transverse fractures, shortening of oblique fractures, and a total lack of control over rotation of diaphyseal fragments, which led to the high rate of failures.

At the beginning of the 1940s, Küntscher [3] proposed the first really rigid intramedullary nail, but a number of them broke (38%), and nailing, then without reaming, sometimes led to diaphyseal splittings. When the nail was introduced, it disturbed the fracture site, which made consolidation uncertain.

In the same period, Steinmann was using a 3-mm section, fully slotted nail. The results registered were 20% pseudarthrosis and sometimes the thread of the nail became embedded in the bone, making it difficult to remove.

Since the 1950s, Street [9, 10] had been using a 4-mm section, square, straight nail, which was placed after reaming and seemed to give better results. The specific anatomical conditions of the forearm and the necessity of obtaining satisfactory rotational control has recently led to the development of new types of implants, for both the radius and the ulna.

Maatz [4] then proposed the ulnar nail, designed with a slotted distal end and an olecranon proximal end fitted with a spring. In fact, the thread still did not offer a sufficient hold in the bone to ensure the necessary interfragmentary compression.

Schiwier [7] used a compression ulnar nail, introduced proximally by the cubital head and screwed in compression at the olecranon level; but the encumbrance of the implant at the elbow became unacceptable for the patients. The necessity to approach the wrist was also unsatisfactory.

All things considered, it is advisable to adapt the implants to the anatomical and physiological conditions of the forearm.

Telescopic Ulna Locking Nail

The ulna is a superficial bone, whose olecranon is not difficult to approach. For an intramedullary approach for osteosynthesis, it requires the following:

1. An implant suited to the anatomy of the bone, being aware that the diaphysis is curvilinear, with several alternate curvatures
2. Achieving control in rotation of each fragment
3. The possibility of compression of the fracture site

The malleable telescopic locking nail with compression distraction fulfills these requirements.

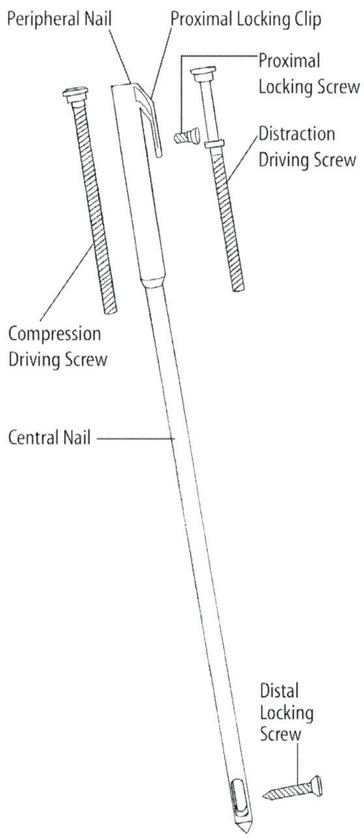

Fig. 13.1. The Ulna Locking Nail

Description and Principles of the Nail

The Implant

The implant (Fig. 13.1) is made of two parts that slide into each other, the 8-mm section, olecranon proximal part being fitted with a vertical slot into which slides a cotter pin that attaches to the 6- or 4.5-mm distal part. The variation of the implant length is 45 mm. The proximal part has a posterior vertical clip intended for proximal locking.

The 4-, 5-, or 6-mm diameter distal part is designed with an oblong hole intended for distal locking. This malleable alloy part allows adaptation of the implant to the various diaphyseal curvatures. The rigid nail remains indicated for the comminuted fractures and the lengthenings.

At the upper end of the proximal part (Fig. 13.2), it is possible to place a one-headed compression screw. The head of this screw rests on the upper end of the proximal part and the whole of the threaded section engages in the distal part. The screwing action leads to a shortening of the whole device, which creates a compression assembly.

At the upper end of the proximal part, it is also possible to place a two-headed distally threaded distraction screw. The second head is blocked in translation by mean of a small transverse screw which crosses the locking clip, the posterior cortex of the bone, and, lastly, the wall of the nail. This locking screw prevents the loosening of the two-headed screw.

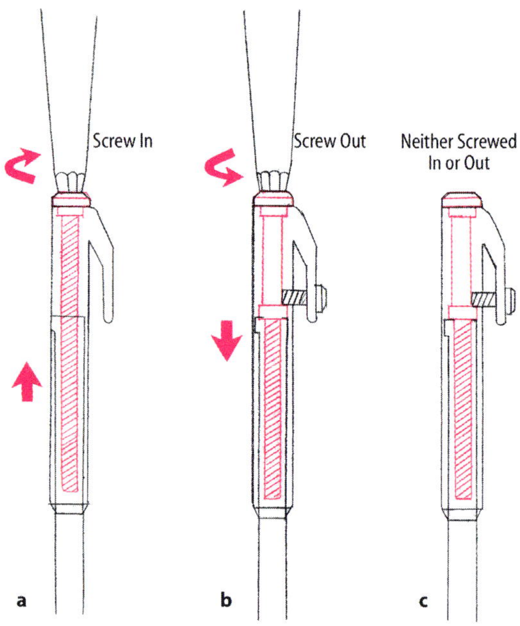

Fig. 13.2 a–c. The three possibilities of mechanical assembly. **a** compression; **b** distraction; **c** neutral

The unscrewing action leads to implant lengthening, creating a distraction assembly. The absence of movement of this two-headed screw leads to no variation in the length of the implant, resulting in a neutral assembly.

Indications

Compression is the most frequently used assembly for the treatment of displaced or unstable shaft fractures, whether they are mid-diaphyseal, proximal or distal, bifocal or trifocal. A compression assembly can also be useful in shortening osteotomies of the ulna, for example after wrist mal-unions with internal overpression syndrome of the wrist. Other indications of a compression assembly include: the *Monteggia* fracture of the olecranon, after segmental resection for tumour involving the shaft with intermediary fibular graft (isolated or vascularised) and, finally, the non-unions (the best field of application of the nail) after conservative treatment or other surgical treatment: wiring, plating, simple nailing or external fixator. The neutral form of assembly is only indicated in comminuted fractures.

Finally, the nail in distraction is indicated in ulna lengthening osteotomies in cases of *Kienböck* disease: among the various proposed methods [8, 9], telescopic nailing is very amenable, the lengthening being easily controlled perioperatively by X-ray because the thread of the screw is of a precise length and it ensures a secure attachment.

Operative Technique

The technique described is the classic technique, used in the absence of the new external reducer of the fractures of both forearm bones and flexible reamers.

1. Pre-operative controls
   The diameter of the medullary canal, which is in part diaphyseal, is measured on the X-ray. For a canal of a diameter of 5 mm or less, the 4–5 mm in diameter nail will be used. For a canal with a larger diameter, the nail of 6 mm will be used.
2. Positioning
   The patient is in a supine position, with a pneumatic tourniquet at the base of the upper limb; the latter rests on a radiotransparent arm table and is free to permit mobilization during the intervention. The image intensifier is positioned parallel to the table on the opposite side of the patient's head, on the side to be operated on (Fig. 13.3).

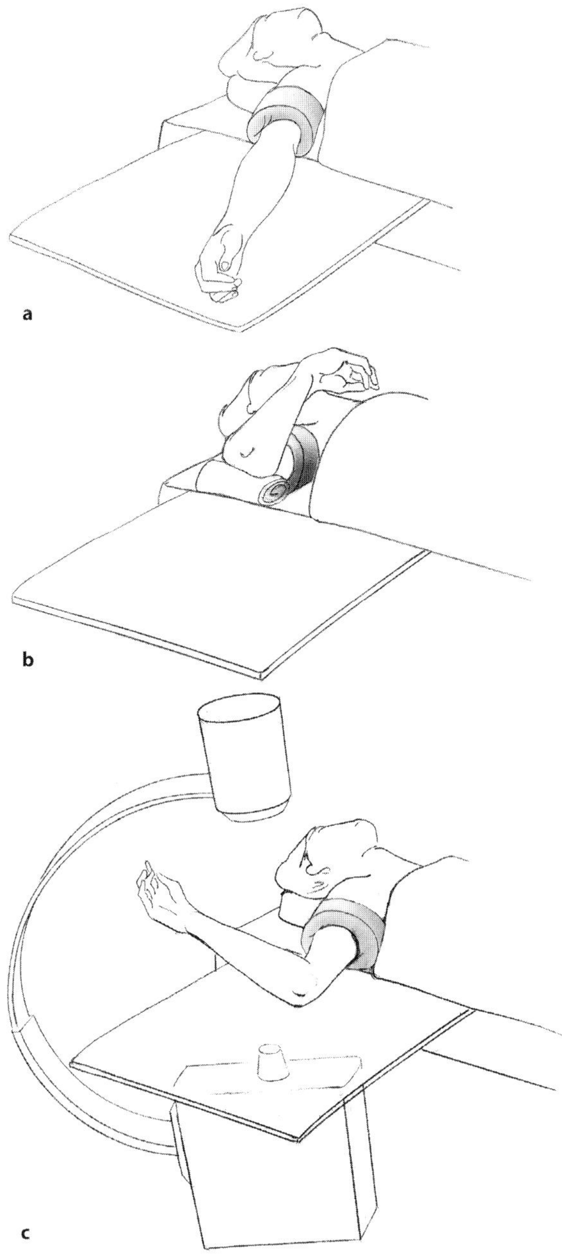

Fig. 13.3 a–c. Patient positioning. **a** Positioning: free upper limb. **b** Positioning for entry point. **c** Positioning for distal locking

3. Pre-operative reduction
   Reduction attempts by axial traction with X-ray control allow precise planning of the reduction, which will be useful during the operative procedure.
4. Draping
   A single drape, pierced in the middle, displays the upper limb up to above the elbow in the operative field.

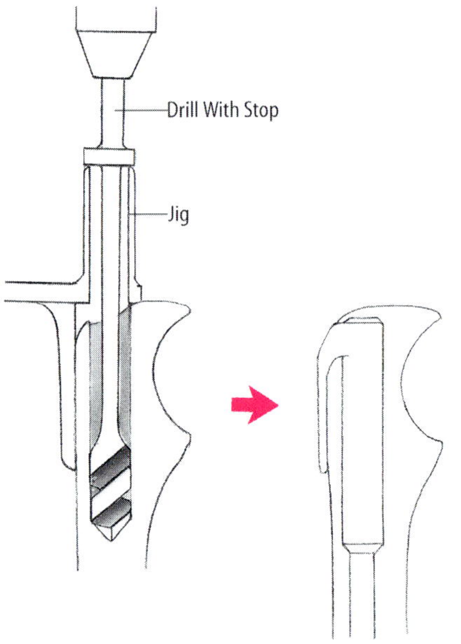

Fig. 13.4. Entry point

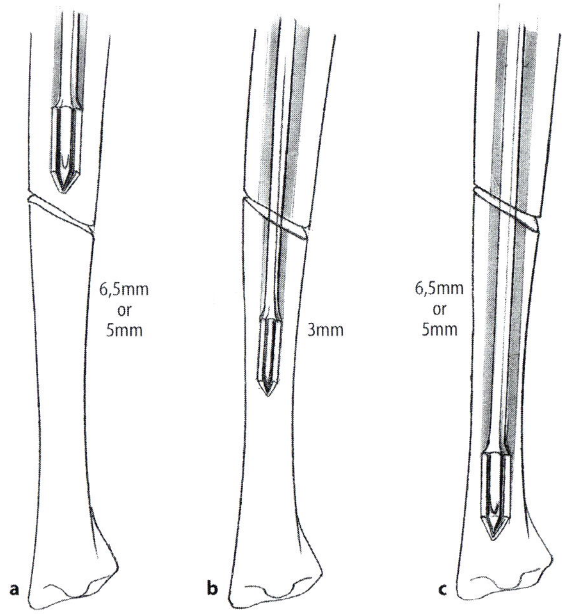

Fig. 13.6 a–c. Reaming procedure

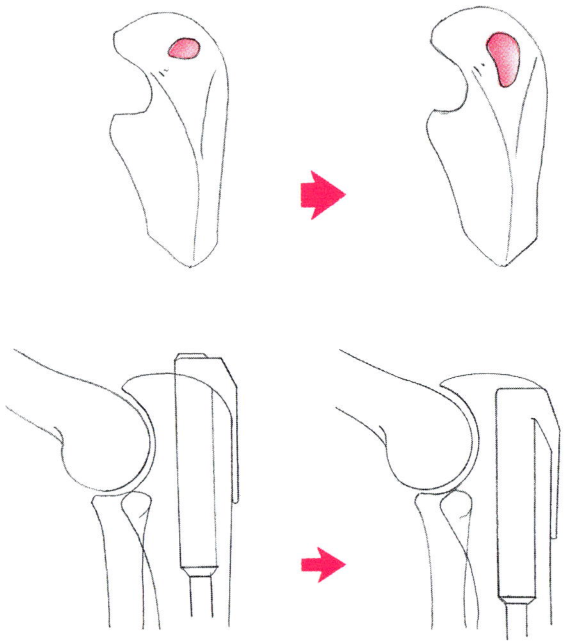

Fig. 13.5. The enlarged entry point with a nibbler allows one to correctly bury the olecranon clip of the nail

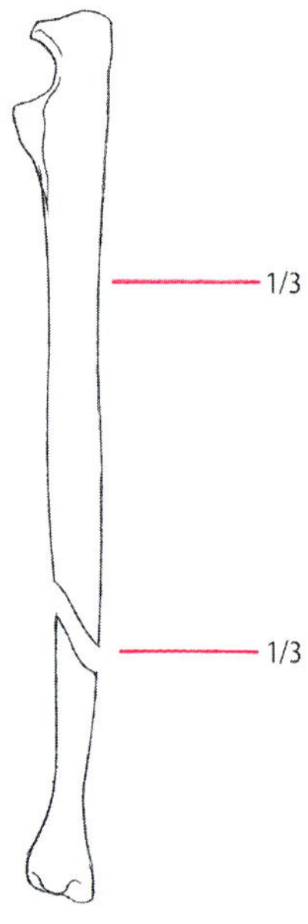

Fig. 13.7. Oblique osteotomy in case of lengthening

5. Approach
   An incision of 3–4 cm starts from the top of the olecranon and goes along the posterior crest of the ulna. The top and the posterior face of the olecranon are prepared with the rasp.
6. Entry point (Fig. 13.4)
   The entry point is determined with the olecranon drilling jig. This ancillary instrument is applied to the olecranon and impacted at the top, guiding a stop drill, 8 mm in diameter. The housing of the olecranon clip of the nail is prepared on a 1-cm surface using the gouge (Fig. 13.4). The implant will then perfectly buried, yielding better patient comfort (Fig. 13.5).
7. Reduction and reaming
   The reaming is progressively carried out using ulna reamers in 0.5-mm increments. We start by reaming the proximal fragment to 0.5 mm above the diameter of the nail

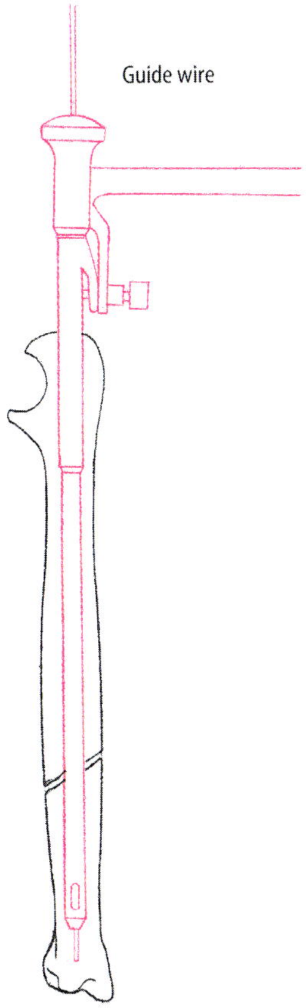

Fig. 13.8. Nailing. Note that the nail is often above the top of the olecranon

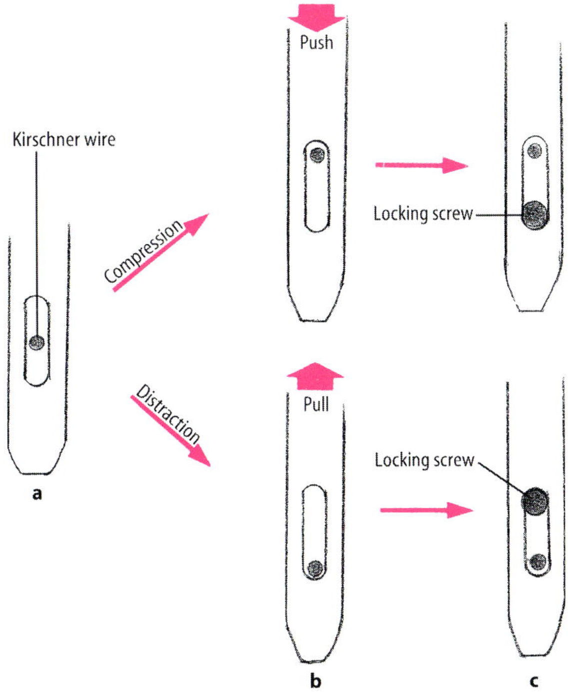

Fig. 13.9 a–c. Current position of the Kirschner wire and screw. **a** Kirschner wire in the middle of the oblong hole. **b** Push the nail for compression, pull the nail for distraction. **c** Correct position of the compression or distraction screw

(Fig. 13.6), which creates enough space to facilitate the passage to the fracture site with a 3-mm reamer. Then we ream the distal fragment, again 0.5 mm above the diameter of the nail. The reduction of the fracture site is then stabilized using the guide wire.
N.B.: In the case of lengthening, a minimal approach is used for the oblique diaphyseal osteotomy at the at the junction of the middle and distal thirds, after reaming (Fig. 13.7).

8. Setting up the nail
The nail is set up on the driving device in a configuration of maximal length (cotter pin below the slot). The whole device is slid along the guide wire using rotation movements. The mallet is not used frequently, usually only during the final stage of nailing. When this stage has been reached, the proximal part of the nail often sticks out the top of the olecranon (Fig. 13.8).
N.B.: To reduce the time of irradiation, it is possible to manually locate the level of the distal end of the implant; just lay a nail from the box of implants along the forearm, locating the upper olecranon limb of the two nails.
9. Distal locking
The upper limb of the patient is positioned in external rotation and abduction of the elbow. The handle for the driving device is kept in a horizontal position, the image intensifier being vertical, the oblong distal hole is then visualized in a lateral profile.
A Kirschner wire, loaded on the drill is placed perpendicular to both cortices in the middle of the oblong distal hole. To check the right position of the wire either on the screen or manually, push up or pull on the nail, which is blocked by the wire (Fig. 13.9).
The following stages are carried out without imaging: the double-barrelled distal targeting device is stabilized along the wire, the handle of the targeting device being kept in the axis of the forearm. After using the awl to drill at 2 mm for a nail of 4.5 mm and at 2.5 mm for a nail of 6 mm, the autothreader screw of 2.7 mm or 3.5 mm is placed across the targeting device with a screwdriver with sleeve.
Lastly, check the correct position of the locking screw, either on the screen or manually by pushing or pulling the nail.

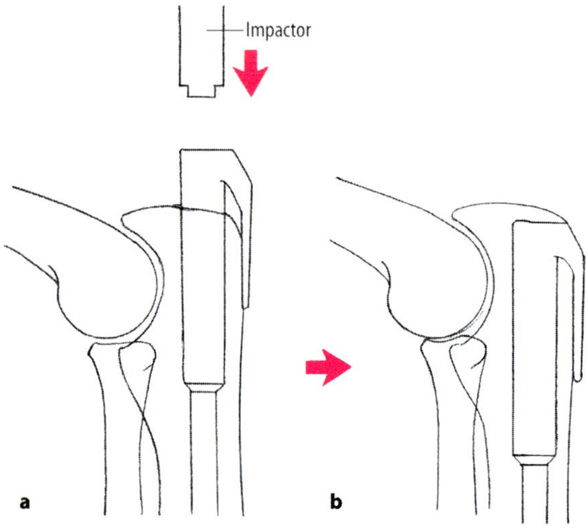

Fig. 13.10. a Insertion of the nail; **b** correct burying of the nail

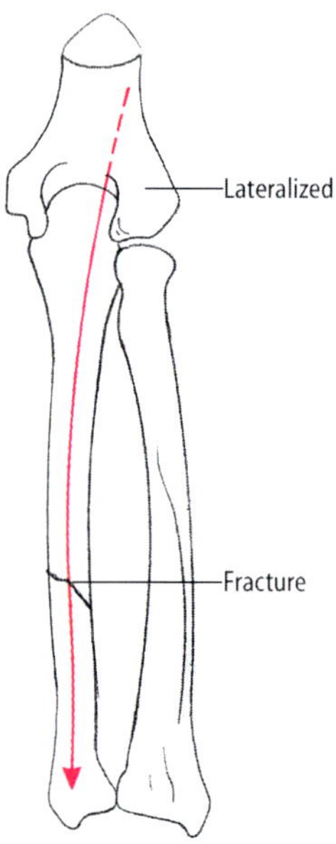

Fig. 13.11. Lateralized entry point

10. Impaction of the olecranon proximal part: proximal locking
    The proximal part of the nail is buried with the final impactor. At this stage, the nail protrudes from the top of the olecranon (Fig. 13.10).
11. Terminal assembly
    a) *Compression*. Simply insert the one-headed slotted compression screw completely. The screwing insertion gives interfragmentary compression. Check, if necessary, the ulna–radial position at the wrist on the monitor. The compression aspect is so effective that it is difficult to check clinically.
    b) *Distraction*. Drill the hole for the locking screw perpendicularly to the clip using the short drill with stop. To correctly place the two-headed distraction driving screw, the upper head *must be in contact* with the proximal part of the nail (screw completely in). Insert the locking screw. To create distraction, screw counter clockwise, which is checked with the image intensifier until an ulna–radial alignment is obtained. The products of reaming, the spongy bone taken from the olecranon, make it possible to graft the distraction site.
    c) *Neutral assembly*. This assembly is similar to the previous one (distraction driving screw + locking screw). Here, the distraction screw is neither screwed, nor unscrewed.
12. Closing
    - Closure of the olecranon incision is done in two layers, with a sub cutaneous suction drainage if needed.
    - Closure of the distal incision is done in one cutaneous layer.

Post-operative Management

In stable fractures, not causing any post-operative concerns, rehabilitation can start immediately. In comminuted fractures, to permit the flexion–extension movements of the elbow and the wrist, axial motion in prono-supination should be delayed for 3–4 weeks.

Errors and Potential Hazards

Entry Point

The entry point has to be lateralized towards the epicondyle. This makes it possible to avoid significant curvatures of the implant and assures that both parts of the implant will slide during the insertion. Moreover, the entry point lateralized towards the epicondyle has the advantage of maintaining a safe distance from the ulnar nerve (Fig. 13.11).

Reaming

- Avoid over-reaming to protect the bone capital
- Do not ream by using too much pressure. Let the head of the reamer automatically centre itself and avoid over-reaming of a cortex.

Nailing

In a distraction assembly, any deformation of the locking clip should absolutely be avoided during the insertion of the nail. Otherwise, it will be impossible to efficiently block the two-headed distraction screw. Do not hesitate to use an osteotome to avoid all risk of clip deformation. The correct use of the olecranon drilling jig avoids this pitfall (Fig. 13.12).

Distal Targeting

If the Kirschner wire is not at the end but in the middle of the oblong hole, do not change the position of the wire. Pull or push the nail to put the wire at one end of the oblong hole instead, thus allowing enough room for the screw.

For a compression assembly, place the wire in the oblong hole *proximally*, the locking screw will be at the correct position (distally) immediately at the end of the compression manoeuvre. Opposite as is done in distraction, place the wire distally and the locking screw will then be proximal, as at the end of distraction (Fig. 13.13).

In the Event of Fracture of Both Forearm Bones

Start by nailing the ulna without using compression, and then complete osteosynthesis of the radius. Compression is then applied to the ulna site.

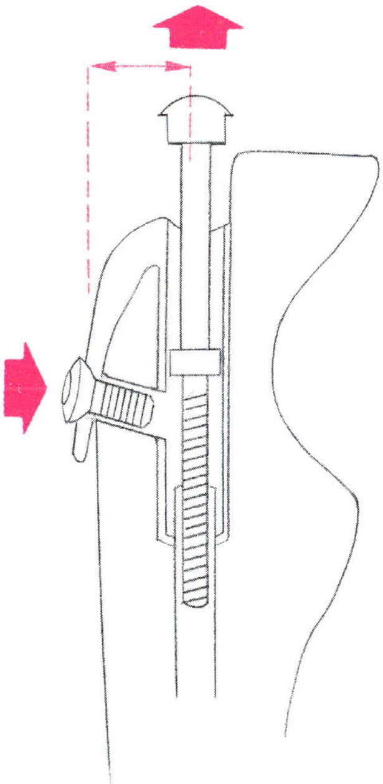

Fig. 13.12. Consequence of the deformation of the locking clip

References

1. Condamine JL (1989) Fracture dipahysaire des deux os de l'avant-bras. In: Encyclopédie Médicale et Chirurgicale – Appareil Locomoteur, Paris, France pp 4–14
2. Kempf I (1978) L'apport du verrouillage dans l'enclouage centro-médullaire des os longs. Rev Chir Orthop 64:635–651
3. Küntscher G (1945) Die Technik der Marknagelung. Thieme, Leipzig

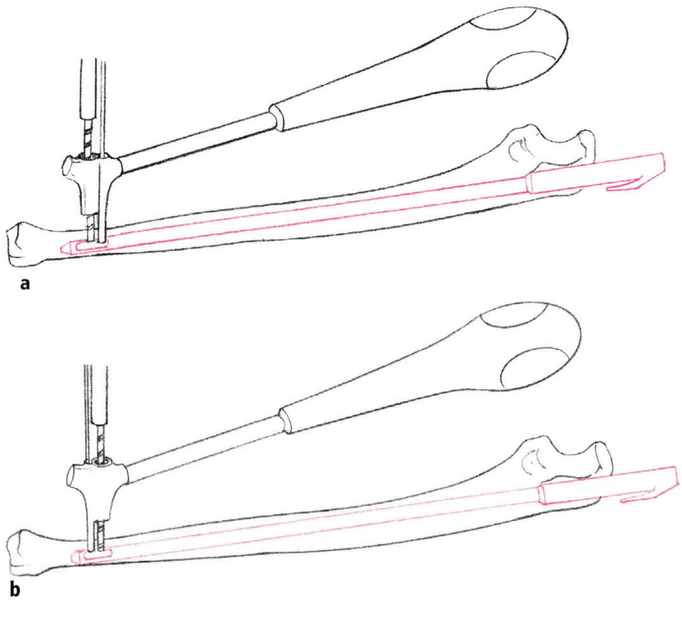

Fig. 13.13. a Distal targeting for compression; **b** distal targeting for distraction

4. Maatz R (1957) L'ostéosynthèse cubitale. Chirurg 28:24–27
5. Rush LV (1937) Reconstruction operation for comminuted fractures of the upper third of the ulna. Am J Surg 38:332–334
6. Shone G (1913) Behandlung von Vorderarmfrakturen mit Bolzung. Munch Med Wochenschr 60:2327–2328
7. Schwier V (1967) Simplification de l'ostéosynthèse par enclouage médullaire du cubitus. Chirurg 38:30–33
8. Seidel H (1989) Humeral locking nail: a preliminary report. Orthopedics 12:219–226
9. Street DM (1986) Intramedullary forearm nailing Clin Orthop 212:219–230
10. Street DM (1987) Intramedullary nailing of the forearm. In: Browner BD, Edwards CC (eds) The science and practice of intramedullary nailing. Lea & Febiger, Philadelphia, pp 325–348
11. Vital JM (1979) Approche des mouvements des deux os de l'avant-bras dans la pronosupination chez le vivant. Anat Clin 2:57–64

CHAPTER 14

Complications of Intramedullary Locked Nailing: Infection and Infected Nonunion

K. Klemm † and D. Seligson

Introduction

The most feared complication in the treatment of fractures is the postoperative development of infection. Infection, as an unexpected outcome of fracture surgery, is particularly dreaded after either plate osteosynthesis or intramedullary nailing. Nonoperative care or the use of an external fixator does not have the same taint, because the extent of the intervention at the fracture site during the operative procedure is less.

It is noteworthy, however, that infection following treatment of a compound fracture is less suspect than infection occurring after osteosynthesis of a closed fracture. The operative consent may be partly responsible. The surgeon explains from the outset the need to debride the compound fracture for the prevention of the infection that will surely result if prompt action is not taken. With compound fractures the patient, the surgeon, and the health care team relate the occurrence of an infection to bacterial contamination at the time of the accident, and the outcome-infection is not felt to be a consequence of the treatment of this injury.

Parenthetically, the facts are quite to the contrary. It is now known that the organisms responsible for the evolution of infection in compound as well as in closed fractures are acquired in most instances at the time and in the place of treatment. At any rate, the patient and family expect, with the development of infection following the treatment of compound fractures, that the surgical team will do the right thing at the right time to minimize the damage caused by the infection and to overcome the problems associated with devitalization of bone and soft tissue by the infectious process.

The case with closed fractures is quite to the contrary. While the treatment of compound fractures is specifically directed toward the prevention of infection, the treatment of closed fractures is expected to take place without the development of infectious complications. Despite ample evidence to the contrary, patients and surgeons have such confidence in modern surgical standards that infection-free wound healing is thought to be the certain outcome of the operative treatment of a closed fracture.

When an infection occurs despite all aseptic measures, this infection is considered to be abnormal, even irresponsible, and quite possibly due to carelessness or even negligence on the part of the surgeon. The doctor, concerned that he may be accused or even sued, tends to develop a defensive posture which hinders him from doing the right thing at the right time. Because of this feeling of guilt, the surgeon does not dare to define the extent of the problem. He resorts to euphemisms and speaks for example of "hematoma," "seroma," or "superficial infection," whereas, quite to the contrary, the entire limb is involved and the treatment will be complex and protracted. Indeed, the single most important concept in the treatment of infection following locked nailing, whether of a closed or an open fracture, is that any prolonged purulent discharge from an operative wound comes from infection of the entire intramedullary implant and the medullary canal. Once this fact is accepted, prompt adequate treatment can be planned and a good outcome insured.

To provide optimal therapy for infection after locked nailing, it is therefore necessary that the physician, the patient, the family, and the medical team accept the reality of a deep infection after intramedullary nailing and that active measures be promptly taken to either cure or at least limit the damage due to this infection.

Pathomechanics – Interaction with Infection

Intramedullary nailing is a complex biological interaction. The nail, prepared sterilely by the implant manufacturer or sterilized by the operating room team, is passed over the operating field and handed to the surgeon in more or less sterile condition. The patient has his or her own resident bioflora. Bacteria may be introduced with the nail into the medullary canal as the nail is passed across the patient's tissues into bone. The bone itself is greatly compromised in its blood supply by the fracture and displacement at the time of injury and may be in part devitalized. Compounding of the fracture may have introduced contamination at the fracture site. In addition, instrumentation of the medullary canal, with or without intramedullary reaming, further compromises the blood supply to bone. Dead bone is, after all, a sequestrum. At the end of the procedure the equation contains an inert implant, a partially vital bone, bacteria, and a host responding to the physiological insult of a trauma.

The inevitable result of intramedullary nailing is the gradual colonization of the implanted intramedullary nail by bacteria. When nailing is successful, the inflammatory reaction at the fracture site subsides and bone repair begins. This occurs at the same time as the host is gradually returning to normal homeostasis. The presence of bacteria and the occurrence of an inflammatory reaction are a part of the process of having fractured a long bone that is treated with an intramedullary nail. At the present time, neither the bacteria nor the inflammatory reaction can be eliminated. The number of bacteria and the extent of the inflammatory response determine whether or not the process at the fracture site is the colonization of the medullary nail or the progression to overt infection. This is a matter of degree. When intramedullary nailing is uncomplicated, as is usually the case, repair is the outcome.

In the infrequent cases where inflammation and bacterial growth become progressive with tissue destruction, then the result without prompt treatment is an infected pseudarthrosis. The presence of dead bone is key to the perpetuation of this pseudarthrosis and the inability to control inflammation and bacterial overgrowth by systemic antibiotics. Thoughtful observation of the X-rays of patients with fractures treated by locked nailing that heal without infectious complications will show the presence of areas of increased bone density in the fracture locus, indicating the presence of dead bone, which is gradually replaced by the normal process of bone turnover. When infection occurs with marked inflammation and an increase in vascularity, these areas of dead bone become all the more evident.

One of the clear advantages of locked nailing compared to Küntscher nailing is that locked nailing provides additional stability at the fracture locus. The locking screws control, to a great extent, rotational and axial forces at the fracture site. This is true even in the presence of infection. On the other hand, the introduction of small caliber locked nails may permit shear forces at the fracture site that would not be present with larger diameter Küntscher nails. With Küntscher nails, the presence of instability generally dictates removal of the intramedullary implant, since the pus which is present at the fracture site further lubricates the surfaces of the bone and the nail and increases motion at the fracture site, which in turn results in greater instability, more inflammation, and progressive pus formation. With a locked nail of adequate size, the nail may not have to be removed prior to fracture healing, since there is adequate stability at the fracture site.

It is worthwhile to consider the different pathomechanics of infection as it develops following locked nailing and plate fixation. Since these methods are entirely different, their biological consequences also differ.

In plate osteosynthesis an incision is made in relation to the fracture and the implant is installed either by direct visualization of the fracture site or by a so-called biological method where the plate is introduced through a short incision away from the fracture site, slid through the fracture locus, and then fixed to the bone through incisions proximal and distal to the fracture. In either the case of a full open incision or in the case of biologic osteosynthesis, the infection is localized to the area of the plate and the fracture site. The infection does not extend proximal and distal to the area of the plate since these areas are not instrumented. There may be devascularization of the bone ends, depending on the extent of trauma and on the extent of the surgical manipulation with dissection of the periosteum, which is of course more extensive if a full open method is selected.

It is not, however, guaranteed that there will be no devascularization of the fracture site by the use of a plate passed percutaneously. Devascularization of bone and of comminuted fracture fragments occurs as a consequence of the accident itself. To some extent, dead bone is always present in every displaced fracture. Subsequent to infection, bone necrosis becomes progressive, and with devascularization, there is a loosening of the screws in the plate and an increase in relative motion between the fracture fragments. This results, finally, in an infected pseudoarthrosis with dead bone, a loose implant, and swollen, infected soft tissues in poor condition.

These circumstances can be aggravated by the presence of a draining sinus, with the additional chemical irritation produced by pus. The therapeutical implications of this process are early removal of the bone plate, and all loose and broken screws, and excision of sequestrated bone fragments and portions of dead bone. A new stabilization of the long bone is performed with an external fixator, and in grossly contaminated cases, the wound is either left open or treated with irrigation-suction. Following the subsidence of gross inflammation and the elimination of significant pus and drainage, an antibiotic-containing implant (such as a gentamicin-PMMA chain) can be placed in the wound; subsequently the bone can be restored by massive cancellous bone grafting or with segmental bone transport to bridge the bone defect created by the sequestrectomy.

The evolution of infection in a comminuted fracture, for example, of the femur treated by locked nailing is entirely different. The intramedullary implant serves as a conduit along which bacteria, pus, and inflammation can spread the entire length of the medullary canal. The infection is never localized to one area (Fig. 14.1). Unlike the situation with formal open plate fracture treatment, the comminuted bone fragments are less likely to be devascularized by dissection, as they are pushed aside when the medullary canal is reamed and instrumented. Unlike the situation in infected plate osteosynthesis, the stability of the bone may be maintained, despite the presence of purulent drainage. This is particularly true if an implant of adequate size has been selected. Furthermore, since callus formation is itself a result of the inflammatory reaction with the presence of stability at the fracture locus, abundant callus formation can be observed as a response to infection. Therefore, with the suppression of infection, no further cancellous bone grafting or segmental transfer may be necessary.

The therapeutic steps necessitated by the presence of infection include early intervention with the installation of irrigation-suction drainage, and appropriate organism-specific systemic antibiotic therapy. This treatment can result in the suppression of infection and avoidance of further abscess formation. Once sufficient callus formation has taken place, so that the bone itself is stable, the locked nail can be removed. Because of the spread of infection up and down the medullary canal, it is nevertheless necessary to ream the intramedullary canal to remove infected endosteal sequestra which cling to its inner walls. Following removal of the implant and reaming, it is advisable either to provide for several days of irrigation-suction of the medullary space or to place a local antibiotic-containing carrier, such as an antibiotic impregnated bead chain, to cure the intramedullary infection.

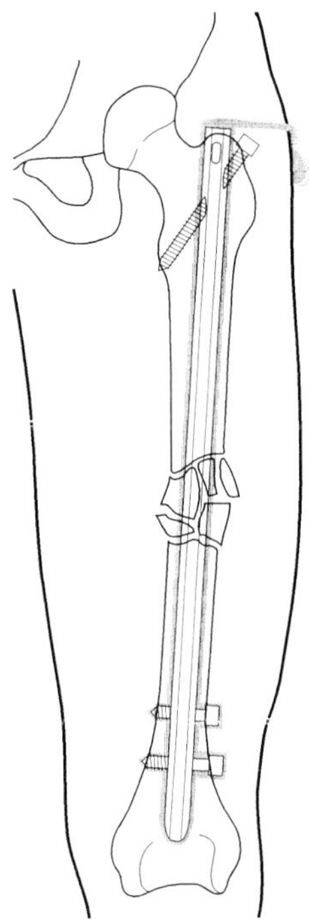

Fig. 14.1. The intramedullary implant is a conduit for bacteria and the infection is never localized to one area

Management of Localized Infection After Locked Nailing

Acute Postoperative Wound Infection

An acute infection can follow any operative procedure. This is true for locked nailing as well. The development of an acute postoperative infection is a special case, because it differs from the general concept that infection following nailing means that the entire nail and entire intramedullary canal are involved. Acute infection following intramedullary nailing has the same early clinical appearance as other acute infections, and is caused by bacterial contamination of the site of soft tissue injury or at one of the surgical wounds. Acute postoperative infections typically develop from 3 to 5 days to 1 to 2 weeks following the initial injury. An acute infection is an emergency and requires prompt surgical treatment because the infection is still localized. This soft tissue infection, however, has the potential to spread to the implant and become an infected nail and bone. The treatment plan consists of an adequate debridement under sterile operative conditions and under anesthesia, a thorough irrigation of the wound, an implantation of gentamicin-PMMA chains (Septopal – Chain, Merck Biomaterials GmbH, Darmstadt, Prof. Kempf, in collaboration with

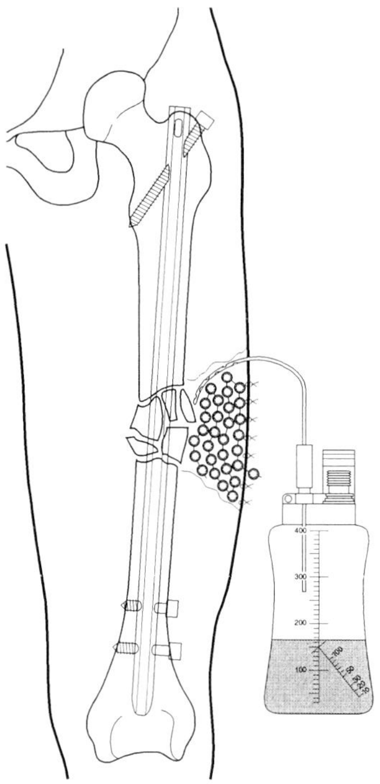

Fig. 14.2. In very early soft tissue infection, local implantation of a gentamicin-PMMA chain can avoid the spread of infection to the implant

Heraeus Kulzer GmbH, Wehrheim/Ts., Germany) to provide high levels of antibiotics in the local area of the infection (Fig. 14.2). Prompt evaluation of the limb, prompt acceptance of the possibility of acute infection, and prompt exploration of the wound are critical steps not only in preventing an intramedullary infection, but also in maintaining patient trust and family confidence.

The judicious use of antibiotics is important. The antibiotic levels can be achieved with locally implanted antibiotic laden carriers, are much greater than the minimal inhibitory concentrations for most common pathogens, and greater than the levels that can be achieved with the parenteral use of antibiotics. Intravenous antibiotics will not achieve high enough local levels to stop an infection in a zone of injury. This is why local implants are crucial. The gentamicin-PMMA chain can be either completely implanted in the wound or can be so placed that a few beads protrude through the skin. When the beads are left subcutaneously, they can be removed without an operative procedure, if they are taken out within the first 7 days after surgery. With the use of gentamicin-PMMA chains, a drain should be placed in the wound, and the surgical wound needs to be closed entirely.

Simultaneous with the local implantation of gentamicin-PMMA chains, intravenous cephalosporins are begun at the time of surgery and continued orally for at least 1 week after the operative treatment of the infection.

The immediate treatment of an acute postsurgical infection without removal of the implant can be successful only if the interlocking is stable and is expected to produce uncomplicated fracture healing. An unstable implant should be revised to a stable nailing when the local wound infection has been suppressed. Under these circumstances, adequate antibiotic coverage should be provided and directed toward organisms that were recovered at the time of the exploration of the acute wound infection.

Acute Medullary Infection After Locked Nailing

In an acute fracture treated by intramedullary nailing, bacteria cause infection by direct spread from a contaminated fracture site, by spread from the entry point or incisions for locking screws, or by direct introduction on the implant. Infection can also follow the treatment of a pseudarthrosis with a locked nail. In the treatment of pseudarthrosis, the situation is more complex, but better preoperative evaluation and patient education is possible. However, the general treatment concepts for the treatment of acute infections after nailings for fresh fractures or for pseudarthrosis are similar.

Once the implant is infected, it is practically impossible to eradicate this infection as long as the nail is in place. In comparison to Küntscher nailing, a locked nail may be stable despite the presence of infection, because the nail is directly fixed to bone by the locking screws. In Küntscher nailing, the lubrication of the intramedullary nail by purulent discharge leads to loss of elastic impingement and loss of multiple contact point jamming, and the osteosynthesis becomes unstable. In an infected nailing with an unlocked device such as a Küntscher nail, an Ender nail, or a Rush pin, the implant becomes an irritating foreign body which itself augments the infection, causes bone resorption, and leads to the development of an infected nonunion.

Local antibiotic implants, such as gentamicin-PMMA chains, cannot be used to treat a generalized infection of a stable locked nail. The gentamicin leached from the implanted bead chain will not reach bacteria over the full length of the nail. The therapeutic options are to try and suppress the infection with the implant in place or to remove the locked nail, debride the infection, and stabilize the fracture site with an external fixator.

If the nail is left in place, then it is anticipated that the fracture will heal in the presence of infection, and finally the nail will be removed and the medullary canal debrided by reaming.

With low-grade infection, it may be possible to open the entrance wound and insert a suction drain hooked up to a vacuum bottle. In stable fractures, a proximal interlocking screw can be removed and the drainage tube slipped down the lumen of the nail. This should not be done if either rotational or axial instability will occur. Once a tract is established, the patient can be sent home with the drainage system. The vacuum bottles can be changed at home by the patient or with home health nursing assistance (Fig. 14.3).

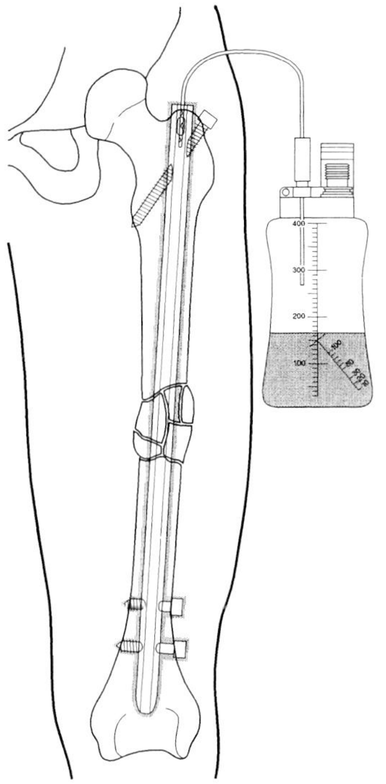

Fig. 14.3. With continuous suction drainage of the infected medullary canal, the infected fracture will consolidate under good stability of the locked nail

The establishment of drainage has to be combined with a program of systemic antibiotic therapy directed at the organisms recovered at the time of surgery. Parenteral therapy is given at first, and as the infection comes under control, if the bacterial sensitivities allow, it can continue as oral medication for some weeks. Once the purulent drainage is minimal, and the clinical signs of infection are reduced or have subsided, the antibiotic therapy can be discontinued. However, the drainage tube should not be removed. It can be cut, so that a few centimeters protrude from the wound. A safety pin passed through the drain prevents the drain from disappearing down the medullary canal. The drain is eventually removed with the nail, when the fracture is united.

Every displaced fracture causes osteonecrosis. The amount of dead bone depends on the extent of periosteal stripping caused by the injury and any further devitalization from the operative procedure. Infection can cause further devitalization of bone, but it can also lead to abundant callus formation because any irritating substance in the marrow space leads to subperiosteal new bone formation. Indeed, this subperiosteal new bone formation is the essential response of bone to injury from whatever source: trauma, tumor, or infection.

With severe, suppurative infection, irrigation-suction drainage may be necessary to prevent sepsis. An ingress tube is threaded into the lumen of the nail proximally. Two liters of saline daily or lactated Ringer's solution (without antibiotics) is either dripped or flushed in 200 cc boluses into the medullary canal. A centrally perforated drain tube is passed as a continuous loop, so its perforations lie at the fracture site (Fig. 14.4). This loop drain can be manipulated to free it from obstructing clots or necrotic tissue without having the drain fall out of the wound. Both ends of this loop drain are connected to low vacuum suction. When the acute phlegmon subsides, the irrigation

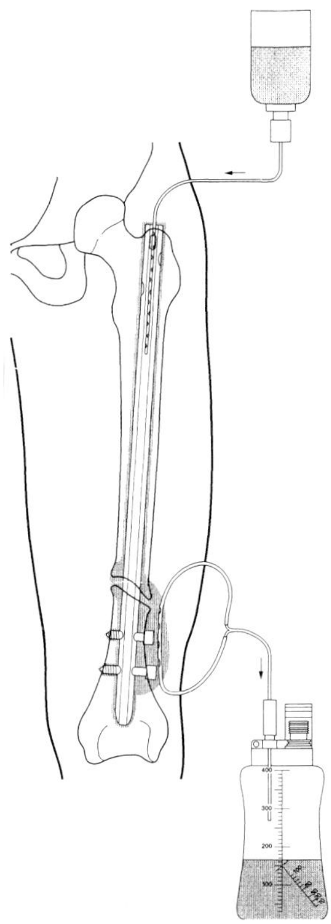

Fig. 14.4. With severe suppurative infection, irrigation-suction is indicated

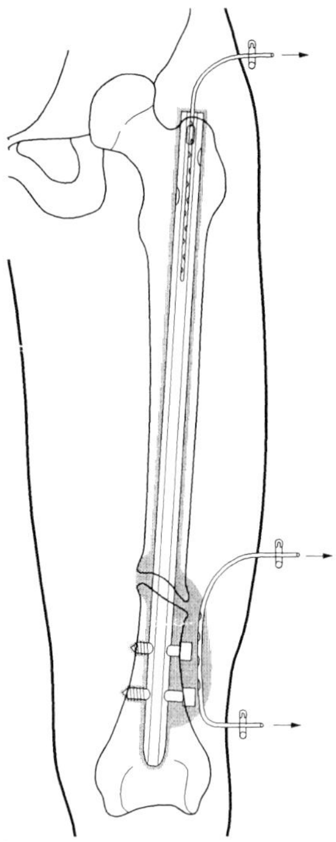

Fig. 14.5. When the acute phlegmon has subsided, irrigation is stopped and the drains are used for passive conduits

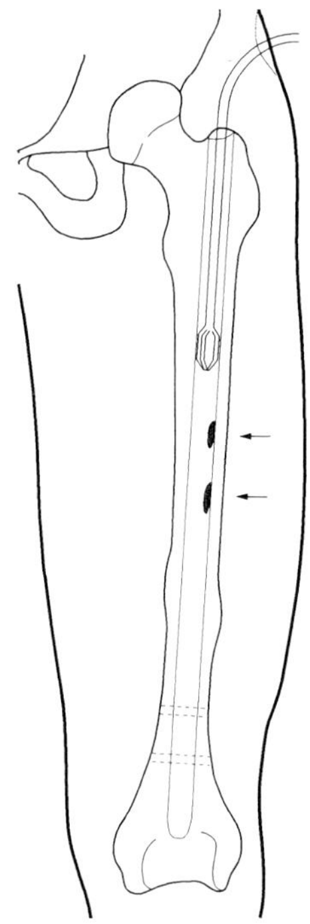

Fig. 14.6. Medullary reaming enables the removal of small lamellar sequestra clinging to the endosteum

can be stopped, and the ingress and egress drains are used, first as suction drains and then as passive conduits to decompress the marrow cavity as described above (Fig. 14.5). Finally, when the fracture union occurs, the infection is controlled by removal of the nail and reaming of the canal, as described below.

Treatment of Residual Infection After Fracture Healing

Once the fracture is sufficiently united and the locked nail is no longer needed for bone stability, the residual infection can be treated. Since dead bone, a foreign body (the nail), and bacteria remain, treatment is necessary to prevent the recurrence of inflammation, additional bone necrosis, drainage, and/or systemic sepsis. Obviously, the nail must be removed. In addition, if significant nonvascular sequestra remain, the injury site should be re-explored and these fragments removed. Finally, it is critical to ream the medullary canal to a diameter 1–2 mm greater than the diameter of the nail that was removed (Fig. 14.6). Reaming removes small infected lamellar sequestra, which are not visible on X-ray, but which nonetheless cling to the endosteum. Reaming should be followed by vigorous irrigation of the medullary canal to flush out these particles. Then a gentamicin-PMMA chain can be placed the length of the medullary canal to provide therapy with a high local dose of antibiotic. This chain is placed using an applicator to pull it down the entire length of the intramedullary canal (Fig. 14.7). A plastic overflow drain is also placed in the medullary canal and connected to a drainage bag. A few beads are left protruding through the skin so that the chain can be removed 5–7 days later without further surgery. However, if the bead chain is left for more than 10 days it becomes encapsulated with the fibrous tissue that forms after the infection has subsided. Then the chain can be impossible to remove without surgical re-exploration of the wound. When a portion of bead chain is left in the canal and the infection has subsided completely, it acts as any other foreign implant, such as a prosthesis. It will be tolerated in an infection-free environment and not cause a clinical problem. However, if residual bacteria become active at a later date and there is a recurrence of infection, then the bone can be windowed, the abscess drained, and remaining portions of implanted bead-chain removed.

At the time of nail removal, bacterial cultures are taken and systemic antibiotics (usually a cephalosporin) are administered for 1–2 days to control the local sepsis which occurs as a consequence of the procedure. If clinical signs of in-

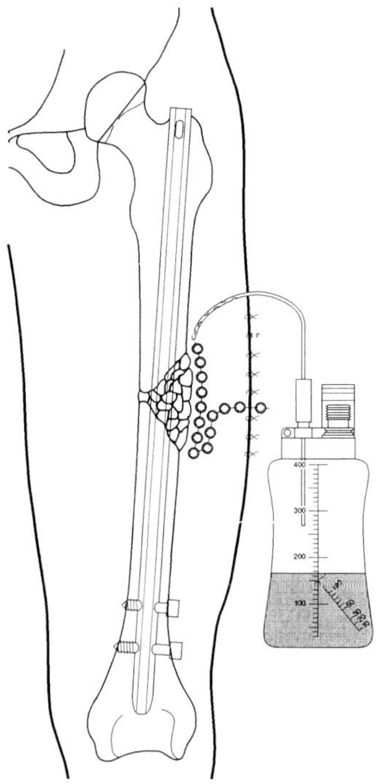

Fig. 14.13. When the infection has subsided, the locked nail can be used for re-osteosynthesis of the nonunion, together with cancellous bone grafting if necessary. A gentamicin-PMMA chain is placed for the prophylaxis of reinfection

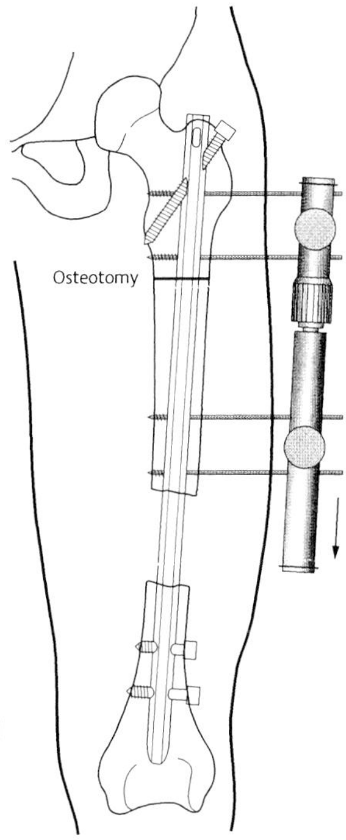

Fig. 14.14. In formerly infected nonunion with substantial bone defect, the locked nail in combination with an external fixator and subtrochanteric osteotomy can be used for bridging the bone defect by callus distraction

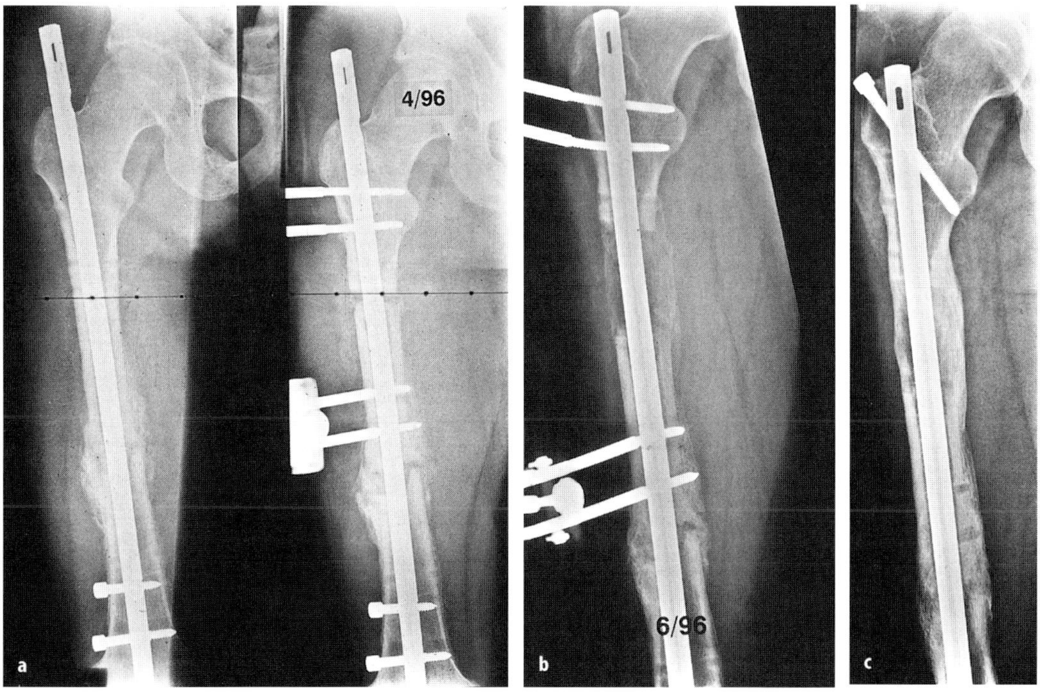

Fig. 14.15 a–c. 16-year-old male. **a** Re-osteosynthesis with a locked nail of a formerly infected nonunion after plating a closed femoral fracture with intentional overlength of the nail for callus distraction. **b** Subtrochanteric osteotomy and mounting of an external fixator for continuous callus distraction of 6 cm. **c** After removal of the external fixator, static locking of the nail to allow full weight bearing

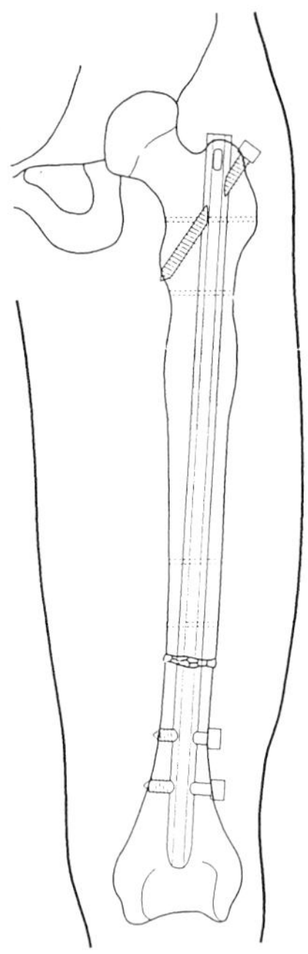

Fig. 14.16. When the defect is bridged by callus distraction, bone grafting may be necessary at the docking area. The external fixator can be removed

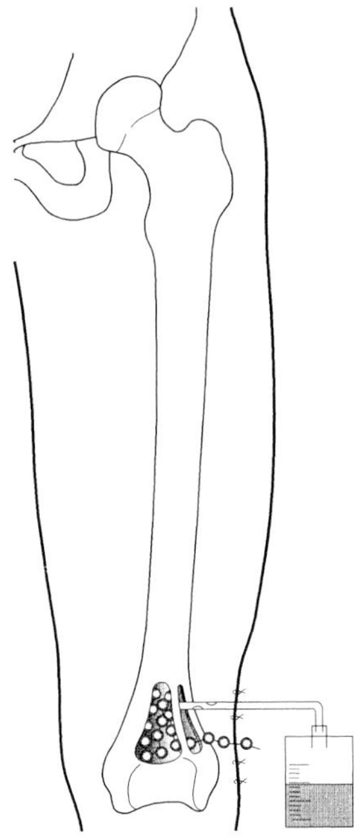

Fig. 14.17. In an isolated intramedullary abscess, the medullary canal is opened at the point of maximum bone scan uptake and the cavity is filled with a gentamicin-PMMA chain

Treatment of Infection Long After Intramedullary Nailing

The isolated intramedullary abscess is a special circumstance which can develop years (even more than 20 years) after intramedullary nailing and subsequent removal of a nail. This condition usually occurs at the distal end of the medullary canal. There are no visual signs of infection. The onset of the condition should be suspected with the onset of pain. This pain is characteristically night pain. It is thought that the condition becomes painful at night, because with bed rest the patient's blood pressure and hence intramedullary pressure are lower. If a soft tissue abscess develops, this occurs late, following perforation of the medullary canal by the abscess with soft tissue abscess and possibly a draining sinus. The diagnosis is made by bone scan, plain X-rays, CT, or MRI, all of which usually show a localized abscess cavity at the distal end of the bone, with obliteration of the medullary canal proximal to the cavity. Chronic inflammation leads to bone sclerosis surrounding the medullary abscess.

The treatment of this condition is operative. The medullary canal is opened at the lateral aspect of the femur at the point of maximum bone scan uptake. The cavity is then curetted and filled with gentamicin-PMMA chains (Fig. 14.17). These chains can be left for a while if no re-infection occurs. If this is the case, the cavity has to be debrided again and refilled with a gentamicin-PMMA chain. Some authors have recommended that the entire medullary canal be re-established by reaming, but this may not be technically possible because of the sclerosing osteomyelitis of the diaphysis of the femur.

Conclusion

In conclusion, it may appear paradoxical that while infection can occur as a consequence of locked nailing of the femur, this method has, from its inception, been used to treat infected nonunion of long bones and has led to the development of the intramedullary locked nail, which is currently in world-wide use for the osteosynthesis of fractures of long bones.

References

1. Klemm K (1972) Die modifizierte Trümmerbruchnagelung zur Stabilisierung der infizierten Pseudarthrosen am Oberschenkel. Hefte Unfallheilk 110:240–243
2. Klemm, K, Schellmann WD (1972) Dynamische und statische Verriegelung des Marknagels. Monatsschr Unfallheilkd 75:568–575
3. Küntscher G (1968) Die Marknagelung des Trümmerbruches. Langenbecks Arch Klin Chir 322:1063–1069

CHAPTER 15

Complications of Centromedullary Nailing (Excluding Infection)

C. Lefèvre and D. Le Nen

Introduction

Unlike techniques of osteosynthesis by open procedures using plates and screws, closed centromedullary nailing requires from the surgeon an entirely different technique approaching the surgical treatment of shaft fractures. Whatever the diaphyseal site involved, the technique of nailing is always subject to the same sequence of successive and identical stages, each dependent on the other. Failure to respect any one of these may be followed by complications of varying gravity, often local, sometimes loco-regional, or even of a systemic nature, when they may be very serious indeed.

This chapter will discuss the various complications, taking as a criterion the moment of the clinical or radiological discovery of the consequences of an error rather than the moment when the technical fault was committed. The various problems will thus be treated in chronological order, depending on whether the complication develops in the intraoperative or the immediate postoperative period, or more remotely after the procedure. For each of these chronological stages the complications specific to each anatomic site of implantation will be discussed: femur, tibia [9], humerus, and ulna. The analysis of each of these complications will be followed either by a repair stratagem or by tricks and devices to prevent their occurrence.

Intraoperative Complications

Positioning

Poor positioning may have serious consequences. The occurrence of a fracture of the upper end of a healthy femur may take place during positioning on the orthopaedic table of an elderly patient with reduced articular mobility. Forced abduction of the unoperated lower limb is the cause of this accident.

The most preserved range of mobility in these elderly patients is always flexion. To prevent this distressing complication, it suffices to position the opposite lower limb with the hip and knee flexed to 90° and without abduction.

Such positioning, apart from the advantage of protecting the unoperated hip, provides an appreciable space between the two lower limbs, thus facilitating manipulation of the image intensifier.

Reduction

Muscular Interposition

Independent of the location of the shaft fracture, reduction sometimes proves impossible. This should suggest the possibility of muscular interposition and avoid the application of heavy traction on the orthopaedic table. On the contrary, it is often necessary to release the traction and to try one's hardest to obtain alignment of the fragments by external manoeuvres, the aim being to avoid recourse to an open approach, which should remain a last resort.

Reduction of the Proximal Femur is Impossible

This is the case with subtrochanteric fractures or fractures of the proximal third of the femur. Despite repeated manoeuvres, the images on the screen stay unchanged: in the frontal view there is a varus tilt of the proximal fragment (due to the action of the gluteal fan) and in the lateral view tilting in flexion (due to the action of the iliopsoas muscle). These types of fracture remain in any case irreducible by external manoeuvres; it is therefore useless and even dangerous to persist in trying to obtain reduction by prolonging the period of irradiation. In cases presenting in this way, supplementary methods of reduction are required, such as a support under the upper thigh which will elevate the distal fragment. If reduction is still not obtained despite this, it is as well not to persist: alignment of the fragment will be obtained during the operation by means of a spatula or a reducing nail, which permits alignment of the two bone fragments by depressing the proximal fragment.

Migration of the Transcondylar Steinmann Pin in the Femur

During the reduction of a fracture of the femoral shaft, it is necessary to avoid excessive traction on the table, which may give rise to intracancellous descent of the Steinmann pin in the condylar block; it has even been seen within the joint! A pin placed too low in an osteoporotic patient may be the cause of this accident. To avoid this pitfall, safety depends on using the following clinical landmarks: placement of the traction pin at a finger's breadth above the upper border of the patella and laterally through the middle of the lateral condyle. Modern tables are usually calibrated. One should never exceed 50 kg of traction to obtain reduction of the femur; if this fails, it becomes imperative to review the positioning in detail, since this is obviously the source of the problem.

Route of Access

The only anatomic risk of the cutaneous approach routes for nailing is the transtendinous infrapatellar approach to the tibia, which may open the knee joint. As soon as the tendinous layer is crossed, the pressure on the scalpel must be reduced, especially on approaching the apex of the patella. In practice, to avoid entering the joint, it suffices to displace the infrapatellar fat pad backwards without traversing it.

Drilling of the Entry Orifice of the Nail

Femur

Difficulty in reaching the apex of the trochanter is always due to faulty positioning. For placement of a gamma nail, inclination of the trunk has the advantage of improving access to the great trochanter. In the case of a shaft fracture, and if this manoeuvre proves insufficient, the lower limb to be operated should then be adducted: inclination of the trunk and adduction of the femur contribute to forming an angle whose trochanteric apex moves outwards and thus becomes more accessible.

Tibia

Effraction of the knee joint is always due to a square tip placed too high, away from the anterior tibial tuberosity. In the first stage, the tip of the AWL should be applied perpendicular to the bony surface to make a preliminary hole just above the tuberosity. Subsequently, the point is directed towards the medullary cavity. By thus embedding the nail, the initially circular bony orifice becomes progressively oval upwards while remaining extra-articular, the plane of security being ensured by the infrapatellar fat pad.

Humerus

During nailing upwards from below, posterior drilling of the distal humerus may give rise to supracondylar fracture. The medullary canal is funnel-shaped: wide proximally, it becomes narrow distally. The distal drilling corresponding to the zone of bifurcation of the two columns proves dangerous. Progressive drilling starting with a fine drill at this level is therefore prudent, performed as much as possible in the axis of the shaft while taking care not to weaken the bone by using drills that are too thick. During nailing from below, drilling of the cartilaginous head of the humerus must be avoided by placing the square tip of the nail in the anatomic neck just medial to the apex of the greater tubercle.

Passage of the Reamer Guide

It is sometimes impossible to cross the fracture site during descent of the guide, which is checked at this level because of the persistence of an incompletely reduced angulation or overlap of the fragments. Rather than repeat a false passage, which always endangers the nerves, it is preferable to adopt one or more of the following solutions:

1. Pre-bend the reamer-guide, either at its extremity to give a small radius of curvature, or in its entirety, which gives a large radius of curvature. In every case attach an American handle to the guide and progress by making small rotary movements of the whole. While pre-bending is helpful in traversing the fracture site, it may be a disadvantage in obtaining centring in the distal shaft of the femur or tibia; what happens is that the pre-bending has the effect of imposing a lateralized course on the guide if one just pushes it, hence the importance of making progress by small movements

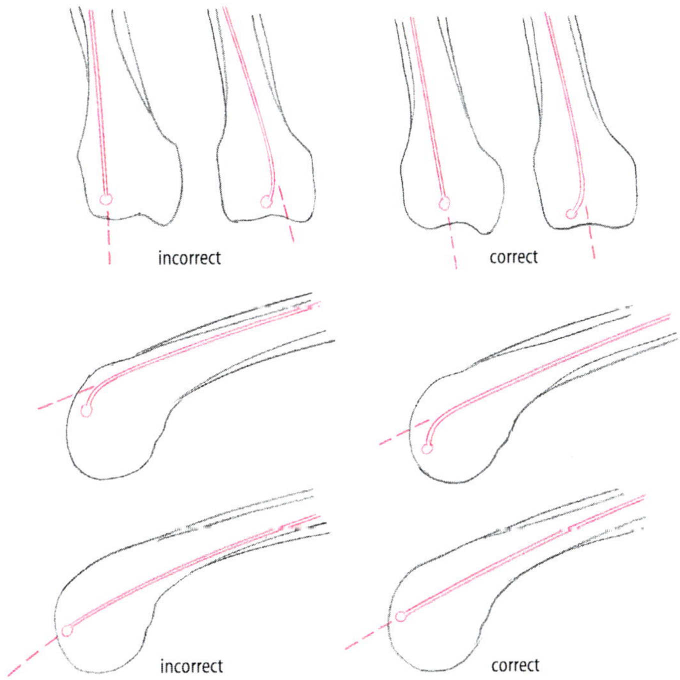

Fig. 15.1. Correct centring. Incorrect centring. Reamer guide centring must be checked frontally and laterally simultaneously

of alternate rotation to control the descent of the guide and then its final centring. Pre-centring distal end to a small radius of curvature should not allow one to forget that the important landmark is the axis of the reamer guide and not its curved extremity (Fig. 15.1).

2. Do not hesitate, in cases of difficulty, to use a sterile towel draped round the thigh or leg at the level of the fracture to obtain correct alignment of the fragments. This manoeuvre is only possible on patients positioned on an orthopaedic table, which is essential for every insertion of a centromedullary nail in the femur or tibia; it has the advantage of reducing the irradiation time considerably, by facilitating the preoperative manoeuvres of reduction and stabilizing this reduction throughout the procedure. Thus, before arranging the drapes, the preoperative reduction of a tibia, and especially a femur, may prove difficult; despite traction, angulation or misalignment of the fragments sometimes persists. One should then ask an assistant to use a bandage passed round the limb at the level of the axial defect to apply traction while regulating its intensity and direction to obtain proper alignment, a manoeuvre that can be used during the operation while respecting the rules of asepsis and which has the advantage of decreasing the period of irradiation.
3. The philosophy of the closed procedure imposes painting the entire circumference of the thigh or leg and keeping the arrangement of drapes at a distance, around the extremities of the limb to be operated: the inguinal region, the root of the thigh and the knee for the femur, the knee above the patella and the ankle below the medial malleolus for the tibia. Nailing of the humerus or forearm calls for complete painting of the upper limb up to the axilla so as to be able to move it freely during the operation. Lastly, a transparent adhesive drape is applied around the entire circumference of the thigh or leg. Such an arrangement guarantees substantial comfort and particularly complete autonomy during operation when modifying or improving the quality of the reduction at any time, thanks to the sterile field around the limb. In practice, one should avoid creating a square field for a closed centromedullary nailing, since if a problem arises, the surgeon may become dependent on persons unhygienically dressed, in trying to obtain an improved reduction at the cost of manoeuvres threatening the respect of the rules of asepsis.
4. Exceptionally, despite careful positioning and good alignment, the reamer guide cannot cross a comminuted fracture site because of an interposed bony fragment acting as a valve and diverting the guide into the soft parts. The solution consists of exerting rotary movements on the guide, pre-bent at its tip, to mobilize the tilted fragment; this manoeuvre usually makes it possible to cross the obstacle.

5. If fractures of the proximal third of the femur are not reducible by simple external manoeuvres; the ideal is to use the so-called small reducer nail method proposed by Küntscher, i.e. in a first stage to ream as far as the fracture site, then pass a small nail (or the specific instrument designed for this purpose) into the proximal fragment, and to slide the guide along it; the nail is then used as a reducing lever and lastly the guide is passed into the distal fragment once alignment of the fragments has been obtained.
6. Finally, as the last resort for a femur or tibia, a square pin inserted percutaneously can help to perfect a reduction and pass the guide, but this manoeuvre is always risky and a possible cause of slippage; it should only be used if there is no alternative.

Reaming

Problem of the Adhesive Drape

Before beginning the first reaming, it is advisable to detach the adhesive drape at the margins of the incision so as to prevent the head of the reamer from dragging folds of the drape into the shaft, a possible source of septic complications.

Aggravation of the Initial Lesions

Aggressive reaming may convert a split into a new fracture isolating one or more fragments. The least suspicion (perceptible or audible at the motor) of such a risk means that the reaming must be stopped.

Obstruction to the Head of the Reamer

Obstruction to the head of the reamer is due to the reamer's having been advanced too rapidly or to the excessively rapid passage of heads of too large a diameter. As soon as a head begins to "bite," increase the size in 0.5 mm stages, ream gently, do not hesitate to withdraw so as to check the state of the heads and clean them if necessary. Once compact bone is burnt, it makes the reamer heads ineffective and causes them to become jammed in the medullary canal. To unblock an impacted head, it usually suffices to exert traction and rotation on the motor in the direction of movement of the motor at the moment it is restarted.

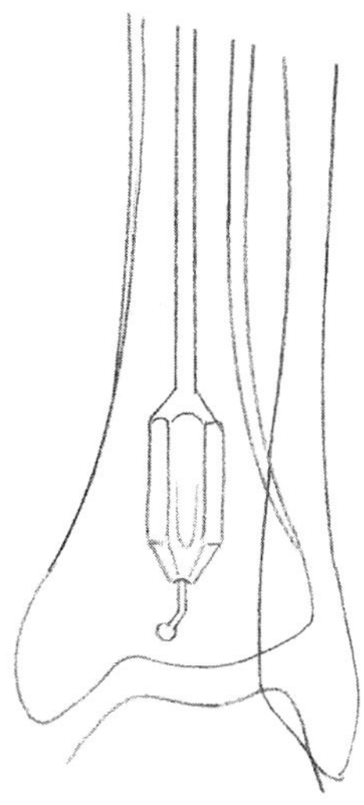

Fig. 15.2. No advantage to over-ream or to ream more distally. Reamer guide with olivary tip allows extraction of a broken reamer

Breakage of the Instrument

Breakage of the instrument (Fig. 15.2) is always due to too rapid and aggressive reaming. It becomes a real complication if care has not been taken to ream over a proper reamer guide with an olivary tip designed to recover a broken reamer head, something that a guide nail with a smooth tip does not allow, for it is imperative to recover the broken instrument.

Over-reaming of a Cortex

Over-reaming of a cortex is avoided by monitoring on the viewing monitor the correct centring of the head of the reamer in the zone to be reamed. Apart from this centring defect, asymmetric over-reaming occurs in narrow medullary zones such as the distal third of the humerus [14], or the distal two-thirds of the ulna, for which full-sized reamers may prove dangerous; an elongated head with its disproportionately high length/diameter ratio may act so as to produce lateralized self-guidance, explaining some cortical effractions during the reaming (Fig. 15.3). Full-sized reamers with short heads should be used or, better still, flexible reamers mounted on the guide, whose smallest diameters of 4.5 mm are perfectly adapted to narrow medullary canals.

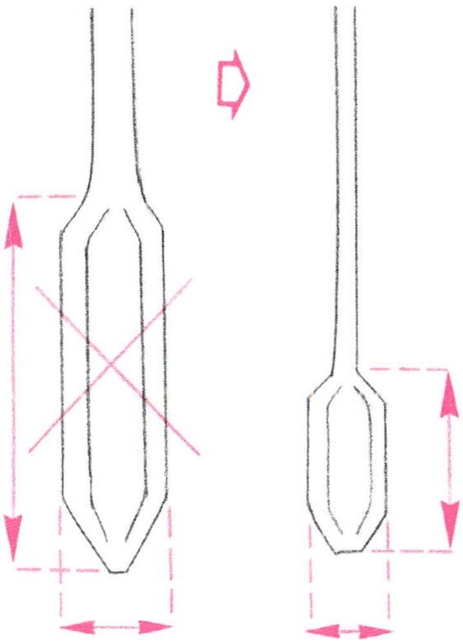

Fig. 15.3. A poorly designed guide head can cause self guid ance and cortical splitting

Heating of the Bone

Though not measurable, heating or even burning of the bone is always dangerous because of the risk of partial necrosis, which may account for some delays in consolidation. One should always avoid pushing on the motor and always insist on the importance of increasing the size of the heads in 0.5-mm stages as soon as the first head begins to "bite" on the cortex.

Reaming of Two-Level Fractures

Reaming of two-level fractures of the tibia and ulna sometimes requires safety measures to prevent rotation of an intermediate fragment dragged by a blocked reamer head, a rotation which irremediably causes its massive necrosis. The solution consists of using a forceps with a claw head embedded in the intermediate fragment percutaneously; the claw must be firmly held during the passage of the reamer head into the intermediate fragment. This type of problem has not been reported with two-level fractures of the humerus. The reaming of a two-level fracture of the femur is likewise without risk because of the powerful muscle insertions along the linea aspera.

Compartment Syndromes and Fat Embolism

Also difficult to assess, an increase in the intramedullary pressure associated with advancement of the reamer head or nail is suspected of causing two serious complications. One is loco-regional, the compartment syndrome, and the other is systemic, fat embolism

Compartment Syndrome

Classically associated with fractures of the leg, compartment syndromes are sometimes the result of badly performed reaming, always associated with an increase of intramedullary pressure, which diffuses within the soft parts around the fracture. As soon as the tissue pressure exceeds the systemic diastolic pressure, an ischemia develops affecting one or more compartments. Clinically, the appearance of a waxy oedema of the leg and diffuse paraesthesiae or hyperaesthesia should lead one to measure the tissue pressures and, in view of the gravity of the prognosis and there being no room for doubt, there should be no hesitation in performing an emergency decompression aponeurotomy and abandoning any idea of an internal osteosynthesis, which would only add to the tissue pressure. Radiologically, the preoperative films are sometimes instructive when, in the context of a high-energy injury, a loss of parallelism or a major gap is noted between the tibial and fibular fragments. This increase of the radiological interosseous space is an index of a rupture of the interosseous membrane, which suggests a major contusion and oedema of the soft parts around the bones, indicated by a diffuse radiological densification of the soft parts around the leg axis.

The classic frequency of compartment syndrome in the leg or forearm is well known, as is their rarity in the thigh or arm; this is linked to the known anatomic features of the proximal and distal segments of the limbs. Compartment syndromes of the forearm have been reported after conservative treatment but also after osteosynthesis by screwed plates; the bulkiness of these systems, added to the post-traumatic and then the surgical oedema of the soft parts, tend to cause the occurrence of this complication; an argument which tends to indicate intramedullary osteosyntheses of the forearm.

Fat Embolism

Undeniably, as shown by intraoperative transesophageal ultrasound studies, the intramedullary pressure associated with reaming displaces and fragments the intra-diaphyseal fatty marrow into disseminated particles giving the striking snowstorm-like image. But this simple migration of fat embolism due to the effect of a phenomenon of hyper-pressure nearly always remains completely asymptomatic [5, 23]. Particularly prevalent after freshly closed fractures of the femur, but also after elongation and shortening osteotomies [10], fat embolism actually occurs in 80% of cases before any osteosynthesis, due to excessive mobilization. This stresses the preventive importance of urgent surgical stabilization in such fractures. Moreover, it seems that multiple traumata combining femoral shaft fracture and severe chest injury with pulmonary contusion increase the risk of developing fat embolism and justify early stabilization all the more, given that there is a priori no significant difference between the different techniques of osteosynthesis [17], except for the patient in a state of shock with an unstable blood pressure, in whom external fixation is to be preferred [17].

In sum, fat embolism and the compartment syndromes appear most often as complications associated with the type of initial injury rather than the intramedullary osteosynthesis. Nevertheless, to minimize the risk of such complications, reamer heads provided with deep grooves to act as vents between the cutting edges should be used, rather than quasi-cylindrical heads, which are actually diaphyseal obturators; recent studies have shown the importance of the design of reamer heads. Furthermore, reaming should always be done gently, without forcing (e.g. pushing on the motor) and there should be no hesitation in making to and fro movements to avoid clogging the head with the risk of blockage, due to heating of the bone [22]. Lastly, reaming the midshaft cortices should always be done moderately; it is no longer necessary, as in the past, to thin the cortices so as to use nails of a very large diameter.

Changing the Guide

The risk involved in changing the guide is one of losing the reduction of the fracture; it is there fore statistically more likely with distal fractures if care is not taken, when changing, to use a temporary hollow guide pushed into the distal epiphysis to bridge the fracture site.

Such a situation makes it necessary to repeat the classic chronological stages: repetition of the reduction using the pre-bent reamer guide, then the passage of the hollow guide until it is well impacted distally, then the removal of the reamer guide, the passage of the guide nail straight to the free extremity, and lastly the removal of the hollow guide. A mistake may be made during insertion of the latter, which becomes blocked at the fracture site. A guide with a bevelled tip should be used, giving it a rotary motion to cross the fracture site; then the apparent remaining length of the hollow guide is determined after the manoeuvre, especially with a distal fracture of the femur, when there is a real risk of losing the reduction in such a long bone.

Breakage of the temporary guide raises the problem of being sure of having recovered all the material. If the break is proximal, it is easier to recover the rest of the tube using a forceps of the type used for removing the cement of a prosthesis. If the breakage is more distal, the reamer guide must be passed again in an attempt to engage its pre-bent expanded tip within the tube, and the guide fragments should be fitted together to make sure they are completely recovered. Using a Teflon guide provided with a radiological marker over its entire length facilitates the recovery manoeuvres. On this point, for forearm fractures, one can use the smaller sheaths of pleural drains or of suction drains as a guide. They have the advantage of having a radiological marker over their entire length. It is important to cut their distal end obliquely to facilitate passage across the fracture site.

Nailing

Cortical Splitting

Whatever the site, cortical splitting always aggravates the initial lesions and necessitates a more complex assembly than initially contemplated. Several factors, sometimes in combination, encourage cortical splitting: the hammer, faulty positioning, and an unsatisfactory entry orifice.

Role of the Hammer

The hammer is undeniably the main culprit [11]. The original Küntscher nails had hollow clover leaf shapes of constant section provided with a longitudinal slot. This configuration gave the intramedullary guide a transverse elasticity dear to Küntscher, which contributed to stabilizing the implant in the medullary canal. Currently, one increasingly sees models of closed nails (hollow tubes without a slot) or even solid nails (actual solid metal rods), totally devoid of transverse elasticity. It can readily be imagined that the use of the hammer to insert such nails can be very dangerous and is to be strongly condemned. The various nails that are now on the market to treat fractures of the trochanteric mass have variable angles of bending in the frontal plane: 10°, 7°, and 5° [21, 23]. Whatever the type of system used, intraoperative splitting, always linked to the use of the hammer, has been described, which demonstrates that a nail of a given type is only an average implant that adapts easily to certain morphotypes of femur, but with more difficulty in other patients.

Whether closed or solid nails are used, it is always essential to prepare the bone properly, not hesitating to continue the reaming as long as the nail cannot be completely inserted solely by hand, without recourse to the hammer. Even for other strictly diaphyseal sites, the present tendency is to nail by hand as much as possible, advancing the nail by means of rotational movements and using the hammer as little as possible. Only by this means will intraoperative splitting become a thing of the past.

The Role of Positioning

The second cause of cortical splitting is associated with defective positioning:

1. For the femur, the risk of internal cortical splitting is linked to an angle of attack between the nail and the shaft axis that is too open. This angle is more open, and therefore more dangerous when the patient is obese or when the operated lower limb is placed in abduction. To facilitate access to the apex of the great trochanter and close this angle of attack, the limb should be adducted and the trunk inclined away from the operated side; in particular, the nail should be kept close to the patient's flank during its descent (Fig. 15.4).
2. For the tibia, the risk is of posterior cortical splitting secondary to an insufficiently flexed knee. The patella, which then remains too far forward, hampers insertion of the nail by again creating an angle of attack between the nail and the shaft axis that is too open and dangerous. To avoid this pitfall, it suffices during positioning of the patient to secure knee flexion of over 90°, which has the advantage of producing recession of the patella and thus facilitates nailing, the axis of the implant approaching that of the proximal shaft (Fig. 15.5).
3. In the humerus, the risk is of posterior cortical splitting in a patient whose shoulder has not been placed in sufficient retropulsion. Because of the presence of the acromion, the reaming is then performed along an axis that is too oblique backwards; hence the risk of posterior splitting of the proximal segment.
4. In the radius, the risk is of anterior cortical splitting, if the entry point chosen is on the posterior aspect of the distal epiphysis and extra-articular in Lister's tubercle. To avoid this risk, the first phase of nailing must be made while directing the concavity of the pre-bent nail upward to facilitate its advancement in the first third of the shaft. Next, when the tip of the nail reaches the middle third of the shaft, the implant is turned so that the pronator curvature of the nail is situated in a frontal plane along the pronator curvature of the radius.

Role of a Poor Entry Orifice

The third cause of cortical splitting is associated with a poor site of entry into the proximal epiphysis.

1. In the femur [1, 13], as has been seen, an entry point that is too lateral tends to cause a medial split (Fig. 15.4, 15.15). The determination of a correct entry point is pre-eminently tactile: the pulp of the index finger of one hand placed against the tip of the square point held in the other serves as a guide. Two planes must then be considered.
   a) Sagittally, the apex of the trochanter is bitubercular like a camel's back; the palpating finger should stop in the middle, between the two humps, in the concavity of the apex of the trochanter.
   b) Transversely, the finger is halted just at the apex of the convexity of the trochanter, neither laterally, because of the risk of lateral cortical splitting mentioned above, nor medially, in the trochanteric fossa within the joint which involves a threefold risk [1]: a secondary fracture of the neck due to its weakening [15], a necrosis of the femoral head due to vascular damage, and lastly, osteoarthrosis of the hip due to secondary articular effraction in cases of diaphyseal osteitis. If there is any doubt, the correct localization of the entry point can be verified by means of the image intensifier.
2. In the tibia, an entry point too near the tibial tuberosity hampers insertion of the nail because of the major thickness of the cortex at this level, again an argument in favour of an open angle of attack on the posterior cortex with a risk of posterior splitting (Fig. 15.5).
3. In the humerus, as seen above, inadequate retropulsion of the patient's arm leads to a very anterior entry point in front of the greater tubercle because of the acromial obstacle. This very anterior entry point will give an oblique course to the reamer guide, and the head of the reamer will then risk creating a posterior cortical split in

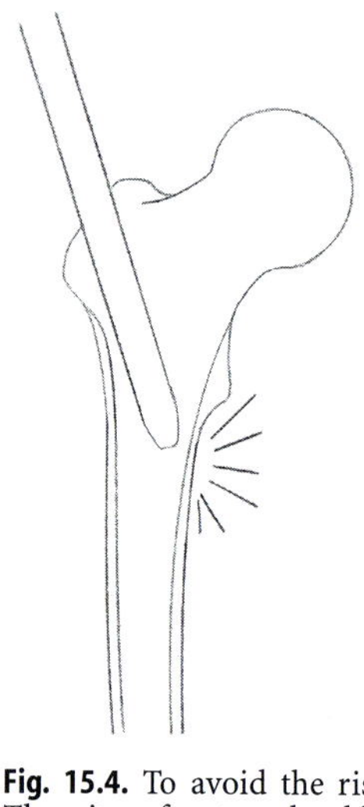

Fig. 15.4. To avoid the risk of internal cortical splitting. (1) The site of entry should be at the apex of the great trochanter and not outside. (2) The nail should be placed against the patient's flank during the initial phase of nailing. (3) Where necessary, the orthopaedic table can be adducted

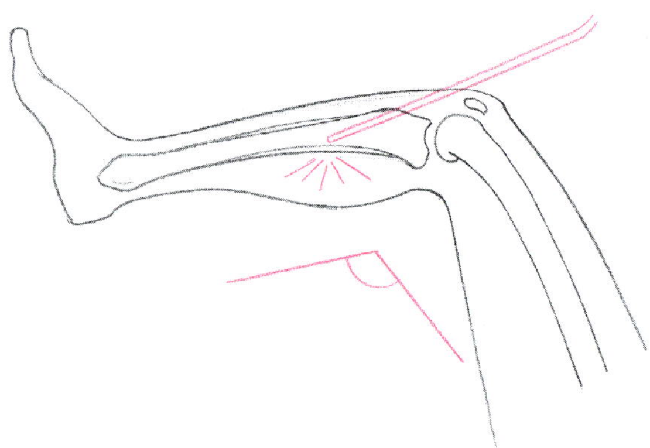

Fig. 15.5. A knee angle exceeding 90° can lead to drawing back the patella, thus avoiding the risk of posterior cortical splitting

the distal fragment. The solution consists of applying frank retropulsion to disengage the apex of the tubercle in front of the acromion. The entry point can then be made in the correct manner, i.e. in the anatomic neck between the cartilaginous head medially and the apex of the greater tubercle laterally.

4. In the ulna, an entry orifice that is too anterior may give rise to a posterior cortical effraction over several centimeters starting from the entry point. To prevent this pitfall, the shaft of the olecranon drilling Jig should be applied well against the posterior aspect of the olecranon; the entry orifice is then correctly centred in relation to the apex, which will always leave a sufficient thickness of posterior cortex.

Bursting of the Diaphysis

Diaphyseal bursting, an extremely grave complication, should no longer be seen. Historically, the very first intramedullary nailings were often complicated by such bursting. In searching for a solution to this problem, Küntscher developed the concept of intradiaphyseal reaming. The regular circular calibration of the constricted mid-shaft portion of the medullary canal thus obtained prepared a cylindrical course for the implant and thus permitted a truly centromedullary nailing without the risk of bursting of the diaphyseal cortices. Unfortunately, for some years now we have seen a veritable resurgence of these diaphyseal burstings in connection with a tendency by certain teams once again to advocate nailing without reaming, considering reaming to be too dangerous. As certain recent publications bear witness [8, 15], failure to ream actually incurs a twofold risk without any possible escape route: one must either use a nail of the right diameter, but insert it with a mallet with the risk of bursting the diaphysis, or one must choose a nail of small diameter, which incurs the risk of breaking the equipment (nail or locking screw).

The charges sometimes made against reaming are fully justified if they relate to invasive and forceful reaming, unnecessarily weakening the diaphyseal cortices and increasing the above-mentioned risks of fat embolism or compartment syndromes. Compared to this, nailing with reaming can retain all its advantages, provided the reaming remains reasonable and there is no longer, as in the past, the intent to black out the medullary canal with large-diameter nails. The philosophy and technique of nailing have evolved; currently, safety considerations advocate reaming less but, on the other hand, locking comes more easily.

Twisting and Blocking of the Nail

Twisting and blocking of the nail are always secondary to aggressive "physical" diaphyseal nailings, where the hammer is once again directly responsible for this type of complication [11]. The classic difference of 1–2 mm between the diameter of the nail to be inserted and that of the last reamer head used must be observed. In practice, the risks of twisting or blockage of the nail are met with mainly in the young adult, whose diaphyseal cortices are usually very elastic; in this case a difference of at least 2 mm seems desirable.

Twisting, which actually occurs only with large hollow femoral nails with a complete slot, has imposed a distal transquadriceps locking in certain situations, without particular consequences. Such twisting has become extremely rare, because the manufacturers of the majority of current hollow nails have eliminated the slot at both ends of the implant.

In conclusion, if one is obliged to resort to the hammer at the start of a diaphyseal nailing, it is best to abandon it and use a nail of lesser diameter: the hammer is meant to be used only for the last few centimeters to fix the implant in the bone of the distal epiphysis.

Blockage of a nail absolutely calls for its removal by means of a nail extractor and recourse to a nail of smaller diameter. We should bear in mind that twisting never occurs naturally with a closed nail without a slot.

Cortical Infringement

The majority of nails currently available on the market are provided with a profiled distal end, eliminating the risks of cortical inpingement described with Küntscher's original nails of constant profile, which could escape from the guide by their longitudinal slot, thus explaining the possibility of infringement of the distal fragment at the fracture site. In principle, modern nails can no longer escape from the nail guide and this type of complication is avoided.

Locking

Locking may be a source of false passages. Two types of case are considered in the following sections.

False Passage and Proximal Jig

False passage occurs with a jig integrated with the nail. The jig sometimes allows locking of the proximal epiphysis of the femur, tibia or humerus, sometimes the more distal locking of a gamma-type nail or perforated nail with several locking orifices. The risk of a false passage is here related to the possibility of divergence by play between the implant and the jig, which are imperfectly joined together. The more one departs from this zone of connection, the greater the risk of a false passage, which justifies the technique of staged locking, always beginning with the most proximal opening, the safest, and leaving the drill in the jig and the nail hole before beginning drilling of the next hole. If the jig is so stabilized, it effectively lessens the risk of error. A false passage requires checking the proper tightening of the jig attached to the nail; in practice, poor tightening giving rise to play between the two components may cause the false passage. If, despite checking, the false passage persists, it then becomes necessary to check the precision of the jig by passing a drill through the jig and the withdrawn nail: the drill should traverse the locking orifice of the nail without difficulty. If this is not the case, the jig has been previously distorted by intemperate hammer blows. We mention here a basic principle before any locked nailing: the instrument nurse should always mount the jig on the nail and check the proper alignment of the orifices of the jig and the nail, by means of a drill. This simple check before inserting the nail prevents subsequent setbacks and wasted time. There are no exceptions to this basic principle, even with teams well versed in nailing techniques who may use equipment of different generations and thus multiply the risks of error.

False Passage and Distal Jig

The other instance of false passage concerns distal locking using indirect methods of aiming, of which the most commonly used remains the free-hand jig held by the surgeon who looks for centring under radioscopic monitoring by means of circular metal markers, which become concentric at the orifice in the nail (Fig. 15.6). The aiming

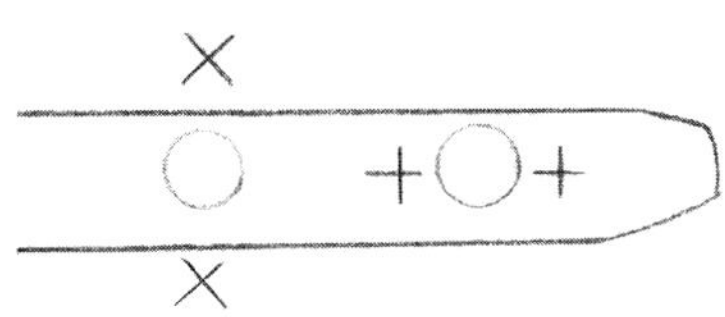

Fig. 15.6. *Upright cross*, common incorrect passage. *Diagonal cross*, exceptional incorrect passage

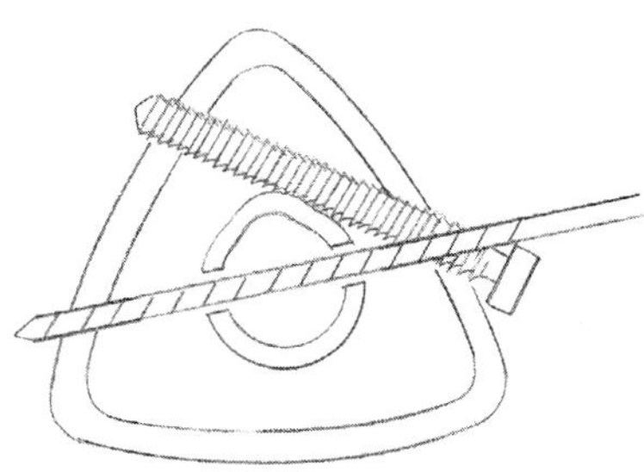

Fig. 15.7. The smaller diameter of the drill compared with that of the screw is used to advantage to rectify an incorrect passage

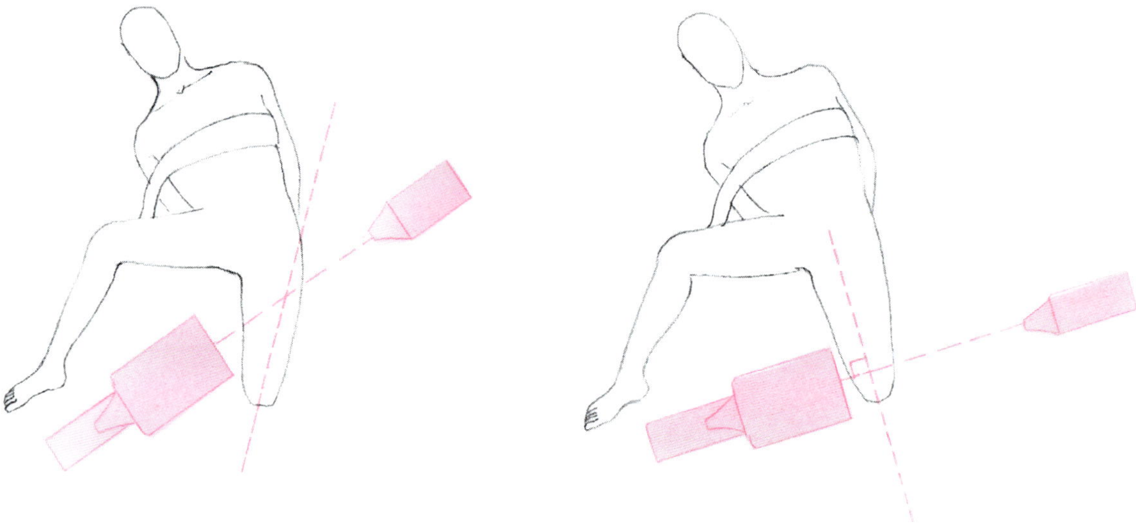

Fig. 15.8. Diaphyseal nailing of the femur. (1) Adduction to expose the trochanter makes nailing easier. (2) Abduction makes distal nailing easier. The lower limb, which is not to be operated on, no longer hinders manipulation of the intensifier

error is always made in the same direction, the screw passing in front of or behind the nail; it is actually rare to find oneself above or below the opening, against the nail. Faced with a false passage, it is best to locate the position of the screw on the monitor, which indicates the course to follow. Thus, if the screw is too anterior, repeat the drilling by the initial superficial cortical orifice while inclining the motor slightly downwards (posteriorly) and drilling slowly (Fig. 15.7). The difference in diameter between the drill and the openings in the nail facilitates this manoeuvre. Thus, by way of the nail openings, one achieves correct drilling of the deep cortex. Of course, the procedure must be reversed for a posterior false passage. The best guarantee for avoiding a distal false passage is to obtain a perfectly circular image of the nail openings on the monitor before the screwing itself. To do this, the intensifier must be strictly perpendicular to the nail. During a femoral nailing, as we have seen above, adduction of the limb to be operated facilitates reaming and nailing; however, before the stage of distal locking, it is very useful to give some abduction by means of the arm of the orthopaedic table. This manoeuvre greatly facilitates manipulation of the lateral view intensifier, which, we repeat, must be perpendicular to the femoral diaphyseal axis. In practice, abduction eases matters by virtue of the gain in space thus obtained and avoids impingement of the apparatus against the opposite lower limb (Fig. 15.8). During centring, it is necessary as a first step to analyse the images obtained carefully, in order to deduce the subsequent plac-

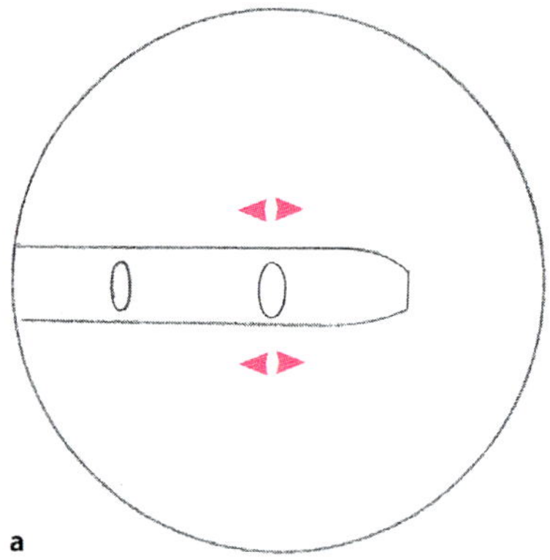

a

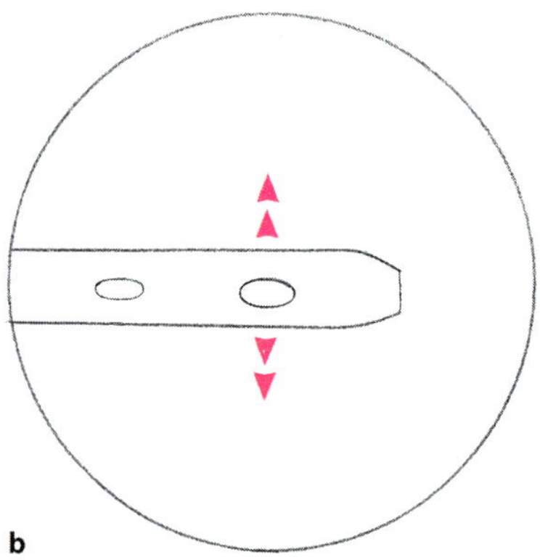

b

Fig. 15.9. a Oval hole with vertical axis. (1) Turn the image intensifier horizontally. (2) Repositioning of the image intensifier perpendicular to the nail. **b** Oblong hole with horizontal axis. (1) C-arm up or down, if not, (2) modify the vertical rotation of the C-arm, if not (3) modify the rotation of the fracture table ing of the intensifier required to obtain a perfectly circular image (Fig. 15.9). At this stage, one must not forget to exploit the possibility of inclining the orthopaedic table laterally. Also, by thus inclining the patient, one can always eventually obtain a perfectly circular image, even though the situation seemed blocked by the intensifier. In this latter case, one must resist the temptation to apply rotation to the limb; a rotational defect at the fracture site will follow, which will be perpetuated by the locking.

Problem of the Elderly Patient with Fragile Cortices

The elderly patient with fragile cortices of the femur or tibia sometimes poses problems concerning the grip of the locking screws. The use of expansive screws of the Vécsei type preserves the mechanical benefits of locking. These screws remain fixed in the openings in the nail, even if they have no grip on the cortices themselves; the effect of the locking is thus maintained.

Value of the Grosse and Lafforque Jig for Femoral and Tibial Aiming

Many jig systems for distal aiming have been brought onto the market, some sophisticated, some onerous, making their purchase difficult in current contexts. However, recent systems of laser aiming appear very useful, as they decrease the duration of irradiation. From experience, the Grosse and Lafforgue type of jig remains inexpensive compared with more recently proposed techniques, more reliable, and especially, by far the least irradiating of all jig systems using the image intensifier. During the centring stage, the team keeps away from the emitting source, an obvious advantage since the dose of radiation is known to decrease as the square of the distance. Naturally, the experience acquired by a skilled manipulator remains the best guarantee of short exposure times.

Problems of Distal Aiming of an Ulnar Nail

The first stage of distal locking of the ulna is the insertion of a Kirschner pin perpendicular to the oval opening in the nail. If the pin is inserted in the middle of the opening, it is impossible to drill and screw using a distal jig; yet it is essential not to remove the pin placed in this way. To be able to do the locking, one must push on the nail (in

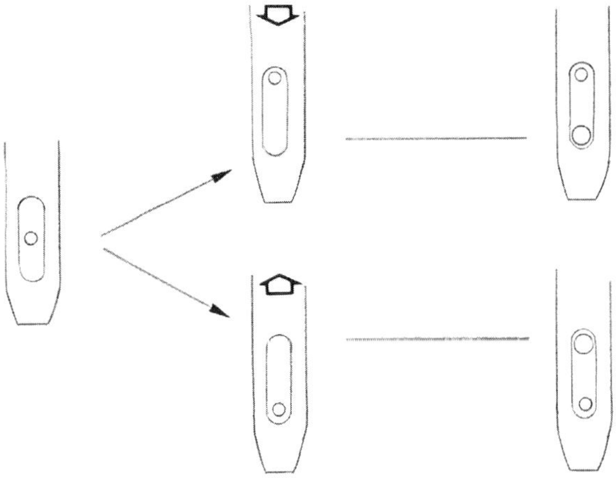

Fig. 15.10. Distal locking of the ulna

the case of assembly with compression); the pin will thus be fixed in the proximal part of the opening, leaving sufficient room for drilling and then screwing in the distal part. Conversely, pulling on the nail to fix the pin in the distal part of the opening allows drilling and screwing in its proximal part in the case of fixation with distraction (Fig. 15.10).

Intraoperative Irradiation

Intraoperative irradiation is always difficult to assess. However, it is of less importance to the patient, who is exposed to it only once, than to the surgeon and his team who accumulate radiation dosage after each procedure using X-rays. This rise in the overall dose increases regularly with the passage of time. Therefore, a few elementary rules to lessen the period of radiation should be mentioned as a reminder. Before radiation, clinical landmarks are always useful: thus the source-intensifier axis should pass accurately through the zone to be investigated radiologically. Furthermore, the distance between the source and the operated limb should always be maximized to avoid radiological magnification and provide an optimal field. Before pressing on the pedal, it is best to wait for the apparatus to stabilize after a manipulation; a fuzzy image is useless. During the irradiation, short exposure times and grid images are important. When choosing an image intensifier, preference should certainly be given to machines equipped with audible signals accompanying the emission of X-rays and with radiation time meters, measures encouraging a lighter foot on the pedal. Lastly, the wearing of a lead apron must be compulsory for the whole team.

Postoperative Complications

Postoperative complications are always discussed in the chronologic order of their usual discovery and are classified into three groups, comprising complications immediately after operation, secondary complications, and lastly, the more remote late complications. Though noted after operation, they are often the outcome of a technical error during the procedure.

Immediate Complications

Once the dressing of the operative wound has been completed, the drapes are removed; the waking patient is transferred from the orthopaedic table onto a stretcher. Clinical examination of the freed operated limb and the immediate postoperative follow-up radiograph may reveal faults, sometimes requiring immediate surgical revision; for this reason, some authors prefer not to waken the patient before viewing the postoperative radiograph [4].

Clinical Aspects

Clinically, attention may be drawn to vascular or neurologic disturbances, sometimes both.

1. A cold, insensitive or hyperaesthetic leg and a tense calf suggest a compartment syndrome, requiring the emergency measures discussed above: measurement of the tissue pressures and even decompression aponeurotomy if there is the least doubt. In this context, we may mention the difficulty created by epidural anaesthesia [12], which temporarily delays the diagnosis and, unfortunately, also the time for surgical decompression.
2. A comparable clinical picture may be associated with an injury of the popliteal vascular pedicle, a dangerous complication of anteroposterior drilling or boring of the proximal tibial epiphysis [1], caused by posterior penetration of the instruments and an incorrectly positioned infra-popliteal support, which flattens the neurovascular structures against the bony plane. This support must be strictly supra-popliteal, at the level of the distal part of the thigh. In practice, anteroposterior screwing of the proximal tibia is only rarely used, as it is very dangerous; diagnostic delays have led to secondary amputations.
3. Asymmetry of the limbs sometimes attracts attention. Sometimes shortening, accompanied by swelling of the leg at the fracture site, is evidence of telescoping of the fragments after release of traction on the table; this situation reflects an imperfect assembly requiring supplementary locking. Sometimes there is elongation of the operated limb, due to a static assembly after excessive traction on the table. Any associated neurologic complication calls for immediate unlocking.
4. Anomalies of rotation sometimes attract attention because of an asymmetry between the bicondylar and bimalleolar axes. Asymmetry is acceptable in a situation with moderate external rotation, but unacceptable if there is even moderate internal rotation; revision or static locking is then necessary.
   These rotation defects are easily prevented by proper positioning of the patient, always using the orthopaedic table every time nailing of the lower limb is performed:
   For a fracture of the femur, the patient is positioned in dorsal decubitus, with the thorax slightly inclined from the side opposite the fracture; the lower limb to be operated, patella facing directly upward, receives traction either classically by a transcondylar Steinmann pin or via the foot inserted in the foot piece of the table. It is useful in this case to use an infra-popliteal support to avoid both slackness of the leg and any metallic superimposition opposite the jointline of the knee,
   For a fracture of the tibia, the patient is in dorsal decubitus; the articulated arm of the orthopaedic table allows positioning of the lower limb with the hip flexed 70°–80° and the knee flexed to 90°–100° (Fig. 15.5). The ankle is stabilized either by a transcalcanean Steinmann pin or by an adhesive bandage fixing the foot to the sole of the footpiece; in either case, monitoring the bimalleolar axis in relation to the bicondylar axis of the knee is made easier.
   Reinders reports that "The procedure does not begin with the skin incision but by positioning the patient on the orthopaedic table. It is for the surgeon to perform this task, in view of the cardinal importance of the position of the patient" [13].
   For a fracture of the humerus, distal and then proximal locking must be done in neutral rotation of the elbow to prevent the risk of excessive internal rotation. As a general rule, during the initial stages of positioning and reduction, before painting the skin and draping, and to avoid subsequent faults in asepsis, care should be taken to see that no metal arm of the table can hinder the imaging of the whole of the

bone to be nailed, in both frontal and lateral views.

5. The neurologic complications give very different clinical pictures, depending on the affected nerve:
   a) Some patients operated on for a femoral fracture complain of perineal paraesthesiae or anaesthesia, later perhaps of troubles in erection, due to compression of the pudendal nerve [2]. These various complications usually disappear in 3 months [2]. Note here again that it is important to apply no more than 50 kg of traction to the lower limb and particularly to treat such fractures as early as possible, which reduces the traction force needed for reduction.
   b) Nailing of the tibia sometimes leads to paresthaesiae in the territory of the common peroneal nerve [20], pressed against a metal popliteal support that is too low, i.e. infrapopliteal. These paresthaesiae usually regress. Remember the safety of a supra-popliteal support.
   c) Proximal anteroposterior locking of a Seidel humeral nail is sometimes the cause of impingement on the axillary nerve. It is known that the contusion of the nerve is associated with the drill or awl, rather than the locking screw, escaping posteriorly, although it is true that the latter must not be too long. However, most important is monitoring the running of the motor while drilling and boring the bone.

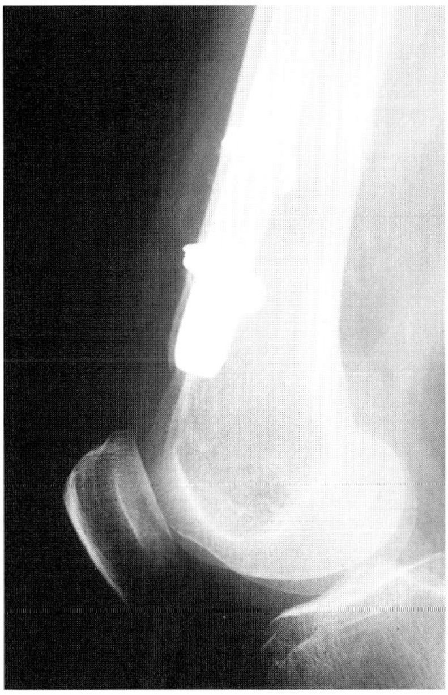

Fig. 15.11. Cortical splitting highlights the importance of checking the centring of the guides and the nail on the intensifier, both frontally and laterally

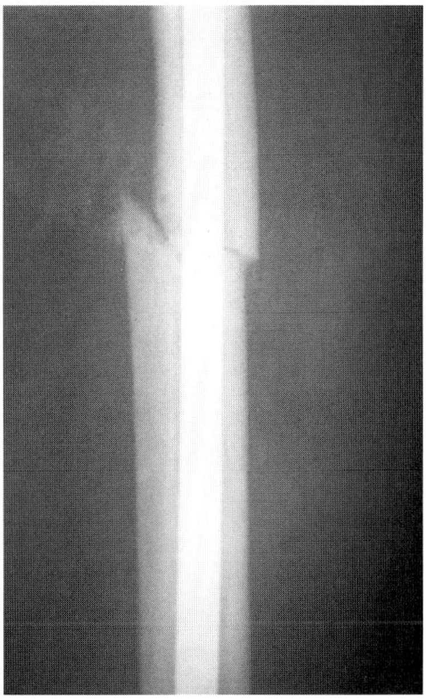

Fig. 15.12. A difference in calibre of the diaphyseal fragments indicates rotation anomalies

Radiological Aspects

The immediate postoperative follow-up radiographs are sometimes sources of unpleasant surprises. The intraoperative monitoring screen shows only limited fields. Moreover, distortions in the screen image may falsify interpretation. The whole of the nailed bone is shown for the first time by the follow-up radiograph.

1. Over-reaming of a cortex is secondary either to an incorrect point of entry or to poor distal entering (Fig. 15.11). Absence of the cortex in one view is always due to an incorrect entry point responsible for over-reaming the cortex, which risks secondarily causing delay in union; this again stresses the importance of a correct entry point, as described above.
2. Sometimes the nail appears too short, which will jeopardize the stability of the assembly. Conversely, the nail may be too long, infringing on the distal joint space; this situation definitively contraindicates any inferior mobilization for fear of seeing the nail become intra-articular.
3. Anomalies of rotation are indicated by a difference in calibre of the shaft fragments on either side of the fracture site, together with a step and an absence of contact of the fibular fragments in leg fractures. To avoid this pitfall,

care must be taken during reduction manoeuvres to obtain on the screen the same calibre of the diaphyseal column and the same thickness of the cortices on either side of the fracture site (Fig. 15.12).

4. Valgus or varus misalignment of the axis in the frontal plane is usually due to poor frontal centring of the reamer-guide in the distal fragment. To avoid this, it is necessary to check that the position of the guide is properly median in the screen image (Fig. 15.13). Positioning in lateral decubitus has been accused of causing an axial defect of the femur in valgus because of the tendency to outward angulation due to the weight of the thigh during the procedure. Though moderate valgus angulation may often be tolerable, a varus deviation is only rarely so, and often calls for surgical revision.
5. Defects of the axis in the sagittal plane in flexion or recurvatum are the result of poor centring of the guide in the lateral view. The sagittal tilt of a distal tibial or femoral fragment rapidly compromises the mechanics of the subjacent joint and again requires surgical revision.
   In the femur, the transcondylar Steinmann pin should be very low and very ventral, to reduce the initial tilt of the condylar mass. Moreover, this position of the pin has the advantage of leaving room for the centromedullary nail. High fractures of the tibia are dangerous to nail because of the major risk of sagittal or frontal tilting of the proximal fragment of the tibia, however experienced the operator is [16, 18]. The nailing of such fractures always calls for special vigilance (Fig. 15.14). Another axial defect in the sagittal plane is sometimes related to the design of some tibial nails, which have a double sagittal angulation, both proximal and distal. The lower angulation is dangerous. If the entry point of the nail is too lateral, the

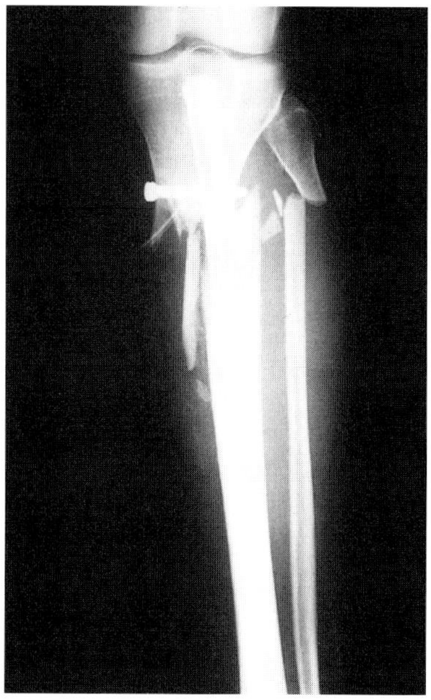

Fig. 15.14. Valgus deviation of a high tibial fracture; nailing is always difficult to perform

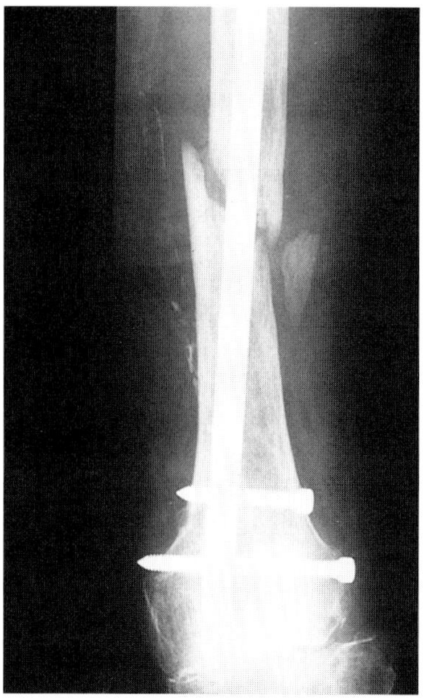

Fig. 15.13. Valgus misalignment is usually due to poor centring of the reamer guide in the distal epiphysis

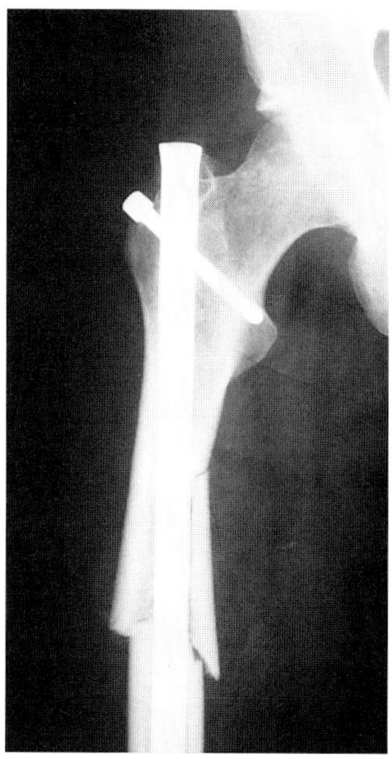

Fig. 15.15. An excessively lateral entry point causing internal cortical splitting and a varus of the proximal fragment

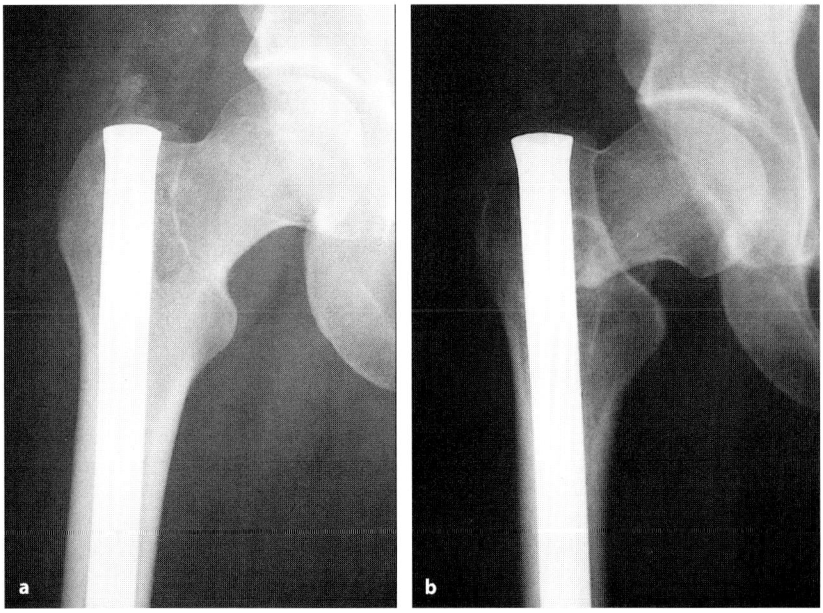

Fig. 15.16. a Immediate postoperative X-ray. **b** Secondary discovery of an associated fracture of the neck, which had initially gone unnoticed

risk is of creating a valgus of the distal fragment; conversely, a too medial entry point may create a varus of the distal fragment.

6. One of the unpleasant surprises in the postoperative follow-up radiograph is finding a split (Fig. 15.15) or an associated fracture, which has gone unnoticed. The classic example is a fracture of the femoral shaft combined with an initially undisplaced fracture of the neck [7, 11] (Fig. 15.16). It may also be secondary to the operative procedure such as a fracture of the femoral neck produced by an incorrect entry point [8, 13]. Intraoperative splitting is usually avoided by non-aggressive reaming and nailing; instruments and implants of too wide a calibre are useless and dangerous.
7. Locking screws can also be the source of problems. Lastly, the immediate postoperative follow-up radiograph may show that the locking screws are too long (and encumbering), too short (not efficient enough) or even to one side of the nail opening and completely ineffective; naturally, their correct repositioning is essential.

Secondary Complications

Haematoma

Haematoma at the operative wound is always due to an absence of drainage. In practice, one should never hesitate to drain every access for nailing, wherever the operative site.

Pain

Pain is often a complication associated with components that are too cumbersome:

1. A femoral nail projecting from the apex of the trochanter brushes against the gluteal muscle at every step, eventually creating a painful bursitis.
2. A tibial nail that is insufficiently embedded irritates the patellar tendon and then becomes a real nuisance for the patient. Ruptures of the tendon have even been described after prolonged irritation.
3. A humeral nail, inserted from above and projecting from the greater tubercle, irritates the rotator cuff and impinges on the acromion at the least movement of abduction, which becomes painful [12]. One should always remain very vigilant during a nailing procedure and absolutely avoid any projection of the nail outside the bone, using an as small an incision as possible on the order of 1 cm in the direction of the fibres of the cuff. Pain in the arm after Seidel nailing suggests a rupture of the long tendon of the biceps by the upper anteroposterior locking screw. To avoid this risk, it is best to use blunt chisels and then a socket carried to be just in contact with the anterior cortex before drilling.
4. An incompletely inserted ulnar nail soon becomes troublesome, the patient complaining of a subcutaneous prominence and pain in the olecranon region on the least contact.
5. Locking screws sometimes become painful [1]; this may be due to the tip of an overlong screw

or to the head of a screw insufficiently embedded in the first cortex (which must be previously enlarged, if necessary, to avoid this risk) or to secondary migration of a screw.
6. Pain in the popliteal region sometimes indicates a false aneurysm of the popliteal artery due to a faulty technique of proximal anteroposterior locking of the tibia.
7. Sometimes the result of premature weight bearing or mobilization, secondary displacements should no longer be seen. They are always due to an initially incomplete assemblage. Usually, there is interfragmentary telescoping or a staggered rotation of a spiral fracture, which then requires osteoclasis and static locked renailing [4].
8. Low fractures must be locked with two screws to stabilize the distal fragment effectively. A single screw serves as a transverse axis of rotation and explains certain secondary tiltings of the lower fragment.
In the case of very low fractures, at the limit of indication for locked nailing, it may be necessary to modify the distal end of the nail. Sawing at the level of the distal extremity of the nail sometimes makes it possible to insert two locking screws distal to the fracture site. It is absolutely essential not to leave a screw in the fracture site (Fig. 15.17). Imaging is imperative after sawing. Rounding off the angles of section of the metal edge will prevent risks of impingement by the nail modified in this way.
9. Fracture below a trochanteric nail noticed during the secondary postoperative period in the absence of a new history of injury suggests an intraoperative cortical split that has gone unnoticed initially and become complete later. Here we must again stress the danger of using the hammer to construct the preliminary hole for the distal locking, since the outer cortex may be very thick at this level.
10. The development of pain accompanied by locally increased skin temperature and congestive oedema of the skin in a febrile context suggests an infective complication and justifies debridement of the infected soft parts together with antibiotic cover; removal of the nail is necessary only in cases of severe septicaemia.

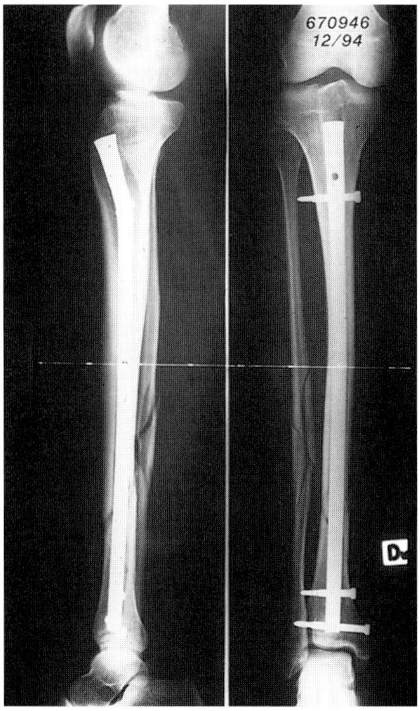

Fig. 15.17. By sawing the nail, it is possible to apply two screws to very distal fractures

Late Complications

Component Rupture

Rupture of components always occurs after prolonged and excessive stress; it is actually evidence of delayed union or pseudarthrosis, bony union not having been able to play its part in withstanding the mechanical stresses [13]. Although these ruptures once seemed to be in marked decline, because of improvements in the design and manufacture of the implants, they have unfortunately reappeared since the use of nails and locking screws of small calibre [7, 8, 19].

Metastatic shaft fractures, usually secondary to lytic lesions, justify recourse to closed ungrooved nails, which are much more resistant. This progress towards nails without a slit parallels the disappearance of the clover leaf shapes dear to Küntscher; the future probably belongs to the closed cylindrical type, which will also be less expensive to manufacture.

Ectopic Calcification

Ectopic calcification is often the cause of painful impingement. Intratendinous calcifications thickening the patellar tendon are a common cause of symptoms.

Some authors have suggested making the bony approach lateral or medial to the tendon, but in fact these lateralized approaches give poor access, hinder reaming and fray the tendon fibres. It is preferable to use a vertical transtendinous approach at the junction of the outer two-thirds

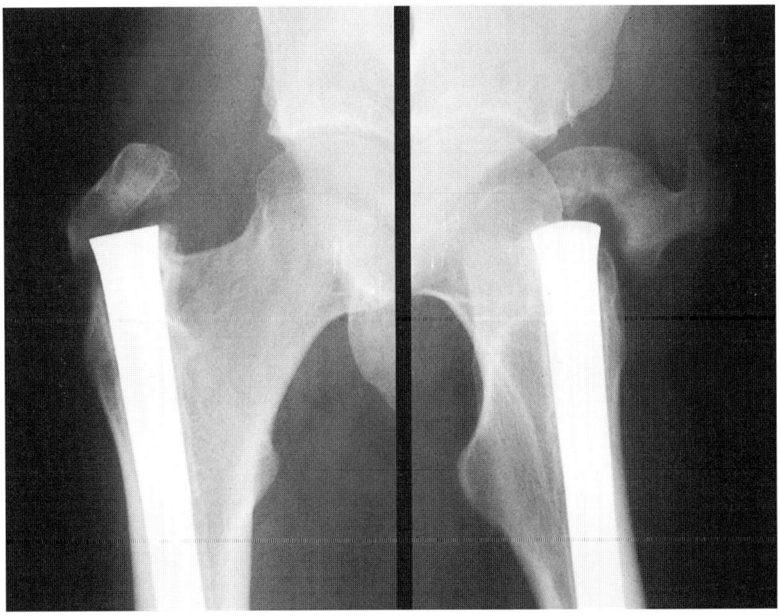

Fig. 15.18. Extensive supratrochanteric calcification, which is functionally hindering and restricts abduction. Repeated irrigation under pressure before closing the original access is recommended

and the inner third, which provides easy posterior access. Supratrochanteric calcification is usually less of a nuisance unless it is very extensive (Fig. 15.18). However, calcification above the greater tubercle of the humerus is very poorly tolerated because of painful restriction of abduction.

It is always possible to remove these various calcifications during removal of the metal, but repeated irrigation under pressure before closing the original access wound remains the best preventive measure.

Malunion

Malunion often causes problems in the lower limb by disturbing its mechanical axis. Progressive displacement with migration of the nail, slow rotation of the soft callus of a spiral fracture, eventually lead to malunion, always secondary to incomplete locking. Hence the importance of performing a static assembly on principle, once the fracture plane becomes oblique or spirally twisted.

Progressive deviations in valgus or rotation have been reported with certain models of centromedullary femoral nails, which are too flexible [1] or too small in calibre [15].

The treatment of angular or rotary defects may be resolved by an intramedullary osteotomy using a closed method and static locked renailing. The accuracy of the derotation is improved by a preliminary CT study.

The technique of extemporaneous intramedullary elongation osteotomy of the femur is also to be considered when the shortening does not exceed 25–30 mm.

Young patients nailed during childhood sometimes pose difficult problems. If a nail has traversed a growth plate that is still active, it creates a virtual epiphysiodesis responsible for a recurvatum of the proximal tibia or unequal length of the lower limbs after femoral nailing. The lengthening induced results from both an "over-anatomic" reduction at the shaft site and an epiphysiodesis of the trochanteric cartilage (varising), leaving the cephalic cartilage active (valgising). This double mechanism adds to the elongation of the femur.

Delayed Union

The appearance of radiological signs of delayed union justifies dynamization, which, outside this context, is not at all essential for bony union, as often noted in clinical practice [3].

Delayed union of the ulna may be resolved by installing simple compression of the nail, bearing in mind the preservation of a radio-ulnar index acceptable to the wrist; if this is not the case, a bone graft will become necessary.

Pseudarthrosis

Pseudarthrosis may be the outcome of cortical over-reaming, leaving an inadequate bony scaffolding that then requires bone grafting. To avoid this complication, measure the calibre of the medullary canal in its midshaft portion on the preoperative radiographs.

If a pseudarthrosis develops despite dynamization, the inadequate mechanical situation should be analysed:

1. A nail that is too short or too flexible allows persistent micro-movements at the fracture site which lead to a hypertrophic pseudarthrosis. Reoperation combining further reaming and a thicker nail will usually deal with this problem [16].
2. Atrophic pseudarthrosis [20] is often associated with a static assembly which needs to be dynamized to restore compression at the fracture site.
3. Pseudarthrosis of the tibia is often due to premature union of the fibula, which then acts as a splint preventing any interfragmentary compression of the tibia. A simple oblique osteotomy of the fibula, often by itself, sometimes combined with renailing, gives excellent results (Fig. 15.19).
4. The particular case of a distal compacted plug of reamed material: in the theoretic situation of dynamic assembly, a proximally locked nail sometimes prevents union by the absence of interfragmentary compression, as in a static set-up. This mechanical situation is actually associated with the presence of reamed material, secondarily compacted by the nailing, leading to the formation of an actual plug of dense cortical bone blocking the distal end of the nail. When possible, removal of the proximal locking screw allows simple resolution of this problem.

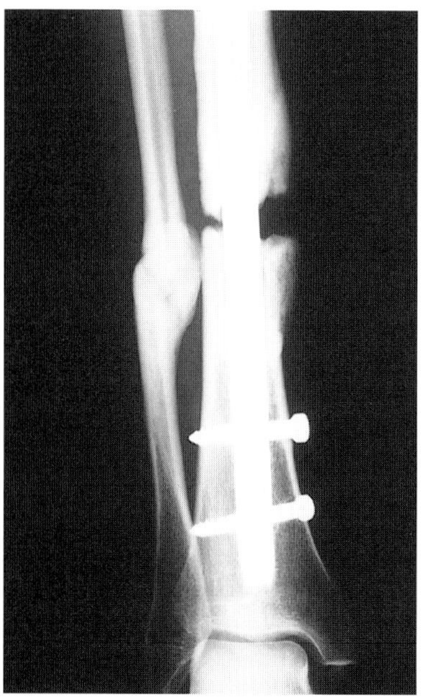

Fig. 15.19. Secondary pseudarthrosis of the tibia due to premature union of the fibula

Delayed Fractures

Delayed shaft fractures have been reported over an old trochanteric nail of the gamma type, occurring as the result of a new injury [21]. These fractures are not to be regarded as weak points of the method, since they can be observed under the same conditions with fixations by screwed plates or prosthetic stems. It is actually a matter of a new and intercurrent accident, to be distinguished from immediate postoperative fractures, which are not intraoperative splittings that have gone unnoticed.

Minimal Compartment Syndrome

Revealed by careful clinical examination, contracture or isolated paresis of a toe indicates a minimal compartment syndrome that has initially gone unnoticed, since the patient has not been troubled or complained of it.

Removal of Components

Removal of the components may be so difficult as to become impossible. This situation is always related to delay in removal, usually in young patients. Apart from the femur, where removal of the nail can be considered at around 18 months after radiological consolidation, the other locations incur a delay of 1 year depending on the same union criteria.

Conclusion

We now know that the prognosis of a fracture is not only associated with the bony problem, but that it largely depends on the quality of the soft parts around the fracture.

Centromedullary nailing by the closed method is a technique of osteosynthesis dealing in principle with both the bone and its muscular setting.

This initial theoretic ideal is marked in clinical practice by excellent long-term results, provided that the indication for the method has been well advised and the operative technique strictly observed. This is the price to be paid for effective prevention of the possible complications of centromedullary nailings, performed by the closed method.

References

1. Browner BD (1986) Pitfalls, errors, and complication in the use of locking Küntscher nails. Clin Orthop 212:192–208
2. Brumback R-J, Ellison T-S, Molligan OJ, Mahaffey S, Schmidhauser C (1992) Pudendal nerve palsy complicating intramedullary nailing of the femur. J Bone Joint Surg Am 74:1450–1455
3. Brumback RJ, Ellison S, Poka A, Bathon GH, Burgess AR (1988) Intramedullary nailing of femoral shaft fractures part III: long-term effects of static interlocking fixation. J Bone Joint Surg Am 74:106–112
4. Brumback RJ, Reilly JP, Poka A, Lakatos RP, Bathon H, Brugess A (1988) Intramedullary nailing of femoral shaft fractures part I: decision-making errors with interlocking fixation. J Bone Joint Surg Am 70:1441–1452
5. Estebe JP (1997) Des embolies de graisse au syndrome d'embolie graisseuse. Ann Fr Anesth Reanim 16:138–151
6. Freedman EL, Johnson EE (1995) Radiographic analysis of tibial fracture malalignment following intramedullary nailing. Clin Orthop 315:25–33
7. Haas NP, Krettek C, Tscherne H (1995) A new solid unreamed tibial nail for shaft fracture with severe soft tissue injury. Injury 26:379–383
8. Hutson JJ, Zych GA, Cole JD, Johnson KD, Ostermann P, Milne EL, Lattal L (1995) Mechanical failure of intramedullary tibial details applied without reaming. Clin Orthop 315:129–137
9. Kempf I, Grosse A, Taglang G (1990) L'enclouage centro-médullaire verrouillé fémur-tibia, matériel technique et indications. In: Enclouage centro-médullaire (monographie des Cahiers d'Enseignement de la SOFCOT no. 39.) Expansion Scientifique Française, Paris, pp 23–37
10. Kenneth JE, Cummings RJ (1992) Fat embolism as a complication of closed femoral shortening. J Pediatr Orthop 12:542–543
11. Khan FA, lkram MA, Badr AA, Kawashki HAL (1995) Femoral neck fracture: a complication of femoral nailing. Injury 26:319–321
12. Morrow BC, Farcsi, Mawhinney IN, Eliott RM (1994) Tibial compartment syndrome complicating an epidural analgesic technique – case report. J Trauma 37:867–868
13. Reinders J, Mockwitz J (1984) Technical faults and complications in interlocking nailing of general and tibial fractures. Acta Orthodox Belg 50:577–590
14. Riemers BL, Foglesong ME, Burke CJ, Butterfield SL (1994) Complications of Seidel intramedullary nailing of narrow diameter humeral diaphyseal fractures. Orthopaedics 17:19–29
15. Strecker W, Suger G, Kinz L (1996) Lokale Komplikationen der Marknagelung. Orthopäde 25:274–291
16. Templeman D, Thomas M, Varecka T, Kyle R (1995) Exchange reamed intramedullary nailing for delayed union and nonunion of the tibia. Clin Orthop 315:169–175
17. Van Os JP, Roumen RMH, Schoots S, Heystraten SMJ, Goris RJA (1994) Is early osteosynthesis safe in multiple-trauma patients with severe thoracic trauma and pulmonary contusion? J Trauma 36:495–498
18. Wende K, Runkel M (1996) Systemische Komplikationen der Marknagelung. Orthopäde 25:292–311
19. Whittle AP, Wester W, Russel TA (1995) Fatigue failure in small diameter tibial nails. Clin Orthop 315:119–128
20. Williams J, Gibbons M, Trundle H, Murray D, Worlocj P (1995) Complications of nailing in closed tibial fractures. J Orthodop Trauma 9:476–481
21. Williams WW, Parker BC (1992) Complications associated with the use of the gamma nail. Injury 23:291–292
22. Wiss DA, Stetson WB (1995) Unstable fractures of the tibia treated with a reamed intramedullary interlocking nail. Clin Orthop 315:56–63
23. Yelton C, Lowe W (1986) Iatrogenic subtrochanteric fracture: a complication of zickel nails. J Bone Joint Surg Am 68:1237–1240

Subject Index

A

B

C

D

M

N

O

P

R

S

Druck- und Bindearbeiten: Stürtz AG, Würzburg